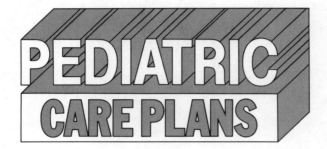

PEDIATRIC CARE PLANS

KATHLEEN MORGAN SPEER, RN, MSN, PhD

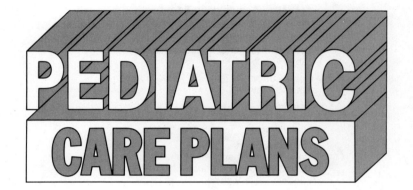

PEDIATRIC CARE PLANS

KATHLEEN MORGAN SPEER, RN, MSN, PhD

Springhouse Corporation
Springhouse, Pennsylvania

Staff

Executive Director, Editorial
Stanley Loeb

Executive Director, Creative Services
Jean Robinson

Director of Trade and Textbooks
Minnie B. Rose, RN, BSN, MEd

Art Director
John Hubbard

Associate Acquisitions Editor
Bernadette M. Glenn

Editors
Kevin Law (editorial manager), Diane Labus

Copy Editor
Jane V. Cray

Designers
Stephanie Peters (associate art director), StellarVisions

Art Production
Robert Perry (manager), Anna Brindisi, Donald Knauss, Catherine Mace, Robert Wieder, StellarVisions

Typography
David Kosten (manager), Diane Paluba (assistant manager), Joyce Rossi Biletz, Robin Rantz, Valerie Rosenberger

Manufacturing
Deborah Meiris (manager), T.A. Landis, Jennifer Suter

Production Coordination
Aline S. Miller (manager), Laurie J. Sander

© 1990 Springhouse Corporation. All rights reserved. No part of this book may be reproduced by any means whatsoever without written permission except for brief quotations embodied in critical articles and reviews. Printed in the United States of America. For information, write Springhouse Corporation, 1111 Bethlehem Pike, Springhouse, Pa. 19477.
PECP-011089

Library of Congress Cataloging-in-Publication Data
Speer, Kathleen Morgan.
  Pediatric care plans/Kathleen Morgan Speer.
    p. cm.
  Includes bibliographical references.
  1. Pediatric nursing.   2. Home Nursing.
  3. Nursing Care Plans.
I. Title.
  [DNLM: 1. Home Care Services.
2. Patient Care Planning.   3. Pediatric Nursing.
WY 159 S7415p]
RJ245.S63 1990
610.73'62—dc20
DNLM/DLC   89-21729
ISBN 0-87434-226-0   CIP

Contents

Appendices

Selected References

Index

Contributors

Marilyn Borgerson, RN, MSN, CPE
Clinical Nurse Specialist (Endocrinology)
Children's Medical Center of Dallas

Mary Breen, RN, MSN
Clinical Nurse Specialist (Craniofacial)
Children's Medical Center of Dallas

Linda Dillon, RN, MSN
Instructor
Baylor University
Dallas

Paula Dimmett, RN, MS
Clinical Nurse Specialist (Cardiology)
Children's Medical Center of Dallas

Michelle Faxel, RN, MS
Director of Nursing Education
The Children's Hospital Medical Center of
Northern California
Oakland

Sally Finical, RN, BSN
Staff Nurse
University of Arizona Medical Center
Tucson

Chris Geyer, RN, MSN
Education Specialist
Children's Medical Center of Dallas

Carol Hines, RN, MN
Clinical Nurse Specialist (General Surgery)
Children's Medical Center of Dallas

Becky Johnston, RN, BSN
Clinical Nurse Specialist
Surgical Services
Children's Medical Center of Dallas

Lynn Kiewel, RN, BSN
Former Staff Nurse
Children's Medical Center of Dallas

Diane Lesh, RN, MSN
Nurse Practitioner
Dallas City Health Department

Kathy Morin, RN, MSN
Clinical Nurse Specialist
Winnipeg (Canada) Children's Hospital

Claudia Odgers, RN, MSN
Quality Assurance Auditor
Blue Cross/Blue Shield
Topeka, Kan.

Nancy Quay, RN, MSN
Former Clinical Nurse Specialist
Children's Medical Center of Dallas

Martha Sanford, RN, PhD
Assistant Professor
Baylor University
Dallas

Bonnie Saucier, RN, PhD
Division Director of Health Sciences
Midwestern State University
Wichita Falls, Tex.

Deborah Schumann, RN, BSN
Neonatal Intensive Care Unit Nurse
Stormont-Vail Regional Medical Center
Topeka, Kan.

Suzanne Schuyler, RN, MSN
Missionary and Former Clinical Nurse
Specialist
Children's Medical Center of Dallas

Maureen Smith, RN, BSN
Assistant Director
Children's Medical Center of Dallas

Kathy Soltis, RN, BSN
Staff Nurse
Children's Medical Center of Dallas

Carolyn Swann, RN, MSN
Director of Nursing Education and
Research
Children's Medical Center of Dallas

Lillian Waring, RN, EdD
Associate Professor
Midwestern State University
Wichita Falls, Tex.

Penny Williams, RN, MSN
Education Specialist
Children's Medical Center of Dallas

Kelly Yager, RN, BSN
Assistant Director
Children's Medical Center of Dallas

Acknowledgments

I give my many thanks to all the contributors of this book. They worked tirelessly from deadline to deadline. My appreciation is also extended to the following persons: Susie Rumsey, my typist and friend, whose skill enabled me to organize this book and bring it to fruition; Bernadette Glenn, associate acquisitions editor, who spent much time answering my many questions; and Barbara Curyea, my sister and fellow nurse, who was my inspiration.

Dedication
This book is dedicated to my daughter, Shannon, and my husband, Gary—I will always treasure your loving support—and to the memory of my beloved parents, Harold and Frances Morgan.

Preface

Children are very different from adults. This is most evident to nurses when treating children diagnosed with illnesses similar to those of adults. Invariably, children respond quite differently. For this reason, nurses need special guidelines when planning the care of pediatric patients.

This care plan book addresses many of the major illnesses affecting pediatric patients. However, it also includes important information on subjects previously not included or difficult to find in most pediatric care plan books—information on home health care, perioperative care, and care of children undergoing radiologic procedures.

Home health care is fast becoming a major trend affecting all aspects of nursing. Providing care in the home requires that nurses work independently and without the immediate support of a hospital setting. Therefore, nurses caring for pediatric patients in the home setting need special knowledge and skills.

Likewise, nurses working with pediatric patients in operating and recovery areas of the hospital also require special knowledge and skills concerning thermoregulation, fluid and electrolyte maintenance, anesthesia induction, and shock. And nurses dealing with children undergoing radiologic procedures must understand the specific procedures and know how to administer proper care before and after the ordeal.

In this book, general care plans are listed alphabetically by medical diagnosis within each body system section. Under each diagnostic head, a description of the illness appears followed by assessment guidelines, which are listed according to body system. A nursing diagnosis, which appears beneath the assessment information, includes a specific goal and a listing of interventions and corresponding rationales. When more than one nursing diagnosis is given for a particular illness, the diagnoses are prioritized according to level of importance. Most care plans also include information on home health teaching to share with the entire family.

Although this book is not meant to be exhaustive, it includes a wealth of information on pediatric care. Nurses at all levels will find this a useful tool when working with children.

Kathleen Morgan Speer, RN, MSN, PhD
Assistant Professor
University of Texas at Arlington;
Research Liaison
Children's Medical Center of Dallas

Introduction

Because children differ greatly from adults—both physiologically and psychologically—pediatric care is considered a specialty. To better respond to children's special needs, many of today's health care facilities are equipped with separate pediatric units in which nurses and other health care professionals can provide treatment based on their patients' individual needs. However, many other health care facilities do not have such highly specialized units. Consequently, in such settings, acutely ill children sometimes do not receive the special attention and care they require—and deserve.

Regardless of the clinical setting, nurses need practical, hands-on information to provide the best possible care for their pediatric patients. One of the best tools available to practicing nurses, as well as students and instructors, is a set of concise, clinically relevant care plans—such as those presented in this book.

Using this book

Pediatric Care Plans includes 78 individual care plans that focus on various aspects of pediatric nursing, including acute illness in the hospital setting, perioperative care, diagnostic studies, and home care. These care plans, arranged alphabetically within each section, provide essential information on specific disorders, treatments, procedures, and problems commonly encountered by nurses working with pediatric patients.

Section I, Common Disorders and Treatments, contains a series of care plans alphabetized within separate body system categories. Each care plan begins with an introduction describing a medical disorder or treatment commonly encountered in pediatric patients. Also included in each care plan is a list of assessment findings, categorized according to body system, as well as a series of NANDA-approved nursing diagnoses with their related interventions and rationales (a complete list of NANDA-approved diagnoses appears in the appendices at the end of the book). Completing each care plan is a documentation checklist specific to the information covered.

Section II, Perioperative Care, consists of a series of care plans dealing with various pediatric problems encountered during the preoperative and postoperative periods. Each care plan includes an introduction describing the problem, assessment findings, nursing diagnoses with related interventions and rationales, and a documentation checklist.

Section III, Diagnostic Studies, focuses on care plans for specific radiographic procedures used in diagnosing illnesses common to pediatric patients. Each care plan begins with an introduction describing the procedure, followed by a list of possible indications for testing. Also included in each care plan are nursing diagnoses with related interventions and rationales as well as a documentation checklist.

Section IV, Home Health Care, contains a series of care plans for treating pediatric patients in the home setting. Similar to the care plans in most other sections, each care plan includes an introduction describing the treatment, a list of assessment findings, nursing diagnoses with related interventions and rationales, and a documentation checklist.

Located in the appendices are several useful, quick-reference charts and graphs essential to nurses working with pediatric patients in any clinical setting.

When using this book, nurses—as well as students and instructors—are urged to keep in mind that each patient is unique and that these care plans are intended only as a general guide to pediatric care. Individual care plans should be adapted to meet the special needs of each patient.

SECTION I

COMMON DISORDERS AND TREATMENTS

RESPIRATORY SYSTEM

Asthma

Introduction

Asthma is a reversible obstructive respiratory process characterized by periods of exacerbation and remission. One of the leading causes of chronic illness in childhood, this condition commonly manifests after age 5 and, before adolescence, affects boys more than girls.

Although commonly caused by allergy (such as to animal dander, pollen, smoke, or dust), asthma also may be precipitated by such factors as illness, stress, fatigue, or exercise. Asthmatic attacks usually result in obstruction of the bronchi and bronchioles, bronchospasms, increased mucus secretions, and mucosal edema.

Treatment usually includes administration of antibiotics and bronchodilators, increased fluid intake, respiratory treatments (such as coughing and deep-breathing exercises and chest physiotherapy), and humidified oxygen. Potential complications of the disorder include pneumothorax, congestive heart failure, respiratory infections, emotional difficulties, and even death. In some cases, the child's condition can improve after adolescence or it can progress to emphysema later in adulthood.

Assessment

Respiratory
• shortness of breath
• wheezing
• retractions
• tachypnea
• cough

Cardiovascular
• tachycardia

Neurologic
• restlessness
• anxiety

Integumentary
• cyanosis

Nursing diagnosis: Impaired gas exchange related to bronchial constriction

GOAL: The child will have improved gas exchange as evidenced by lack of wheezing and retractions, pinkish skin color, and a capillary refill time of 3 to 5 seconds.

Interventions

1. Encourage the child to perform coughing and deep-breathing exercises every 2 hours. Instruct him to take three or four deep breaths, then cough while in a sitting position.

2. Suction the child, as needed, to remove mucus from the airway.

3. Perform chest physiotherapy three or four times each day.

4. Assess the child's respiratory rate and auscultate for lung sounds.

Rationales

1. Coughing helps to clear mucus from the lungs, and deep breathing facilitates oxygenation. Sitting upright facilitates the coughing process.

2. Suctioning helps to remove secretions that the child cannot clear on his own.

3. Chest physiotherapy—a combination of postural drainage, chest percussion and vibration, and coughing and deep-breathing exercises—helps to loosen and eliminate secretions, reexpand lung tissue, and promote efficient use of respiratory muscles. (See *Performing chest physiotherapy,* page 4.)

4. This provides data to assess changes in breathing before and after treatment.

Nursing diagnosis: *Fatigue related to hypoxia*

GOAL: The child will exhibit decreased restlessness and fatigue as evidenced by decreased agitation, uninterrupted sleep periods, no signs of respiratory distress, and increased ability to perform activities.

Interventions

1. Assess for signs and symptoms of hypoxia or hypercapnia, including restlessness, agitation, cyanosis, increased heart rate, and increased respiratory rate.

2. Monitor serum theophylline levels at least every other day (normal levels should be between 8 and 20 μg/ml). If levels are above 20 μg/ml, notify the doctor, who will probably lower the dosage before the next administration.

3. Place the child in a supine position with the head of the bed elevated 45 degrees.

4. Provide adequate rest and quiet time.

Rationales

1. The early detection and prompt treatment of hypoxia and hypercapnia help to prevent restlessness and fatigue.

2. Theophylline, the drug of choice for treating asthma, causes restlessness and agitation when blood drug levels are too high.

3. Placing the child in this position increases the lungs' ability to expand and facilitates increased oxygenation, thereby decreasing restlessness.

4. Resting and quiet time decrease the child's activity level, thereby decreasing his respiratory effort and lessening fatigue.

Nursing diagnosis: *Altered nutrition: less than body requirements related to GI distress*

GOAL: The child will have decreased GI distress as evidenced by decreased nausea and vomiting and improved nutritional intake (ingestion of at least 80% of each meal).

Interventions

1. Serve the child small, frequent meals (five or six per day) consisting of foods he prefers.

2. Provide nonspicy foods with a low fat content.

Rationales

1. Small, frequent meals require less energy to digest and do not overfill the stomach and decrease lung expansion. Providing the child with some of his favorite foods helps ensure adequate intake.

2. Spicy foods and foods with a high fat content cause GI distress and are not easily digested.

Nursing diagnosis: *Fluid volume deficit related to loss of fluid from the respiratory tract*

GOAL: The child will maintain adequate hydration as evidenced by good skin turgor and a urine output of 30 ml/hour.

Interventions

1. Assess the child's skin turgor, and monitor his urine output every 4 hours.

2. Encourage the child to drink at least 3 to 8 glasses (750 to 2,000 ml) of fluid per day, depending on his age.

Rationales

1. Such assessment and monitoring helps to determine the level of hydration and the need for additional fluids.

2. Adequate amounts of fluids are necessary to maintain hydration.

PERFORMING CHEST PHYSIOTHERAPY

Chest physiotherapy, which involves auscultation, postural drainage, chest percussion and vibration, coughing and deep-breathing exercises, and evaluation of the therapy's effectiveness, enhances the removal of excessive secretions in children with respiratory conditions.

To perform chest physiotherapy, proceed as follows:
• Check the doctor's order for the location of the affected lung area and prescribed type and sequence of procedures.
• Explain the procedure to the child, provide privacy, and wash your hands.
• Perform *auscultation* of the child's lung fields to determine baseline respiratory status.
• Perform *postural drainage*.
  □ Position the child, as ordered.
  □ Instruct the child to remain in each position for 10 to 15 minutes. During this time, perform percussion and vibration, as ordered.
• Perform *percussion*.
  □ Instruct the child to breathe slowly and deeply, using the diaphragm, to promote relaxation.
  □ Hold your hands in a cupped shape, with fingers flexed and thumbs pressed tightly against your index fingers.
  □ Percuss each segment for 1 to 2 minutes by alternating your hands in a rhythmic manner. Listen for a hollow sound on percussion to verify correct performance of the technique. (For young infants, use a padded medicine cup to percuss the lung fields.)
• Perform *vibration*.
  □ Ask the child to inhale deeply and then to exhale slowly through pursed lips.
  □ During exhalation, firmly press your hands flat against the chest wall. Tense your arm and shoulder muscles in an isometric contraction to send fine vibrations through the chest wall.
  □ Vibrate during five exhalations over each chest segment.
• Instruct the child in *coughing* to remove loosened secretions.
  □ Tell the child to inhale deeply through his nose and then to exhale in three short huffs.
  □ Then have him inhale deeply again and cough through a slightly open mouth. (Three coughs usually are effective. An effective cough sounds deep, low, and hollow; an ineffective cough sounds high-pitched.
  □ Repeat the exercise two or three times.
• Auscultate the child's lung fields to *assess effectiveness of therapy*.
• Instruct the child to perform *deep-breathing exercises*, depending on his age.
  □ Place the child in a sitting position to promote optimal lung expansion. Then have him place one hand on the middle of his chest and the other on his abdomen, just below the ribs to feel the rise and fall of the diaphragm.
  □ Tell the child to inhale slowly and deeply, pushing his abdomen out against his hand to provide optimal distribution of air to the alveoli.
  □ Then tell him to exhale through pursed lips and to contract his abdomen. (Exhalation through pursed lips improves oxygen diffusion, encourages a deep, slow breathing pattern, and puts back pressure on the airways so that they stay open longer and expel a greater amount of stale air. Abdominal contraction pushes the diaphragm upward, exerts pressure on the lungs, and helps to empty them.)
  □ Instruct the child to perform exercises for 1 minute and then to rest for 2 minutes. Gradually progress to a 10-minute exercise period four times a day.

Nursing diagnosis: *Noncompliance related to treatment regimen*

GOAL: The child will comply with medical treatment and nursing care as evidenced by taking all medications and participating in routine treatment.

Interventions

1. Allow the child to participate in decisions concerning his routine treatment, such as times for chest physiotherapy and meals.

2. Explain to the child all procedures, such as laboratory workups, chest physiotherapy, and the reason he needs medication. Explain that chest physiotherapy helps loosen lung secretions to help him cough more effectively and breathe easier. Also explain that laboratory workups allow the doctors and nurses to evaluate the effectiveness of medications.

Rationales

1. Allowing the child to have some control over simple routines increases his feeling of self-control and aids in compliance with the overall treatment regimen.

2. Explanations help decrease fear and feelings of loss of control.

Nursing diagnosis: *Knowledge deficit related to home care*

GOAL: The child and parents will verbalize an understanding of home care instructions.

Interventions

1. Explain the physiology of the disease to the child and parents.

Rationales

1. Understanding the disease process may help the child and parents to comply with the treatment regimen.

Interventions

2. Based on the child's history, teach about possible precipitating factors that lead to asthma attacks, such as allergens, infections, exercise, weather changes, and stress.

3. Teach the child and parents about signs and symptoms of respiratory infection, including fever, respiratory distress, wheezing, and tachypnea.

4. Teach the child and family about the importance of taking all prescribed medications and about their possible adverse effects. Explain that:
• theophylline (a bronchodilator) may cause nausea, vomiting, restlessness, abdominal pain, and fever
• terbutaline (a bronchodilator not usually recommended for children under age 12) may cause tachycardia and some GI distress
• metaproterenol (a bronchodilator) may cause some GI distress
• albuterol (a bronchodilator) should cause no adverse effects
• corticosteroids (anti-inflammatory agents) may cause GI distress, altered immune response, and water retention.

5. Teach the importance of maintaining activity levels appropriate for the child's condition.

Rationales

2. Such teaching may help decrease the number of future attacks.

3. Early detection and treatment of respiratory infection may prevent or lessen the respiratory distress associated with asthma attacks.

4. Compliance with the medication regimen is necessary to ensure consistently stable blood drug levels, thereby ensuring control over asthma attacks.

5. Maintaining physical fitness is important to the child's normal development. Unless he is having an acute asthma attack, the child should maintain his usual activity level.

Documentation checklist

During the hospitalization, be sure to document the following:

___ the child's status and assessment findings upon admission
___ any changes in the child's status
___ pertinent laboratory and diagnostic findings
___ fluid intake and output
___ nutritional intake
___ the child's response to treatment
___ the child's and parents' reaction to chronic illness and hospitalization
___ patient and family teaching guidelines
___ discharge planning guidelines.

Bronchiolitis

Introduction

Bronchiolitis, an inflammatory viral infection of the bronchioles, results in decreased gas exchange in the alveoli. Commonly caused by respiratory syncytial virus (RSV), this disorder usually occurs in children age 2 to 12 months, especially during the winter and early spring.

The infection is characterized by mucosal edema, increased mucus secretions, bronchiolar obstruction, and overdistention of the alveoli.

Assessment

Respiratory
• increased respiratory rate
• retractions
• nasal flaring
• decreased breath sounds
• crackles
• wheezing
• prolonged expiration

Cardiovascular
• tachycardia

Neurologic
• irritability

Gastrointestinal
• feeding difficulty

Integumentary
• elevated temperature

Nursing diagnosis: *Impaired gas exchange related to bronchiolar edema and increased mucus production*

GOAL: The child will have improved gas exchange as evidenced by ease of respiration and pinkish skin color.

Interventions

1. Provide a high-humidity environment by placing the child in a mist tent or Croupette.

2. Administer oxygen by face mask, nasal cannula, or oxygen tent, as ordered.

3. Position the child with his head and chest elevated and neck slightly extended.

4. Perform chest physiotherapy every 4 hours, as ordered.

5. Administer bronchodilators, as ordered.

6. Suction the child, as needed, to remove secretions.

7. Administer antiviral agents, as ordered.

8. Promote adequate rest by decreasing the noise level, dimming the lights, and providing warmth and comfort.

Rationales

1. Cool mist from a mist tent or Croupette helps liquefy secretions and decreases bronchiolar edema.

2. Oxygen helps relieve the restlessness associated with respiratory distress and hypoxia.

3. This position maintains an open airway and eases respiration by decreasing pressure on the diaphragm.

4. Chest physiotherapy helps loosen and ease the removal of mucus that may be blocking the small airways. (See *Performing chest physiotherapy*, page 4.)

5. Although commonly used to treat muscle spasms, bronchodilators are effective in treating bronchiolar edema. They work by relaxing the smooth muscles of the bronchi and bronchioles, allowing oxygen to pass to the lungs more freely.

6. Removing secretions helps clear the bronchioles and thereby improves gas exchange.

7. Antiviral agents, such as ribavirin, are used to treat RSV, the most common causative agent in bronchiolitis.

8. Adequate rest decreases the respiratory distress associated with bronchiolitis.

Interventions	**Rationales**
9. Assess the child's respiratory rate and rhythm hourly. If the child has increased respiratory distress, auscultate for breath sounds, perform chest physiotherapy, and inform the respiratory therapist of the child's condition.	9. Frequent assessments ensure adequate respiratory function.
10. Monitor the child's apical pulse. If the pulse rate is above 150 beats/minute, notify the doctor immediately.	10. Tachycardia—a possible sign of hypoxia or an effect of bronchodilator use—can be revealed by the apical pulse rate.

Nursing diagnosis: *Potential fluid volume deficit related to increased water loss through exhalation and decreased fluid intake*

GOAL: The child will maintain fluid balance as evidenced by a urine output of 30 ml/hour and good skin turgor.

Interventions	**Rationales**
1. Administer I.V. fluids, as ordered.	1. I.V. fluids are used to hydrate the child until the crisis has passed.
2. Ensure that the child receives adequate rest.	2. Resting allows the child's respiratory rate to return to baseline levels, thereby decreasing the amount of water lost through exhalation.
3. Monitor the child's fluid intake and output carefully.	3. Careful monitoring ensures adequate hydration. If the child experiences decreased urine output, he may require additional fluids.
4. Assess for signs and symptoms of dehydration, including weight loss, pallor, poor skin turgor, dry mucous membranes, oliguria, and increased pulse rate.	4. Evidence of dehydration suggests that the child is not receiving enough fluids.
5. Increase the child's oral fluid intake when the acute period has subsided.	5. Fluids help to liquefy secretions.

Nursing diagnosis: *Ineffective thermoregulation related to hyperthermia*

GOAL: The child will have no evidence of fever as evidenced by a lack of increased temperature.

Interventions	**Rationales**
1. Maintain a cool environment by using lightweight pajamas and covers and maintaining the room temperature between 72° and 75° F. (22.2° and 23.9° C.).	1. A cool environment helps to reduce body temperature through radiant heat loss.
2. Administer antipyretics, as ordered.	2. Antipyretics, such as acetaminophen, effectively reduce fever.
3. Monitor the child's temperature every 1 to 2 hours for sudden elevation.	3. Sudden elevation in temperature may result in a seizure.
4. Obtain a sputum specimen for culturing.	4. Treatment of bronchiolitis depends on identifying the causative agent through culturing.
5. Administer antimicrobials, if ordered.	5. Antimicrobials may be ordered to treat the underlying causative organism. Antibiotics usually are not ordered to treat RSV.
6. Give the child tepid sponge baths to relieve fever.	6. Sponge baths with tepid water effectively cool the body through conduction.

Nursing diagnosis: *Impaired social interaction related to isolation*

GOAL: The child will maintain social contacts despite being isolated because of his respiratory condition.

Interventions

1. Explain to the child and parents the purpose and nature of isolation, including details about unfamiliar surroundings and the use of masks and gowns.

2. Introduce yourself upon entering the child's room.

3. Provide a means of communication with a call system.

4. Assess the child at least hourly for any changes in his condition.

5. Provide diversional activities, such as toys, books, television, and music.

6. Encourage parental presence and participation in caregiving activities.

Rationales

1. Such explanations are necessary to avoid frightening the child.

2. The child and parents often have difficulty distinguishing staff personnel because of the required isolation clothing.

3. A call system is necessary to enable the child and parents to communicate the need for assistance.

4. Frequent assessments are necessary despite the fact that the child is in isolation.

5. Such diversions are necessary to keep the child stimulated and distracted when in isolation.

6. Parents provide a major source of socialization for the child in isolation.

Nursing diagnosis: *Fatigue related to respiratory distress*

GOAL: The child will rest at least 1 hour in the morning and evening.

Interventions

1. To help decrease the child's fatigue, provide rest periods every 2 hours. Also, bathe the child, change the bed linens, and perform neuro checks during the same visit to allow for uninterrupted periods of rest.

2. Provide a quiet environment.

Rationales

1. The child needs adequate rest, as fatigue increases respiratory distress.

2. Unnecessary noise and activity may tire the child and result in increased respiratory distress.

Nursing diagnosis: *Altered nutrition: less than body requirements related to the disease process*

GOAL: The child will have improved nutritional intake as evidenced by consuming at least 80% of each meal.

Interventions

1. Provide small, frequent meals that include foods the child prefers.

2. Provide a diet high in calories and protein.

Rationales

1. Small, frequent meals require less energy expenditure and respiratory use. Providing favorite foods helps ensure that the child will eat more of each meal.

2. A high-protein, high-calorie diet is necessary to meet the child's increased metabolic needs.

Nursing diagnosis: *Anxiety (child and parent) related to lack of knowledge about the child's condition*

GOAL: The child and parents will be less anxious as evidenced by verbalizing an understanding of the child's condition.

Interventions

1. Assess the child's and parents' understanding of the child's condition and prescribed treatment regimen.

2. Allow the parents to stay with the child.

3. Explain all procedures in developmentally appropriate terms.

4. Provide emotional support to the parents during the hospitalization.

Rationales

1. Such assessment serves as a basis on which to begin teaching.

2. Staying with the child allows the parents to provide support.

3. Anxiety related to misunderstanding and lack of knowledge can be lessened if explanations are provided beforehand and throughout the hospitalization.

4. Hospitalization poses a crisis situation. Listening to the parents' concerns and feelings helps them to deal with the crisis.

Nursing diagnosis: *Knowledge deficit related to home care*

GOAL: The parents will verbalize an understanding of home care instructions.

Interventions

1. Teach the parents and child (if appropriate) how and when to administer medications, including details about dosages and adverse effects.

2. Explain the signs and symptoms of respiratory distress and infection, including fever, dyspnea, tachypnea, yellowish or greenish sputum, and wheezing.

3. Explain the importance of the child's receiving adequate rest.

4. Teach the importance of adequate nutrition and hydration, stressing the need for plenty of fluids and a diet high in calories.

5. Teach the importance of providing a humidified environment with cool mist.

Rationales

1. Understanding the importance of maintaining a consistent medication regimen may help the parents to comply with the child's overall treatment. Knowing what adverse effects to expect should prompt the parents to call for assistance, when needed.

2. Such knowledge should prompt the parents to seek medical advice and attention, when needed.

3. After infection, the child requires frequent rest periods to aid recovery and prevent a relapse of the infection.

4. Fluids help to liquefy secretions. A diet high in calories helps to replace calories expended in fighting the disease.

5. Humidified air helps to thin secretions. Cool, humidified air from a mist tent is safer than the warm air of a vaporizer, as it won't cause burns.

Documentation checklist

During the hospitalization, be sure to document the following:

___ the child's status and assessment findings upon admission

___ any changes in the child's status

___ pertinent laboratory and diagnostic findings

___ fluid intake and output

___ nutritional intake

___ the child's response to treatment

___ the child's and parents' reaction to the illness and hospitalization

___ patient and family teaching guidelines

___ discharge planning guidelines.

Bronchopulmonary Dysplasia

Introduction

Bronchopulmonary dysplasia (BPD) is a chronic, progressive pulmonary condition of unknown etiology characterized by pulmonary edema and a prolonged need for oxygen. BPD often occurs in premature infants with respiratory distress syndrome who have undergone endotracheal intubation, administration of high concentrations of oxygen, and high positive-pressure ventilation for prolonged periods.

Treatment is supportive, usually focused on managing the symptoms, as no cure exists. Potential complications include chronic respiratory disease and frequent respiratory infections.

Assessment

Respiratory
• respiratory distress
• retractions
• dyspnea
• crackles
• rhonchi
• wheezing

Cardiovascular
• poor capillary refill time

Gastrointestinal
• difficulty feeding
• weight gain or loss

Musculoskeletal
• fatigue

Integumentary
• pallor
• circumoral cyanosis

Nursing diagnosis: *Impaired gas exchange related to difficulty in expectorating mucus and fluid retention in the lungs*

GOAL: The child will have improved gas exchange as evidenced by lack of wheezing, decreased retractions, pink skin color, and a capillary refill time of 3 to 5 seconds.

Interventions

1. Assess the child's respiratory and fluid status, noting skin color, respiratory effort, retractions, capillary refill time, breath sounds, secretions, vital signs, and edema every hour for 4 hours. Report any deviations from baseline data.

2. Perform chest physiotherapy every 4 hours for 15 to 20 minutes and gentle suctioning 4 times daily or as needed (see *Performing chest physiotherapy,* page 4).

3. Administer oxygen, as ordered. Monitor transcutaneous oxygen levels, if necessary.

4. Administer bronchodilators, as ordered.

5. Monitor the child's fluid intake and output carefully.

6. Administer diuretics, as ordered.

7. Monitor electrolyte levels.

Rationales

1. Monitoring is essential because children with BPD are susceptible to lower respiratory infections, development of hypertension, and respiratory failure.

2. Chest physiotherapy helps loosen mucus in the lungs and assists with expectoration. Suctioning eliminates excess mucus from the airway.

3. BPD may cause intermittent or persistent hypoxia, necessitating oxygen therapy.

4. Bronchodilators may be ordered to treat acute respiratory infections or for maintenance therapy to improve the passage of air to the alveoli.

5. Monitoring fluid intake and output is essential to determine whether the child is adequately hydrated, as adequate hydration is necessary to help liquefy secretions.

6. Diuretics, which may be given routinely, help improve respiratory function by decreasing fluid retention and the risk of pulmonary edema.

7. Such monitoring is essential, especially if diuretics are given; hypokalemia may occur.

Interventions	Rationales
8. Increase the child's fluid intake if not contraindicated.	8. Increased fluid intake helps liquefy secretions.

Nursing diagnosis: *Altered nutrition: less than body requirements related to increased metabolic rate and high caloric demands*

GOAL: The child will maintain caloric requirements as evidenced by weight gain.

Interventions	Rationales
1. Weigh the child daily at the same time (usually before the morning meal), without clothes and preferably with the same scale.	1. Weighing the child on a daily basis is necessary to monitor any weight gain or loss.
2. Consult the hospital dietitian when planning the child's meals, especially with regard to high-calorie supplements and formulas.	2. A dietitian can help with determining the child's nutritional needs based on age-appropriate developmental data. To increase the caloric intake, the dietitian may recommend feeding the child small, frequent meals of high-calorie supplements and formulas, such as MCT Oil in formula, rather than increasing the total volume consumed.
3. Supplement oral feedings with nasogastric feedings as needed and during the night.	3. If the child cannot consume the appropriate amount of calories through oral feedings, nasogastric feedings may be necessary to ensure he maintains weight.
4. Spend extra time with the child during feedings, as needed, to allow for frequent burping and resting.	4. Children with BPD sometimes experience fatigue during feedings and require extra time to complete feedings.

Nursing diagnosis: *Altered growth and development related to chronic illness, prematurity, or prolonged hospitalization*

GOAL: The child will achieve developmental milestones despite his prematurity or chronic illness.

Interventions	Rationales
1. Assess the child's developmental status using standardized developmental tools, such as the Washington Guide or Denver Developmental Screening Test. Consult a child development expert, if available.	1. Children with BPD are at risk for developmental delays and require careful assessment to identify any lags. Child development experts can assist in assessing delays and planning therapy.
2. Ensure that the child is provided with consistent caregivers, such as consistent nursing staff, when possible.	2. Children are more likely to progress developmentally if consistently exposed to the same caregivers.
3. Develop an individualized plan that includes visual, auditory, tactile, and social stimulation. Post or hang the developmental plan at the child's bedside for all caregivers to see.	3. A specialized plan is necessary to meet the child's unique developmental needs. Posting or hanging the plan ensures that all personnel who come in contact with the child can provide consistent stimulation to help the child progress developmentally.
4. Observe the child for signs and symptoms of hearing or vision impairment by assessing the child's response to sound and to color and shapes at varying distances. Report any evidence of such impairment immediately.	4. Because developmental delays can be caused by hearing or vision impairment, early detection is essential.

Nursing diagnosis: *Altered parenting related to the child's chronic illness*

GOAL: The parents will bond effectively with the child as evidenced by verbalizing positive feelings and demonstrating positive interactive behaviors, such as touching, stroking, holding, and making direct eye contact.

Interventions

1. Encourage parental participation in caring for the child.

2. Provide positive feedback for positive interactive behaviors.

3. Discuss the child's individuality with the parents. Allow them to express their concerns about the child's illness.

4. Help the parents to identify stressors and solve problems. Refer them to appropriate social agencies, as needed.

Rationales

1. Direct parental participation in the child's care should help facilitate bonding.

2. Positive reinforcement encourages continued positive behaviors.

3. Viewing the child as an individual helps to increase the bonding between the parents and their child. Expressing their concerns helps them to ventilate feelings and cope with the situation.

4. Because stressors may be overwhelming, the parents may need assistance in dealing with certain pressures brought on by the child's illness. Referral may be necessary to provide emotional and financial support.

Nursing diagnosis: *Potential for impaired skin integrity related to irritation from nasogastric (NG) feedings secondary to BPD*

GOAL: The child will maintain skin integrity as evidenced by pinkish, intact skin around the nares and cheeks.

Interventions

1. Apply a skin barrier, such as Stomahesive, to both cheeks and secure tape to the barrier and cannula.

2. Assess and cleanse the skin by removing the skin barrier, as needed.

3. Change the child's body position every 2 hours.

Rationales

1. The skin barrier serves as a protection from irritation caused by the application of tape directly to the child's skin.

2. The skin barrier should be removed periodically to assess and cleanse the skin, thereby preventing skin breakdown.

3. Changing the child's body position helps to prevent skin breakdown.

Nursing diagnosis: *Anxiety (parent) related to fear and lack of knowledge concerning the child's illness*

GOAL: The parents will be less anxious as evidenced by demonstrating increased verbalization about the child's condition and decreased fearfulness of procedures.

Interventions

1. Assess the parents' understanding of their child's condition and prescribed treatment.

2. Provide explanations about all treatments, procedures, and equipment.

3. Provide emotional support to the parents during the hospitalization.

Rationales

1. Such assessment provides a basis on which to begin teaching.

2. Anxiety related to lack of knowledge and misunderstanding can be lessened if explanations are provided beforehand and throughout the child's hospitalization.

3. Because hospitalization poses a crisis situation, providing emotional support helps the parents to better deal with the situation.

Nursing diagnosis: *Knowledge deficit related to home care*

GOAL: The parents will verbalize an understanding of home care instructions.

Interventions

1. Explain to the parents the importance of exposing the child to cool, humidified air.

2. Teach the parents the signs and symptoms of respiratory distress, including dyspnea, tachypnea (over the normal rate), cyanosis, and retractions.

3. Provide instruction on oxygen administration, including details on the rate and frequency.

4. Teach the parents how and when to administer medications, including information on dosages and adverse effects.

5. Teach the parents how to give cardiopulmonary resuscitation.

6. Teach the parents how to administer NG feedings if the child is discharged with an NG tube. Include specific information about tube placement and feeding solutions.

Rationales

1. Humidified air liquefies secretions and facilitates breathing. Cool, humidified air from a mist tent is safer than warm air from a vaporizer, as it won't cause burns.

2. Knowing such signs and symptoms should prompt the parents to seek medical advice and attention, when needed.

3. Children with BPD usually require continuous oxygen. Parents must have firsthand knowledge to provide appropriate care.

4. Parents need to know specific information regarding how to administer medications consistently and safely. Such knowledge also helps ensure compliance with the medication regimen.

5. Because children with BPD are at increased risk for respiratory distress, parents must know how to provide prompt care in an emergency.

6. Because children with BPD are prone to aspiration, they often require feedings by an NG or, in some cases, a gastrostomy tube. Parents must know how to initiate feedings and monitor their progress.

Documentation checklist

During the hospitalization, be sure to document the following:
___ the child's status and assessment findings upon admission
___ any changes in the child's status
___ pertinent laboratory and diagnostic findings
___ fluid intake and output
___ nutritional intake
___ the child's response to treatment
___ the child's and parents' reaction to the illness and hospitalization
___ patient and family teaching guidelines
___ discharge planning guidelines.

RESPIRATORY SYSTEM

Croup

Introduction

Also known as laryngotracheobronchitis, croup is an infection of the upper and lower airways that sometimes results in respiratory distress (laryngospasm, dyspnea, and barking cough), stridor, retractions, and cyanosis. It usually follows an upper respiratory tract infection.

Typically affecting children between ages 3 months and 3 years, croup can be life-threatening if not treated. Treatment usually includes administration of antibiotics and fluids and exposure to humidified air to maintain respiration. If the child's respiratory status is severely compromised, intubation or tracheostomy may be required.

Assessment

Respiratory
• history of cold symptoms lasting 1 to 2 days
• signs and symptoms of respiratory distress

• dyspnea
• retractions
• cyanosis
• barking cough
• whooping sound on inspiration

Cardiovascular
• tachycardia

Neurologic
• altered level of consciousness
• anxiety

Integumentary
• elevated temperature

Nursing diagnosis: *Ineffective breathing pattern related to upper airway edema and thickened secretions*

GOAL: The child's airway will remain patent as evidenced by relief of respiratory distress.

Interventions

1. Assess the child's respiratory status frequently or continuously for signs and symptoms of increased respiratory distress and obstruction, including increased respiratory rate, stridor, and retractions; nasal flaring; prolonged expirations; cyanosis; confusion; restlessness; decreased breath sounds; tachycardia; and barking cough.

2. Provide cool, humidified air via a mist tent, Croupette, or face mask.

3. Administer oxygen, as ordered.

4. Administer aerosolized racemic epinephrine, as ordered.

5. Place the child in high-Fowler's position.

Rationales

1. Signs and symptoms of increased respiratory distress may indicate that the obstruction is worsening. A rapid, rising respiratory rate with an increased heart rate may be the first sign of hypoxia.

2. Cool mist helps to liquefy secretions.

3. Oxygen may be ordered to alleviate hypoxia and restlessness. However, because oxygen use may mask the early signs of hypoxia and increasing obstruction with subsequent hypercapnia, it should only be used to treat known hypoxia.

4. Racemic epinephrine reduces swelling of the subglottic mucosa. Because of the drug's short-term effect, children should be observed for evidence of rebound obstruction.

5. This position facilitates increased lung capacity by decreasing diaphragmatic pressure on the lungs.

Nursing diagnosis: *Potential fluid volume deficit related to decreased oral intake*

GOAL: The child will maintain fluid balance as evidenced by good skin turgor and a urine output of 30 ml/hour.

Interventions

1. Assess the child's ability to tolerate fluids.

2. Administer and monitor I.V. fluids, as ordered.

3. Carefully monitor the child's fluid intake and output.

4. Assess the child for signs and symptoms of dehydration, including poor skin turgor, dry mucous membranes, sunken fontanels, and sunken eyes.

Rationales

1. The child's tolerance of fluids may be complicated by throat discomfort, increased respiratory rate, or vomiting.

2. I.V. fluids may be ordered to decrease the physical effort associated with oral feeding. Oral fluids are contraindicated in children with severe respiratory distress because of the risk of aspiration and vomiting.

3. Careful monitoring is essential because decreased urine output may indicate early dehydration.

4. The child's fluid intake may need to be adjusted if signs of dehydration are apparent.

Nursing diagnosis: *Anxiety (child) related to respiratory distress and hospitalization*

GOAL: The child will be less anxious as evidenced by restful sleep periods and a stable respiratory status.

Interventions

1. Allow the child to assume a comfortable position during treatment with humidified air or oxygen.

2. Postpone any nonurgent tests until the child's respiratory status has improved.

3. Encourage the parental presence.

4. Provide familiar objects, such as toys and blankets, for the child to keep with him in the mist tent or Croupette.

Rationales

1. The child should be made as comfortable and secure as possible to alleviate anxiety during treatment, as discomfort may result in increased respiratory rate and stridor. A mist tent or Croupette often is better tolerated than a face mask.

2. Because the child's anxiety level may already be high as a result of his increased respiratory distress, testing may compound the problem further.

3. Parental presence helps reduce anxiety and, consequently, helps stabilize the child's respiratory rate.

4. Familiar objects provide a sense of security and help relieve some of the anxiety associated with the new and strange environment.

Nursing diagnosis: *Anxiety (parent) related to fear and lack of knowledge concerning the child's condition*

GOAL: The parents will be less anxious as evidenced by verbalizing an understanding of the child's condition and demonstrating decreased fearfulness of procedures.

Interventions

1. Assess the parents' understanding of their child's condition and the prescribed treatment.

2. Explain to the parents all procedures, treatments, and equipment.

Rationales

1. This knowledge serves as a basis on which to begin teaching.

2. Anxiety related to lack of knowledge or misunderstanding can be lessened if explanations are provided beforehand and throughout the child's hospitalization.

Interventions	**Rationales**
3. Provide emotional support to the parents during the hospitalization.	3. Hospitalization poses a crisis situation for parents; emotional support helps them deal better with the crisis.

Nursing diagnosis: *Knowledge deficit related to home care*

GOAL: The parents will verbalize an understanding of home care instructions.

Interventions	**Rationales**
1. Teach parents how and when to administer medications, including information about dosages and adverse effects.	1. Understanding the medication regimen may help parents to comply with the child's overall treatment. Knowing the adverse effects associated with medications should prompt parents to seek medical advice and attention, when necessary.
2. Explain to the parents the signs and symptoms of respiratory distress and infection, including fever, dyspnea, tachypnea, yellowish or greenish sputum, and wheezing.	2. Parents should know this information so that they can seek medical advice and attention when necessary.
3. Explain the importance of the child's receiving adequate rest.	3. After infection, the child needs frequent rest periods to aid recovery and prevent relapses.
4. Teach about the importance of adequate hydration and nutrition. Explain that the child will need to drink 2 to 4 glasses (500 to 1,000 ml) of fluids daily (depending on the child's renal and cardiovascular status) and to eat high-calorie meals.	4. Fluids help liquefy secretions. A diet high in calories helps replace calories expended to fight the disease process.
5. Teach about the importance of providing a humidified environment using cool mist.	5. Humidified air helps to thin secretions. Cool, humidified air from a mist tent is safer than the warm air of a vaporizer because it won't cause burns.

Documentation checklist

During the hospitalization, be sure to document the following:
___ the child's status and assessment findings upon admission
___ any changes in the child's status
___ pertinent laboratory and diagnostic findings
___ fluid intake and output
___ nutritional intake
___ the child's response to treatment
___ the child's and parents' reaction to the illness and hospitalization
___ patient and family teaching guidelines
___ discharge planning guidelines.

RESPIRATORY SYSTEM

Cystic Fibrosis

Introduction

Cystic fibrosis, the most common life-threatening genetic disease of white children in the United States, affects the functioning of the respiratory and other body systems from increased, thickened secretions produced by the mucous-secreting exocrine glands. Typically, these thick secretions block the ducts of such organs as the lungs, pancreas, and liver, resulting in difficult breathing, chronic respiratory infections, nutritional deficits, and cirrhosis.

The disease, which varies in severity, is associated with many complications, including chronic respiratory infections, meconium ileus, rectal prolapse, and infertility. Treatment includes pulmonary therapy, administration of pancreatic enzymes and vitamins, and a diet high in calories and protein. Although many children are surviving into adulthood, more males survive than do females.

Assessment

Respiratory
• wheezing
• nonproductive cough
• dyspnea
• barrel chest
• bronchitis
• digital clubbing

Gastrointestinal
• failure to thrive
• foul-smelling, bulky, loose stools or chronic diarrhea
• increased appetite
• rectal prolapse
• ulcers
• intestinal obstruction

Genitourinary
• infertility (detected later in life)
• vaginal infections

Integumentary
• bruising
• cyanosis
• salty-tasting skin

Nursing diagnosis: *Impaired gas exchange related to increased mucus production*

GOAL: The child will have increased mobilization of mucus secretions as evidenced by decreased respiratory distress, cyanosis, and coughing.

Interventions

1. Perform chest physiotherapy every 4 hours (see *Performing chest physiotherapy,* page 4).

2. Administer humidified oxygen.

3. Assess the child's respiratory status every 4 hours.

4. Instruct the child to perform deep-breathing exercises every 4 hours.

5. Administer expectorants and bronchodilators, as ordered.

Rationales

1. The positioning and chest percussion and vibration performed in chest physiotherapy facilitates mobilization of secretions. The breathing exercises help to maintain lung capacity and increase oxygenation.

2. Humidity loosens and thins secretions; oxygen increases tissue aeration. Because the child's stimulus to breathe often depends on low oxygen levels, highly concentrated oxygen should not be used.

3. Frequent respiratory assessments allow for early detection of changes in the child's condition.

4. Deep-breathing exercises help to increase lung expansion.

5. These agents help promote the thinning of secretions and lung expansion.

Nursing diagnosis: *Potential for infection related to increased mucus production*

GOAL: The child will have no signs of infection as evidenced by lack of fever, chills, and increasing respiratory distress.

Interventions	Rationales
1. Administer antibiotics, as ordered.	1. Antibiotics may be ordered to help fight infection.
2. Assess vital signs for evidence of increased respiratory rate, dyspnea, tachypnea, and cyanosis.	2. These changes in vital signs indicate a worsening of infection.
3. Monitor the white blood cell (WBC) count.	3. An elevated WBC count is an indication of infection.

Nursing diagnosis: *Altered nutrition: less than body requirements related to reduced absorption of nutrients*

GOAL: The child will have an improved nutritional status as evidenced by minimal weight loss, good skin turgor, and increased intake (eating over 80%) of meals.

Interventions	Rationales
1. Weigh the child at the same time each day, using the same scale.	1. Daily weights aid in assessing the child's nutritional status.
2. Administer pancreatic enzymes before meals and with snacks.	2. Pancreatic enzymes aid in digestion to enable absorption of nutrients.
3. Provide a diet high in calories, protein, and carbohydrates.	3. This type of diet helps replace nutrients lost through decreased absorption in the gastrointestinal tract.
4. Avoid giving respiratory treatments after meals.	4. Respiratory treatments may cause coughing and vomiting after meals.
5. Provide foods appropriate for the child's age and developmental level that are within the child's dietary specifications.	5. Appropriate foods, such as finger foods for toddlers, aid in the child's developmental growth.

Nursing diagnosis: *Potential for injury related to electrolyte imbalances*

GOAL: The child will maintain stable electrolyte levels.

Interventions	Rationales
1. Provide salt with each meal.	1. Table salt allows for replacement of sodium lost through the skin. If not replaced, sodium imbalance may occur.
2. Provide adequate hydration.	2. Maintaining adequate fluid levels is necessary for proper functioning of the circulatory and renal systems.

Nursing diagnosis: *Anxiety (child) related to respiratory distress and hospitalization*

GOAL: The child will have a decreased anxiety level as evidenced by restful sleeping periods and a stable respiratory status.

Interventions	Rationales
1. Allow the child to assume a comfortable position.	1. If the child is forced into a specific position, he may experience increased anxiety and, consequently, increased respiratory distress.

Interventions

2. Postpone all testing until a patent airway is ensured.

3. Encourage parental presence and participation in the child's care.

Rationales

2. Laboratory tests and procedures may increase the child's anxiety level, thereby increasing respiratory distress.

3. Every effort should be made to decrease the child's anxiety. Parental presence and participation provides security and reduces anxiety.

Nursing diagnosis: *Anxiety (parent) related to lack of knowledge concerning the child's condition*

GOAL: The child's parents will be less anxious as evidenced by their ability to support the child and explain the condition.

Interventions

1. Assess the parent's understanding of the child's condition and prescribed treatment.

2. Provide explanations about the medical condition, procedures, and required treatments.

3. Provide emotional support to the parents during the hospitalization.

Rationales

1. Such assessment serves as a basis on which to begin teaching.

2. Anxiety related to lack of knowledge and misunderstanding can be lessened if explanations are provided beforehand and throughout the child's hospitalization.

3. Hospitalization poses a crisis situation. Listening to the parents' concerns and feelings helps them to deal with that crisis.

Nursing diagnosis: *Knowledge deficit related to home care*

GOAL: The parents will verbalize an understanding of home care instructions.

Interventions

1. Teach the parents about antibiotic administration and its potential adverse effects, including rash, GI distress, vomiting, and respiratory distress.

2. Teach the parents the signs and symptoms of respiratory distress, including dyspnea, tachypnea, cyanosis, wheezing, and tachycardia.

3. Stress the importance of encouraging the child to drink 2 to 4 glassess (500 to 1,000 ml) of fluids each day (depending on the child's renal and cardiovascular status).

4. Teach the importance of providing the child with a diet high in calories, protein, and carbohydrates.

Rationales

1. Parents need to know how to administer medications safely and consistently. Knowing the potential adverse effects associated with medications should prompt them to seek medical advice and attention, when necessary.

2. Recognizing the signs and symptoms of respiratory distress should prompt parents to seek medical advice and attention, when necessary.

3. Adequate fluids are essential to replace water lost through the lungs, as dehydration can result in electrolyte imbalances.

4. Such a diet helps replace some of the nutrients lost through nonabsorption.

Documentation checklist

During the hospitalization, be sure to document the following:

___ the child's status and assessment findings upon admission

___ any changes in the child's status

___ pertinent laboratory and diagnostic findings

___ fluid intake and output

___ nutritional intake

___ respiratory therapy

___ medication administration

___ the child's response to treatment

___ the child's and parents' reaction to the illness and hospitalization

___ patient and family teaching guidelines

___ discharge planning guidelines.

RESPIRATORY SYSTEM

Epiglottitis

Introduction

Epiglottitis is an obstructive airway infection characterized by rapidly occurring acute respiratory distress and inflammation of the epiglottis. The infection, which often is caused by *Hemophilus influenzae* type b, has a rapid onset. Typically, the child exhibits no symptoms at bedtime, but awakens with swallowing difficulty and a sore throat.

This condition usually affects children between ages 2 and 8 and may be life-threatening if not treated immediately. Treatment includes mechanical ventilatory support or tracheostomy. Antibiotics also may be used. The prognosis is generally good if the child receives immediate treatment.

Assessment

Respiratory
• history of sore throat with sudden onset of respiratory distress (dyspnea, tachypnea, retractions, wheezing)

Cardiovascular
• tachycardia

Neurologic
• anxiety

Gastrointestinal
• drooling
• inability to swallow

Musculoskeletal
• erect, chin-thrust posturing

Integumentary
• elevated temperature

Nursing diagnosis: *Altered breathing pattern related to upper airway edema*

GOAL: The child's airway will remain patent as evidenced by no signs of acute respiratory distress.

Interventions

1. Assess the child for signs and symptoms of respiratory distress, including dyspnea, tachypnea, cyanosis, drooling, and wheezing.

2. Assess for increased swelling of the airway, which indicates an emergency. Notify the doctor immediately if this occurs.

3. Avoid direct stimulation of the airway with a tongue depressor, culture swab, suction catheter, or laryngoscope.

4. Allow the child to assume a comfortable position other than the horizontal position.

5. Assess the child's skin color, respiratory status, and heart rate continuously until a patent airway is ensured.

6. Keep emergency intubation equipment at the child's bedside at all times.

Rationales

1. Such assessment is necessary to determine the severity of the child's condition and to prevent complete respiratory failure.

2. Early recognition of increased swelling is essential because swelling, which occurs rapidly, is sometimes fatal. The doctor must be available for endotracheal tube placement.

3. Any manipulation of the epiglottis may cause laryngospasm and swelling, possibly causing complete obstruction.

4. Allowing the child to assume his own comfortable position helps ease anxiety and decreases the risk of developing increased respiratory distress. Placing the child in a horizontal position may cause rapid tissue deterioration.

5. Continuous observation is mandatory because increasing edema can cause complete obstruction at any time.

6. Emergency intubation equipment should be on hand for the doctor's use in case complete obstruction occurs.

Nursing diagnosis: *Ineffective airway clearance related to placement of artificial airway*

GOAL: The child's airway will remain patent and secure as evidenced by no signs or symptoms of respiratory distress.

Interventions

1. Assess the adequacy of the child's respirations, noting especially any sign of increased respiratory rate, rhonchi, wheezing, retractions, and restlessness.

2. Restrain the child with soft wrist or elbow restraints. Be sure to check the circulation in the hands and fingers every 4 hours. Also, administer sedatives, as ordered.

3. Maintain the tube's placement by taping the tube securely to the child's maxilla.

4. Maintain the child's head and neck in a neutral position (with the head and neck in complete alignment). During positioning, move the head and trunk together as a unit.

5. Carefully suction the child, as needed, when secretions appear in the airway.

6. Administer humidified oxygen by face mask or a nasal cannula, as ordered.

Rationales

1. Such changes in the respiratory status usually indicate respiratory distress.

2. Restraints may be necessary to prevent the child from pulling out the endotracheal tube, as reintubation can be difficult, traumatic, and potentially life-threatening. Sedatives may be necessary to prevent agitation and anxiety.

3. Proper taping will ensure minimal movement and decrease the incidence of extubation.

4. This ensures minimal movement of the tube in the trachea, thereby decreasing the risk of trauma and later stenosis.

5. Frequent suctioning may be necessary because the artificial airway interferes with the child's ability to clear secretions. This should be done carefully to avoid causing increased trauma to the airway, which could lead to hypoxia and atelectasis.

6. Humidified oxygen is necessary to prevent secretions from drying and thickening in the airway.

Nursing diagnosis: *Potential fluid volume deficit related to decreased fluid intake*

GOAL: The child will maintain fluid balance as evidenced by good skin turgor, adequate urine output, and a capillary refill time of 3 to 5 seconds.

Interventions

1. Avoid giving the child oral fluids before intubation.

2. Administer and monitor I.V. fluids, as ordered.

3. Carefully monitor the child's fluid intake and output.

4. Assess the child for signs of dehydration, including poor skin turgor, dry mucous membranes, and sunken fontanels and eyes.

Rationales

1. Oral intake should be avoided before intubation because of swallowing difficulty and the risk of aspiration.

2. I.V. fluids are used to hydrate the child.

3. Decreased urine output may be an early indication of dehydration.

4. Dehydration indicates that the child's fluid intake needs to be readjusted.

Nursing diagnosis: *Ineffective thermoregulation related to hyperthermia secondary to infection*

GOAL: The child will have no elevation in fever.

Interventions

1. Monitor the child's temperature every 2 to 4 hours for elevation.

2. Administer antipyretics, as ordered.

3. Administer tepid sponge baths if the child is unresponsive to medication.

4. Obtain blood cultures, as ordered.

5. Administer antimicrobials, as ordered.

Rationales

1. Temperatures greater than 101.3° F. (38.5° C.) usually are associated with *Hemophilus influenzae,* the most common causative agent in epiglottitis.

2. Antipyretics help reduce fever and allow the child to rest more comfortably.

3. Tepid sponge baths cool the body surface, constrict blood vessels, and lower the overall metabolism, thereby lowering the body temperature.

4. Cultures are necessary to identify and treat septic infections, which occur in up to 70% of all children with epiglottitis.

5. Antimicrobials, such as cefuroxime, ampicillin, and chloramphenicol, are effective against *Hemophilus influenzae.*

Nursing diagnosis: *Anxiety (child) related to respiratory distress and hospitalization*

GOAL: The child will be less anxious as evidenced by restful sleeping periods and a stable respiratory status.

Interventions

1. Allow the child to assume a comfortable position.

2. Postpone all testing until a patent airway is ensured.

3. Encourage parental presence and participation in the child's care.

4. Explain all procedures and treatments to the child in terms he can understand.

5. Provide the child with familiar objects, such as toys and blankets.

Rationales

1. If forced into a specific position, the child may have increased anxiety, resulting in increased respiratory distress.

2. Testing may further compound the child's already anxious state, thereby increasing respiratory distress.

3. Every effort should be made to make the child as comfortable as possible to decrease his anxiety. Parental presence and participation provides the child with a sense of security.

4. Explanations offered beforehand can help lessen the anxiety associated with certain procedures and treatments.

5. Familiar objects help the child feel more secure in the strange hospital environment.

Nursing diagnosis: *Anxiety (parent) related to lack of knowledge concerning the child's condition*

GOAL: The parents will be less anxious as evidenced by their ability to support their child and explain his condition.

Interventions

1. Assess the parents' understanding of the child's condition and prescribed treatment.

Rationales

1. Such assessment will serve as a basis on which to begin teaching.

Interventions

2. Provide explanations about the medical condition, procedures, and prescribed treatment.

3. Provide emotional support to the parents during the hospitalization.

Rationales

2. Anxiety related to lack of understanding or misunderstanding can be lessened if explanations are provided beforehand and throughout the child's hospitalization.

3. Hospitalization poses a crisis situation. Listening to the parents' concerns and feelings helps them to deal with that crisis.

Nursing diagnosis: *Knowledge deficit related to home care*

GOAL: The parents will verbalize an understanding of home care instructions.

Interventions

1. Teach about antibiotic administration, including information about such potential adverse effects as gastrointestinal distress, rash, and respiratory distress (dyspnea, tachypnea, cyanosis, wheezing, and tachycardia).

2. Explain the importance of encouraging the child to drink 2 to 4 glasses (500 to 1,000 ml) of fluid each day.

Rationales

1. Parents need to know how and when to administer antibiotics safely and consistently. Knowing the potential adverse effects should prompt them to seek medical advice and attention, when necessary.

2. Fluids are necessary to replace water lost through the lungs and to help with difficult swallowing. Inadequate fluid intake can lead to dehydration and eventual electrolyte imbalance.

Documentation checklist

During the hospitalization, be sure to document the following:
___ the child's status and assessment findings upon admission
___ any changes in the child's status
___ pertinent laboratory and diagnostic findings
___ intubation efforts
___ fluid intake and output
___ the child's response to treatment
___ the child's and parents' reaction to the illness and hospitalization
___ patient and family teaching guidelines
___ discharge planning guidelines.

RESPIRATORY SYSTEM

Pneumonia

Introduction

Pneumonia is an inflammation of the lungs usually caused by bacterial (*Staphylococcus*) or viral (respiratory syncytial virus) infection. Occurring as a primary disease or as a complication of another illness, pneumonia is characterized by thick exudate that blocks the alveoli and decreases oxygen exchange. Onset may be rapid in the bacterial or viral form.

Common in infants and young children, pneumonia may occur at any age. Treatment includes primary respiratory support for the viral form and antibiotics and respiratory support for the bacterial form.

Assessment

Respiratory
• increased respiratory rate
• retractions
• crackles
• decreased breath sounds
• nasal flaring
• cyanosis
• cough

Cardiovascular
• tachycardia

Gastrointestinal
• decreased appetite

Musculoskeletal
• restlessness

Integumentary
• elevated temperature

Nursing diagnosis: *Impaired gas exchange related to exudate accumulation and increased mucus production*

GOAL: The child will have improved gas exchange as evidenced by ease of respiration, improved skin color, and decreased restlessness.

Interventions

1. Allow the child to assume a comfortable position.

2. Provide cool mist environment via face mask, oxyhood, or oxygen tent.

3. Administer oxygen by face mask, oxygen hood, or oxygen tent, as ordered.

4. Encourage the child to cough and deep-breathe every 2 hours.

5. Suction the child, as needed.

6. Perform chest physiotherapy every 4 hours, as ordered (see *Performing chest physiotherapy,* page 4).

7. Assess the child's respiratory status for evidence of dyspnea, tachypnea, wheezing, crackles, rhonchi, and cyanosis.

8. Encourage oral fluid intake, if not contraindicated. However, do not give milk or full-strength formula.

9. Provide frequent rest periods.

Rationales

1. Assuming a comfortable position, such as a semierect position, helps make breathing easier.

2. Cool mist humidifies the airways, helps thin secretions, and reduces bronchial edema.

3. Administration of oxygen helps decrease the restlessness associated with respiratory distress and hypoxemia.

4. Coughing aids in the removal of secretions; deep-breathing encourages lung expansion.

5. Suctioning may be necessary to maintain airway patency, especially if the child's cough is ineffective.

6. Chest physiotherapy helps loosen exudate and secretions for easy removal through coughing and suctioning.

7. These signs indicate that the treatment may be ineffective and that the child's condition may be worsening.

8. Although fluids generally liquefy secretions, milk and formula thicken secretions.

9. Frequent resting is necessary to conserve energy to fight infection.

Nursing diagnosis: *Ineffective thermoregulation related to hyperthermia secondary to infection*

GOAL: The child will have no signs of fever.

Interventions

1. Maintain a cool environment.

2. Administer antipyretics, as ordered.

3. Monitor the child's temperature every 1 to 2 hours for sudden elevation.

4. Obtain a sputum specimen for culturing.

5. Administer antimicrobials, as ordered.

6. Administer tepid sponge baths, as needed, to relieve fever.

Rationales

1. A cool environment helps to reduce temperature through radiant heat loss.

2. Antipyretics usually reduce fever effectively.

3. Sudden elevation in temperature may cause a seizure.

4. A sputum specimen is necessary to help identify the causative agent.

5. Antimicrobials are used to treat the causative organism.

6. Tepid sponge baths cool the body surface through conduction.

Nursing diagnosis: *Potential fluid volume deficit related to fluid loss through hyperthermia or hyperpnea (or both)*

GOAL: The child will maintain fluid balance as evidenced by adequate urine output, good skin turgor, and a capillary refill time of 3 to 5 seconds.

Interventions

1. Carefully monitor the child's fluid intake and output.

2. Assess the child for increased respiratory rate and fever every 1 to 2 hours.

3. Assess the child for signs and symptoms of dehydration, including oliguria, poor skin turgor, dry mucous membranes, and sunken fontanels and eyes.

4. Administer I.V. fluids, as ordered.

5. Encourage oral fluid intake every 2 hours, if not contraindicated by the child's condition.

Rationales

1. Careful monitoring is essential because decreased urine output may indicate dehydration.

2. Such monitoring is essential to detect fluid loss, which typically increases with increases in respiratory rate and temperature.

3. Because fluid loss may be greater than expected, fluid intake may need to be adjusted accordingly.

4. I.V. fluids may be necessary to keep the child adequately hydrated.

5. Increased fluid intake is necessary to prevent dehydration and to liquefy secretions.

Nursing diagnosis: *Ineffective airway clearance related to respiratory distress*

GOAL: The child's respiratory difficulty will be lessened as evidenced by restful sleeping periods and decreased respiratory and heart rates.

Interventions

1. Monitor the child for signs of increased airway swelling and impending obstruction, including dyspnea, tachypnea, wheezing, and drooling.

2. Avoid direct stimulation of the airway with a tongue depressor, culture swab, suction catheter, or laryngoscope.

Rationales

1. Early recognition of these signs is essential because swelling usually progresses rapidly and can be fatal.

2. Any manipulation of the airway tissue may cause laryngospasm and swelling, possibly leading to complete obstruction.

Interventions	**Rationales**
3. Allow the child to assume a comfortable position, excluding a horizontal position.	3. A horizontal postion may cause rapid tissue deterioration, possibly leading to complete obstruction.
4. Monitor the child's respiratory status and vital signs continuously until a patent airway is ensured. Keep emergency intubation equipment at the bedside.	4. Continuous monitoring is mandatory because increasing edema can cause complete obstruction at any time, requiring emergency intubation.

Nursing diagnosis: *Fatigue related to sleep-pattern disturbance*

GOAL: The child will have decreased fatigue as evidenced by increased periods of alertness and play activity.

Interventions	**Rationales**
1. Make sure the child has frequent scheduled periods of uninterrupted rest.	1. Decreased stimulation and activity help conserve energy and ensure a stable respiratory rate.
2. Maintain a calm, restful environment.	2. As the child's respiratory rate stabilizes, he will be able to sleep more soundly. A calm, restful environment promotes sleep.

Nursing diagnosis: *Altered nutrition: less than body requirements related to increased metabolic needs*

GOAL: The child will have improved nutritional intake as evidenced by increased intake (eating 80%) of meals.

Interventions	**Rationales**
1. Maintain the child on a high-protein, high-calorie diet.	1. A diet high in protein and calories is necessary to meet the child's increased energy needs.
2. Serve the child small, frequent meals that include foods he prefers.	2. Small, frequent feedings decrease respiratory effort. Serving favorite foods helps ensure that the child will eat most of each meal.

Nursing diagnosis: *Impaired social interaction related to possible isolation*

GOAL: The child will socialize with his family and significant others.

Interventions	**Rationales**
1. Explain the purpose and nature of isolation to the child and parents, including details on requirements for wearing hospital gowns and masks.	1. Such explanations are necessary to prepare the child for unfamiliar equipment and sights, such as people wearing masks.
2. Introduce yourself upon entering the child's room.	2. Because of the required isolation clothing, it may be difficult for the child and parents to distinguish hospital staff.
3. Provide the child with a means of communication, such as a call system.	3. The child and parents must be able to communicate the need for assistance easily.
4. Monitor the child's vital signs every 1 to 2 hours.	4. Monitoring is essential and should be ongoing, even though the child is in isolation.
5. Provide the child with diversional activities, such as toys, books, television, and music.	5. Such activities stimulate the child and provide a means of distraction during isolation.

Interventions	**Rationales**
6. Encourage parental presence and participation in the child's care.	6. Parents represent the major source of socialization for a young child.

Nursing diagnosis: *Anxiety (parent) related to lack of knowledge about the child's condition*

GOAL: The parents will be less anxious as evidenced by their ability to support the child and explain his condition.

Interventions	**Rationales**
1. Assess the parents' understanding of the child's condition and prescribed treatment.	1. Such an assessment provides a basis on which to begin teaching.
2. Allow the parents to stay with the child throughout the hospitalization.	2. Allowing the parents to stay provides the child with support.
3. Explain all procedures to the child and parents.	3. Anxiety related to lack of knowledge or misunderstanding can be lessened if explanations are provided beforehand and throughout the hospitalization.
4. Provide emotional support to the parents throughout the hospitalizaion.	4. Hospitalization poses a crisis situation. LIstening to the parents' feelings and concerns helps them to deal with the crisis.

Nursing diagnosis: *Knowledge deficit related to home care*

GOAL: The parents will verbalize an understanding of home care instructions.

Interventions	**Rationales**
1. Instruct the parents on how and when to administer medications, including details on dosages and adverse effects.	1. Understanding the importance of consistent medication administration may help the parents to comply with the medication regimen. Knowing the potential adverse effects should prompt them to seek medical advice and attention, when necessary.
2. Explain the signs and symptoms of respiratory distress and infection, including fever, dyspnea, tachypnea, yellowish or greenish sputum, and wheezing.	2. Knowing the signs and symptoms should prompt the parents to seek medical advice and attention, when necessary.
3. Instruct the parents on the importance of adequate rest.	3. After infection, the child requires frequent rest periods to aid in recovery and prevent a relapse.
4. Explain the importance of encouraging fluids and maintaining the child on a high-calorie diet.	4. Fluids help liquefy secretions; a diet high in calories helps replace calories expended to fight the disease.
5. Instruct the parents to provide a humidified environment with a cool mist humidifier.	5. Humidified air helps to thin secretions. Cool air is safer than warm air because it won't cause burns.

Documentation checklist

During the hospitalization, be sure to document the following:
___ the child's status and assessment findings upon admission
___ any changes in the child's status
___ pertinent laboratory and diagnostic findings
___ fluid intake and output
___ nutritional intake
___ the child's response to treatment
___ the child's and parents' reaction to the illness and hospitalization
___ patient and family teaching guidelines
___ discharge planning guidelines.

Respiratory Disorders of the Newborn

Introduction

Various respiratory disorders can occur during the neonatal period, including respiratory distress syndrome (RDS, formerly known as hyaline membrane disease), transient tachypnea, meconium aspiration syndrome, pneumonia, pneumothorax, and persistent pulmonary hypertension. Although both term and premature infants are susceptible to these disorders, prematurity usually is the primary precipitating factor.

RDS is the leading cause of neonatal death, usually resulting from the immaturity of the infant's lungs and their inability to sustain normal and stable respiratory functioning. In some cases, the infant may exhibit normal breathing patterns initially after birth but quickly develops signs and symptoms of RDS.

Complications often include congestive heart failure, intraventricular hemorrhage, and necrotizing enterocolitis. Bronchopulmonary dysplasia also may occur in infants exposed to high levels of oxygen therapy for prolonged periods.

Treatment is aimed at providing respiratory support and correcting the problems that can complicate RDS, including hyperthermia or hypothermia, metabolic acidosis, infection, and hypertension or hypotension. Diuretics, vitamin E, and antibiotics also may be used.

Assessment

Respiratory
- cyanosis
- tachypnea (more than 60 respirations/minute)
- expiratory grunting
- costal retractions
- nasal flaring
- apnea
- diminished breath sounds
- crackles
- rhonchi

Cardiovascular
- bradycardia
- heart murmur
- shift in point of maximal impulse

Musculoskeletal
- hypotonia
- asymmetry of the thoracic cavity

Integumentary
- pallor
- cyanosis
- elevated or lowered temperature

Nursing diagnosis: *Impaired gas exchange related to inadequate surfactant levels*

GOAL: The infant will have improved gas exchange as evidenced by arterial blood gas (ABG) levels within the normal range.

Interventions

1. Assess the infant's respiratory status every hour by auscultating lung fields, evaluating the degree and symmetry of lung expansion, and monitoring ABG levels.

2. Observe for evidence of nasal flaring and retractions. If noted, administer oxygen and perform chest physiotherapy, as ordered.

3. Schedule nursing interventions to minimize stress and help conserve the infant's energy.

4. Perform chest physiotherapy every 4 hours, as tolerated (see *Performing chest physiotherapy,* page 4).

5. Assess the infant for signs and symptoms of RDS, and implement the prescribed treatment mode (see *Treatment for respiratory distress syndrome*).

Rationales

1. Continual updates on the infant's respiratory status are essential to evaluate improvement or deterioration in lung disease.

2. Nasal flaring and retractions indicate that the infant is in respiratory distress.

3. Scheduling helps limit the frequency of care measures, thereby reducing the infant's stress and energy expenditure.

4. Percussion, vibration, and positioning increase the mobilization of secretions and decrease the risk of pneumonia.

5. Early assessment and prompt treatment ensure optimal oxygen exchange.

TREATMENT FOR RESPIRATORY DISTRESS SYNDROME

Treatment for an infant with respiratory distress syndrome (RDS) requires vigorous respiratory support. Warm, humidified, oxygen-enriched gases are administered by oxygen hood or, if such treatment fails, by mechanical ventilation. Severe cases may require mechanical ventilation with positive end-expiratory pressure or continuous positive airway pressure (CPAP), administered by a tightly fitting face mask or, when necessary, endotracheal intubation.

Treatment also includes the following:
• a radiant infant warmer or Isolette for thermoregulation
• I.V. fluids and sodium bicarbonate to control acidosis and maintain electrolyte balance
• tube feedings or total parenteral nutrition to maintain adequate nutrition if the infant is too weak to eat.

If using an oxygen hood, follow these guidelines:
• Calibrate the oxygen analyzer every 8 hours to ensure accurate readings.
• Administer warm, humidified, oxygen-enriched gases to prevent cold stress and drying of the mucous membranes.
• Avoid fluctuations in the FIO_2 or O_2 Sat levels, adjusting as needed to maintain PaO_2 levels (O_2 Sat levels should remain above 90%). Such fluctuations may result in poor oxygen perfusion to the tissues.
• Monitor and document hourly FIO_2 levels, monitor readouts, oxygen temperature, skin color, and the quality of respirations.
• Assess the infant's oxygen status through blood gas levels taken every 4 to 6 hours (or every 20 to 30 minutes after changes in FIO_2 levels).
• Gently suction the infant's oropharynx and nares, as needed to maintain airway patency.
• If the infant is in a supine position, place a small blanket roll under his neck and shoulders to hyperextend the neck slightly and maintain airway patency.
• Notify the doctor about any changes in the infant's clinical status.
• Maintain the infant's body temperature, as decreased temperature results in increased respiratory rate and effort.

If using CPAP, note the following additional measures:
• Avoid excess humidity in the ventilatory tubing to prevent the possibility of the pooled water's emptying into the infant's airway.
• Clean nasal prongs every 2 hours to prevent airway obstruction.
• Auscultate lung fields hourly and note any deviation in the point of maximal impulse. Also, continually observe chest symmetry and excursion. This is done to evaluate air movement, assess for bilateral equality, and rule out pneumothorax.
• Insert an open orogastric tube to help prevent abdominal distention.
• Clean the nares and mouth, as needed. Also, apply glycerin to the mouth and lips to prevent drying and cracking of the mucous membranes.

If using a mechanical ventilator, keep in mind the following additional measures:
• Be alert to signs of extubation, including an audible cry, decreased breath sounds, and sudden deterioration in skin color and heart rate.
• Suction the endotracheal tube, as needed, to maintain airway patency. Use sterile technique to minimize the risk of infection.
• Check ventilator readouts hourly to maintain proper functioning within the designated parameters.
• Keep an Ambu bag and infant mask at the bedside in case of ventilator malfunction or accidental extubation.
• Administer muscle relaxants, as ordered, to promote relaxation of the pulmonary vascular bed and thereby improve gas exchange. (Muscle relaxants usually are given to restless infants who fight mechanical ventilation. Before administration, be sure you know the correct dosage and potential adverse effects of the medication and assess the tube for proper location. After administration, monitor the infant closely, maintain all alarms, and change the infant's position periodically.)

Nursing diagnosis: *Altered nutrition: less than body requirements related to respiratory distress*

GOAL: The infant will have improved nutritional intake as evidenced by good skin turgor and maintained or increased weight.

Interventions

1. Provide parenteral nutrition until the infant's respiratory status stabilizes.

2. When the respiratory status has stabilized, begin feeding the infant sterile water to assess his tolerance to oral feedings.

3. If the infant does not have a strong sucking, gag, or swallow reflex or is at risk for aspiration, provide feedings through a nasogastric (NG) tube.

Rationales

1. Parenteral feedings are necessary to prevent aspiration, which may occur during oral feedings when the infant is in respiratory distress. Such feedings also help conserve the infant's energy, allowing for improved respiratory status.

2. Because sterile water is not as thick as formula, the infant is less likely to develop aspiration pneumonia if he aspirates the feeding.

3. An NG tube provides direct access to the stomach, thereby preventing the risk of aspiration.

Nursing diagnosis: *Altered growth and development related to hospitalization*

GOAL: The infant will progress developmentally during the hospitalization.

Interventions

1. Encourage the parents and other caregivers to touch and stroke the infant.

2. Move the infant's arms and legs gently, bending each extremity at the joint.

3. Place black and white stripes along the sides of the crib.

4. Place a music box or tape recording in the infant's crib.

Rationales

1. Because touch is essential to normal development, the infant needs frequent touching and stroking to progress developmentally.

2. Moving the extremities helps develop muscle tone and prevents muscle wasting and contractures.

3. Black and white stripes provide visual stimulation and allow the infant to begin focusing.

4. Music provides the child with auditory stimulation.

Nursing diagnosis: *Potential for altered parenting related to separation from the infant*

GOAL: The parents will maintain interest and parental attachment as evidenced by touching and talking to the infant and asking questions about his condition.

Interventions

1. Answer the parents' questions about the infant's condition.

2. Encourage the parents to touch and talk to the infant.

3. Maintain phone contact with the parents if they cannot visit the infant in the hospital.

Rationales

1. Answering questions helps decrease fear and anxiety, which may be impairing the parent-child relationship.

2. Such encouragement may alleviate the fear the parents may have about harming or becoming too attached to their sick child.

3. Phone contact helps maintain parental ties when the parents cannot visit the infant because of financial, family, or logistical reasons.

Nursing diagosis: *Anxiety (parent) related to lack of knowledge about the infant's condition*

GOAL: The parents will be less anxious as evidenced by verbalizing fears and interacting with the infant.

Interventions

1. Assess the parents' understanding of the child's condition and prescribed treatment.

2. Provide explanations about the medical condition, procedures, and treatment.

3. Provide emotional support to the parents during the infant's hospitalization.

Rationales

1. Such assessment provides a basis on which to begin teaching.

2. Anxiety related to lack of knowledge or misunderstanding can be lessened if explanations are provided beforehand and throughout the hospitalization.

3. Hospitalization poses a crisis situation. Listening to the parents' feelings and concerns helps them to deal with the crisis.

Nursing diagnosis: *Knowledge deficit related to home care*

GOAL: The parents will verbalize an understanding of home care instructions.

Interventions

1. Instruct the parents on the signs and symptoms of respiratory distress, including tachypnea, dyspnea, cyanosis, wheezing, and tachycardia.

2. Explain the importance of feeding the infant a formula that is high in calories and protein.

3. Instruct the parents to provide stimulation through use of bright colors, developmentally suitable toys, talking, and moving the infant's extremities.

4. Provide instruction on apnea monitoring devices and chest physiotherapy.

Rationales

1. Knowing the signs and symptoms of respiratory distress should prompt parents to seek medical advice and attention, when necessary.

2. An infant with a respiratory disorder, especially one who is premature, requires increased calorie and protein intake because of his increased respiratory effort.

3. Stimulation is essential to help the infant progress developmentally.

4. The infant may require chest physiotherapy and home monitoring with an apnea monitor.

Documentation checklist

During the hospitalization, be sure to document the following:
___ the child's status and assessment findings upon admission
___ any changes in the child's status
___ pertinent laboratory and diagnostic findings
___ fluid intake and output
___ nutritional intake
___ growth and development status
___ ventilator settings
___ the parents' reaction to the illness and hospitalization
___ family teaching guidelines
___ discharge planning guidelines.

Congenital Heart Defects

Introduction

Congenital heart defects, the second leading cause of death in infancy, are caused by abnormal cardiovascular development during fetal life resulting in obstructions or altered blood-flow patterns. Defects are classified as either cyanotic or acyanotic.

In cyanotic defects, blood is shunted from the right to the left side of the heart, where unoxygenated blood flows from the left ventricle to all parts of the body, resulting in cyanosis. In acyanotic defects, oxygenated blood is shunted from the left to the right side of the heart but is not mixed with unoxygenated blood in the systemic circulation.

Below is a listing of the major defects affecting infants:

• *Ventricular septal defect (VSD)*, the most common of all congenital heart defects, refers to an abnormal opening in the ventricular septum that allows shunting of oxygenated blood from the left ventricle to mix with unoxygenated blood in the right ventricle. Usually, VSD requires surgical repair.

• *Coarctation of the aorta* refers to the narrowing of the aorta near the remnant of the fetal ductus arteriosus. Usually, this defect requires surgical repair.

• *Transposition of the great vessels* is a defect in which the pulmonary artery and the aorta are in reversed positions: the aorta is attached to the right ventricle, and the pulmonary artery is attached to the left ventricle. This creates two separate circulatory systems that are incapable of sustaining life. Surgery is necessary to correct the defect.

• *Atrial septal defect (ASD)* refers to an opening in the septum of the atria that allows blood to shunt from the left to the right. If ASD does not close spontaneously, surgery is necessary.

• *Patent ductus arteriosus (PDA)* is a persistent opening between the aorta and the pulmonary artery that failed to close at birth. Although PDA, which predominantly affects premature infants, may close spontaneously, surgery may be necessary.

• *Tetralogy of Fallot* consists of four separate defects— VSD, overriding aorta, pulmonary stenosis, and right ventricular hypertrophy—requiring surgical repair.

Assessment
VSD
Cardiovascular
• mild defect: holosystolic murmur at the left lower sternal border

• moderate to severe defect: holosystolic murmur (same as for mild defect), signs and symptoms of congestive heart failure (CHF) (tachypnea, tachycardia, restlessness, increased central venous pressure, weight gain, decreased urine output, diaphoresis), and failure to thrive

COARCTATION OF THE AORTA
Cardiovascular
• mild: 1+ or absent femoral, popliteal, and pedal pulses; mild hypertension (detected bilaterally in the arms)
• moderate: absent femoral, popliteal, and pedal pulses; moderate to severe hypertension (detected bilaterally in the arms)
• severe: same as for moderate defect, plus signs and symptoms of CHF

TRANSPOSITION OF THE GREAT VESSELS
Cardiovascular
• heart murmur (if VSD is present)
• egg-shaped heart on X-ray
• 3+ or 4+ pulses (depending on whether ductus arteriosus is patent)
• no increase in oxygen saturation with oxygen administration

Integumentary
• severe cyanosis

ASD
Cardiovascular
• quiet diastolic rumble murmur (best heard by a highly trained practitioner)

Respiratory
• increased incidence of upper respiratory tract infections

PDA
Cardiovascular
• mild: 4+ bilateral peripheral pulses, wide pulse pressure, and a continuous murmur in the left upper anterior midclavicular thorax
• moderate: signs and symptoms of CHF

Respiratory
• frequent upper respiratory tract infections (with mild defects)

TETRALOGY OF FALLOT
Cardiovascular
- holosystolic murmur along the lower left sternal border
- boot-shaped heart on X-ray
- normal peripheral pulses
- tendency toward cyanotic spells (dyspnea, deep sighing respirations, bradycardia, fainting, seizures, and loss of consciousness)

Hematologic
- polycythemia
- elevated hemoglobin and hematocrit levels

Integumentary
- cyanosis

Nursing diagnosis: *Anxiety (parent) related to child's congenital heart defect*

GOAL: The parents will have decreased anxiety as evidenced by verbalizing feelings, asking appropriate questions about the child's condition, and continuing to interact with the child.

Interventions

1. Explain the heart defect using an illustration, and answer any questions the parents may have.

2. Update the parents regularly on the child's condition.

3. Allow the parents to hold or cuddle the child as soon and as often as possible.

Rationales

1. Explaining the defect and answering the parents' questions helps reduce anxiety by allowing them to visualize and better understand the defect.

2. Regular updates allow the parents to maintain some contact with the child, thereby alleviating some anxiety.

3. Holding and cuddling promote bonding and a sense of security, thereby alleviating anxiety.

Nursing diagnosis: *Knowlege deficit related to impending surgery and hospitalization*

GOAL: The parents and child (if appropriate) will demonstrate an understanding of the impending surgery and hospitalization as evidenced by verbalizing the purpose of surgery and asking appropriate questions.

Interventions

1. Assess the parents' and child's knowledge of the impending surgery and hospitalization and the child's developmental level (see Appendix A: Normal Growth and Development).

2. Instruct the child and parents on the perioperative events requiring their direct participation, including the following:
- bathing the child with povidone-iodine solution or hexachlorophene the night before surgery
- touring the intensive care unit before surgery
- making sure the child has nothing by mouth before surgery (the actual time will depend on the child's age)
- attending teaching sessions on the purpose and use of postoperative procedures and equipment, such as chest tubes, oxygen masks, incentive spirometers, dressings, endotracheal tubes, I.V. lines, central venous pressure and arterial monitoring, ECG monitors, and postural drainage.

3. Teach the child coughing, deep-breathing, and splinting techniques, if age-appropriate.

Rationales

1. Such assessment serves as a basis on which to begin teaching.

2. The child and parents need to anticipate the preoperative and postoperative events surrounding the surgery. The surgeon will explain the actual procedure and associated risks to the parents.

3. Coughing, deep breathing, and splinting help to loosen and remove secretions from the respiratory tract and increase oxygenation. Familiarization with these techniques promotes compliance postoperatively.

Nursing diagnosis: *Potential injury related to positioning, electrical current, blood loss, and surgical procedure*

GOAL: The child will suffer no injuries during the surgical procedure.

Interventions

1. Assess the child's pressure points hourly during the surgical procedure for evidence of skin breakdown. Assess for redness, blanching of the skin, abrasions, or open wounds.

2. Turn the child's head hourly during the surgical procedure.

3. Calculate the child's total fluid volume.

4. If the child is undergoing surgery to repair coarctation of the aorta, monitor the blood pressure in the leg during the surgery.

5. Monitor the child's heart rhythm. Have temporary pacing wires and a temporary pacemaker available in case of an emergency.

6. Check Bovie pad and ECG electrode sites for evidence of burns.

Rationales

1. Skin breakdown, which can occur within 1 hour after the start of surgery, places the child at risk for infection.

2. Turning the head helps prevent skin breakdown.

3. This information is necessary to estimate the child's fluid intake and expected blood loss for fluid volume replacement to maintain cardiac output.

4. During surgery to repair coarctation, an aortic cross clamp is required. Monitoring the blood pressure in the leg helps assess the proper return of bloodflow to the lower body.

5. Monitoring the heart rhythm is essential because the surgical procedure may temporarily or permanently interrupt the normal conduction of the heart.

6. Electrical grounding at these sites may cause first-degree burns.

Nursing diagnosis: *Altered cardiac output: decreased related to surgical procedure*

GOAL: The child will maintain adequate cardiac output postoperatively as evidenced by stable heart and respiratory rates and a pinkish skin color.

Interventions

1. After surgery, assess the child's cardiac status hourly by taking the following measures:
• Measure and record hourly the child's hemodynamic monitor readings (arterial line, central venous pressure line, intracardiac catheter, thermistor cardiac output).

• Monitor laboratory blood studies, including prothrombin time, arterial blood gas (ABG) measurements, and complete blood count.

• Assess the child for signs and symptoms of CHF.

• Assess the child's heart sounds for muffling or a friction rub.

Rationales

1. Surgery can cause severe trauma to the child's body.
• Hemodynamic instability may result from the trauma of surgery. Specifically, changes in central venous pressure can indicate right-sided heart failure, changes in arterial line pressure can indicate changes in blood pressure, and changes in cardiac output can indicate CHF.

• Cardiac bypass can damage the blood cells and cause hemolysis of red cells, possibly leading to anemia. Anticoagulants may be ordered to prevent clots. ABG measurements indicate the level of oxygen perfusion in the blood.

• Because of the stress of surgery, the child may be at risk for CHF from the increased work load of the heart and increased sodium and water retention.

• Bleeding may occur in the pericardial sac and restrict the heart's ability to function. Muffled heart sounds may indicate cardiac tamponade. Friction rub may indicate postpericardiotomy syndrome (delayed pericardial or pleural reaction characterized by fever, chest pain, and signs of pericardial or pleural inflammation).

Interventions

2. Assess the child's renal function by taking the following measures:
• Measure and record fluid intake and output hourly (normal output should be greater than 1 ml/hour).
• Monitor specific gravity with every void or every 2 to 4 hours if a catheter is in place.

• Monitor blood urea nitrogen (BUN) and serum creatinine levels.

3. Assess the child's fluid and electrolyte status by taking the following measures:
• Monitor electrolyte levels.

• Measure and record fluid intake and output hourly.

• Assess for edema and poor skin turgor.

• Weigh the child daily.

4. Assess the child's respiratory status by taking the following measures:
• Monitor and record the child's respiratory rate and patterns, breath sounds, skin color, and capillary refill time. Also monitor ventilator settings, intracardiac catheter and oximeter readings, and carbon dioxide levels.
• Assess for endotracheal (ET) tube patency by checking tape security and noting tube placement on X-ray.
• Monitor and record the amount of chest tube drainage hourly (normal output is less than 3 ml/hour). Also check for excessive bleeding.
• Monitor ABG levels every 4 to 8 hours.

• Ventilate the child with 100% oxygen for 1 minute before and after ET suctioning.

5. Assess the child's neurologic status, noting pupillary reactions, muscle tone, and reflexes (grasp, sucking, and swallow).

Rationales

2. Surgery may compromise normal renal functioning.

• Measuring and recording the fluid intake and output helps determine fluid status and kidney functioning.
• Specific gravity measurements serve as an assessment of hydration status and the kidneys' ability to concentrate urine.
• Decreased BUN and creatinine levels may indicate kidney failure.

3. Surgery may cause fluid and electrolyte imbalances.

• Monitoring electrolyte levels helps determine the child's hydration status and potassium level. (Decreased potassium levels may result in dysrhythmias.)
• Measuring intake and output helps determine fluid status and kidney functioning and helps prevent fluid overload.
• Evidence of edema and poor skin turgor may indicate poor hydration and CHF.
• Weight gain is an early sign of CHF.

4. Surgery may compromise the child's respiratory status.
• Immobility, pain, and the use of anesthetic gases alter normal pulmonary function.

• Malposition of the ET tube can hamper respiratory function.
• Excessive drainage may indicate hemorrhage.

• ABG levels directly measure the effectiveness of respiratory status.
• Ventilation with 100% oxygen relaxes the alveoli and prevents severe hypoxia and respiratory arrest.

5. Impaired neurologic status can occur as a result of decreased cardiac output, hypoxia, acidosis, electrolyte imbalance, or cerebral thrombosis.

Nursing diagnosis: *Potential for infection related to immobility and numerous wound entries*

GOAL: The child will have no signs of infection as evidenced by lack of fever, a stable white blood cell count, and no change in vital signs.

Interventions

1. Assess wound and I.V. sites hourly for evidence of bleeding, erythema, infiltration, and excess drainage.

2. Monitor the child's temperature and check for leukocytosis.

Rationales

1. The child's immunologic system has already been stressed by surgery. Any further stress caused by wound infection could lead to septic shock. Fluid loss by infiltration or bleeding could alter cardiac output.

2. Elevated temperature and leukocytosis may indicate infection.

Interventions	**Rationales**
3. Assess the child's pressure points hourly for the first 2 or 3 hours, then every 2 hours thereafter.	3. Such assessments are necessary to avoid skin breakdown.
4. Administer antibiotics, as ordered.	4. Antibiotics may be prescribed to help fortify the immunologic system.
5. Change dressings, as ordered, using sterile technique.	5. Sterile technique aids in preventing the introduction of bacteria into the incision.

Nursing diagnosis: *Potential for injury related to indomethacin administration (in premature infants with patent ductus arteriosus)*

GOAL: The infant will demonstrate no signs of injury as evidenced by stable heart and respiratory rates and adequate urine output.

Interventions	**Rationales**
1. Administer indomethacin, as ordered. Be sure to check, then double-check all dosages before administering the medication.	1. Indomethacin constricts the ductus to promote closure. Double-checking dosages helps prevent the risk of overdosage.
2. Assess and record the infant's cardiac, respiratory, renal, gastrointestinal, and neurologic status every 4 hours; if unstable, assess every 1 to 2 hours.	2. Such assessment is necessary to detect any possible complications (such as hemorrhage or adverse reactions to anesthesia) after indomethacin administration.

Nursing diagnosis: *Altered cardiac output: decreased related to spasm of pulmonary infundibulum (in children with tetralogy of Fallot)*

GOAL: The child will have no evidence of cyanotic spells.

Interventions	**Rationales**
1. Recognize the signs and symptoms of cyanotic spells, including dyspnea, deep sighing respirations, bradycardia, fainting, seizures, and eventual loss of consciousness.	1. Early recognition allows for intervention before the anoxia becomes severe enough to cause loss of consciousness.
2. Place the child in a prone knee-to-chest position.	2. This position decreases the work load on the heart.
3. Speak in quiet tones and gently rub the child's back.	3. Soothing tones and touch comfort the child and help relax the spasm.
4. Ventilate the child with 100% oxygen via face mask, nasal cannula, or a blow device.	4. Ventilation with 100% oxygen increases the amount of oxygen in inspired air and in the circulation.
5. Administer morphine sulfate I.M., as ordered.	5. Morphine helps relax the spasm.
6. Teach the parents how to perform interventions 1 through 4.	6. Knowing how to perform these interventions helps parents to cope with the crisis brought on by the spasm and allows them to participate in the child's care.
7. Teach the parents how to administer beta-blocker medication, such as propranolol hydrochloride.	7. Beta blockers interrupt the mechanism involved in spasms of the pulmonary infundibulum. Teaching parents how to administer such medications helps promote home compliance with the regimen.

Nursing diagnosis: *Potential for infection (bacterial endocarditis) related to high-flow shunt (in children with VSD)*

GOAL: The child will have no signs of bacterial endocarditis and bacteremia.

Interventions

1. Explain to the parents the causes of bacterial endocarditis, including dental and surgical procedures, which release enormous amounts of bacteria that can attach to the cardiac valve via high-pressured ventricular blood flow. Also explain that, to prevent infection, antibiotic therapy usually is ordered.

2. Provide the parents with written instructions for antibiotic therapy usually prescribed for specific procedures.

Rationales

1. Knowing this should promote compliance with the prescribed antibiotic therapy.

2. Such information should promote compliance with the medication regimen, if necessary.

Nursing diagnosis: *Anxiety (child) related to ICU environment, separation from parents, parental anxiety, surgery, and immobility*

GOAL: The child will be less anxious as evidenced by cooperating with the procedures and treatment and demonstrating age-appropriate play.

Interventions

1. Encourage the parents to visit the child and participate in his care as often as possible.

2. Explain to the child and parents each step in the postoperative care.

3. Consult a child-life worker or play therapist about providing the child with toys and activities appropriate for his developmental level.

Rationales

1. Parental contact provides the child with feelings of safety and security.

2. Familiarity with procedures and nursing measures promotes decreased anxiety and increased cooperation.

3. Toys and activities help divert the child's attention from his environment and provide developmental stimulation.

Nursing diagnosis: *Knowledge deficit related to home care*

GOAL: The parents will verbalize an understanding of home care instructions.

Interventions

1. Instruct the parents on the signs and symptoms of wound infection, including purulent drainage, fever, and a foul-smelling odor.

2. Teach the parents how to administer medications while the child is still hospitalized.

3. Teach the parents how to monitor the child's pulse rate and to report persistent deviations of 15 to 20 beats above or below the baseline level.

4. Instruct the parents to feed the child small, frequent meals.

Rationales

1. Because infection can occur as late as 3 weeks after surgery, parents need to know which signs and symptoms to report.

2. Practice promotes comfort with the procedure and ensures compliance with the regimen. Having the parents practice while the child is still hospitalized enables the nurse to assess the parents' ability to administer medications correctly.

3. Monitoring the pulse rate enables parents to report any significant changes that could indicate complications.

4. Small, frequent meals decrease the work load on the heart, thereby decreasing fatigue.

Interventions

5. Instruct the parents on the signs and symptoms of postpericardiotomy syndrome, including fever, chest pain, and dyspnea.

Rationales

5. Postpericardiotomy syndrome, a potentially life-threatening condition, can occur up to 3 weeks after major heart surgery. Parents need to know which signs and symptoms to report in case of an emergency.

Documentation checklist

During the hospitalization, be sure to document the following:
___ the child's status and assessment findings upon admission
___ any changes in the child's status
___ pertinent laboratory and diagnostic findings
___ fluid intake and output
___ nutritional intake
___ growth and development status
___ the child's response to treatment
___ the child's and parents' reaction to the illness and hospitalization
___ patient and family teaching guidelines
___ discharge planning.

Congestive Heart Failure

Introduction

Congestive heart failure (CHF) develops when the heart cannot pump sufficient amounts of blood into the systemic circulation to meet work demands. Usually differentiated into left- or right-sided failure, CHF is commonly caused by congenital heart defects during infancy.

Complications associated with this disorder include hepatomegaly, ascites, and cyanosis. Treatment may include administration of diuretics (to treat edema and prevent the reabsorption of sodium) and digitalis (to increase cardiac contractility and slow the heart rate), a low-sodium diet, fluid restrictions, and decreases in activity level and stress.

Assessment

INFANTS

Cardiovascular
• mild: resting tachycardia
• severe: decreased peripheral pulses (1 + or 2 + ; if patent ductus arteriosus is cause, 4 +)

Respiratory
• mild: resting tachypnea
• compensatory: excessive respiratory effort, including resting tachypnea, substernal and intercostal retractions, nasal flaring, crackles, and dry cough

Gastrointestinal
• mild: slow weight gain

Genitourinary
• severe: decreased urine output (less than 1 ml/hour)

Musculoskeletal
• mild: fatigue with feedings

Integumentary
• mild: diaphoresis (head and face)
• compensatory: orbital edema, peripheral edema

CHILDREN AND ADOLESCENTS

Cardiovascular
• mild: resting tachycardia
• severe: decreased peripheral pulses (1 + or 2 + ; if patent ductus arteriosus is the cause, 4 +)

Respiratory
• mild: resting tachypnea, exertional dyspnea
• compensatory: excessive respiratory effort (including resting tachypnea, substernal and intercostal retractions, nasal flaring, crackles, and dry cough), wheezes

Gastrointestinal
• mild: loss of appetite, rapid weight gain ("water weight")

Genitourinary
• severe: decreased urine output (less than 1 ml/hour)

Musculoskeletal
• mild: exertional fatigue

Integumentary
• mild: diaphoresis (forehead)
• compensatory: orbital edema, dependent edema of the arms and legs

---

Nursing diagnosis: *Altered cardiac output related to increased blood flow to the lungs (as in ventricular septal defect, patent ductus arteriosus, atrioventricular fistula, cardiac valvular insufficiency, renal failure, or excessive I.V. fluid administration)*

GOAL: The child will maintain a stable cardiac status as evidenced by stable heart and respiratory rates and no crackles or rhonchi.

Interventions

1. Assess and record the child's cardiovascular status by noting apical heart rate and rhythm, peripheral pulses, blood pressure, capillary refill time, and skin changes (mottling, edema, increased or decreased temperature, diaphoresis).

2. Use a cardiac monitor to assess the child's status. Assess his vital signs and notify the doctor immediately if any significant changes are noted.

Rationales

1. Such assessment provides essential data on changes in the child's cardiac status, including tachycardia, bradycardia, hypotension, and irregular heart rate—all indications of cardiac decompensation.

2. Cardiac monitoring provides immediate detection of changes in the child's heart rate and rhythm, such as tachycardia (an early sign of CHF) and dysrhythmias (a possible adverse effect of some CHF medications).

Interventions	Rationales
3. Administer digoxin (the drug of choice) or other cardiovascular medications, as ordered.	3. Such medications slow and strengthen heart contractions.
4. Provide frequent rest periods.	4. Frequent rest decreases the heart's work load.
5. When treating the child, approach him in a calm manner, provide consistency in care, and perform procedures that may seem threatening in a treatment room, not in the child's room.	5. These interventions can help decrease stress and anxiety, thereby decreasing the heart's work load.

Nursing diagnosis: *Impaired gas exchange related to pulmonary edema*

GOAL: The child will maintain adequate oxygenation as evidenced by pinkish skin color and mucous membranes and a capillary refill time of 3 to 5 seconds.

Interventions	Rationales
1. Assess and record the child's respiratory status by: • noting the rate, character, and regularity of respirations • auscultating breath sounds • noting the presence and character of cough.	1. This information provides essential data on changes in the child's respiratory status, such as evidence of respiratory distress (dyspnea, crackles, tachypnea, retractions, cyanosis).
2. Place the child in semi-Fowler's position.	2. Semi-Fowler's position enables gravity to pull down the inner organs to relieve pressure on the heart and lungs.
3. Administer oxygen by face mask, oxygen hood, or nasal cannula, as ordered.	3. This increases the amount of oxygen in inspired air, as oxygen exchange in the alveoli is impaired with pulmonary congestion.
4. Administer diuretics, as ordered.	4. Administration of diuretics encourages tissues to release fluid and the kidneys to flush out the excess fluid.
5. Monitor serum electrolyte levels.	5. Electrolyte imbalances may occur as a result of edema or diuretic use.
6. Monitor oximeter readings.	6. An oximeter can measure increases and decreases in the child's oxygenation, which can become compromised because of pulmonary congestion and impaired gas exchange at the alveoli.

Nursing diagnosis: *Altered nutrition: less than body requirements related to decreased energy reserves*

GOAL: The child will maintain adequate nutritional intake as evidenced by increased intake (eating 80% of all meals), stable weight, and good skin turgor.

Interventions	Rationales
1. Schedule feedings or meals after rest periods, and provide a calm environment.	1. Scheduling feedings and meals after rest periods ensures the child's maximum energy level for the work of sucking, swallowing, and chewing. A calm environment induces relaxation and promotes improved intake.
2. Serve small, frequent feedings or meals (five to six per day).	2. Small, frequent meals eliminate the possibility of stomach distention from eating too much at one time and allow the child to rest between feedings, as energy reserves are quickly depleted during the eating process.

Interventions	**Rationales**
3. Place the child in semi-Fowler's position during feedings.	3. Semi-Fowler's position facilitates easier swallowing. Gravity helps relieve pressure on the heart and lungs.
4. Feed the child his favorite formula or meals that include some of his favorite foods.	4. Feeding the child his favorite formula or foods helps ensure improved intake.
5. If ordered, administer oxygen during feedings.	5. Because pulmonary congestion has decreased the child's oxygen uptake, increasing the oxygen concentration of inspired air will help increase the child's energy reserves.
6. Increase the child's caloric intake by offering high-calorie formulas or foods.	6. The child's caloric intake must be increased to meet the increased metabolic demands resulting from tachypnea, tachycardia, and respiratory distress.
7. Begin the child on nasogastric feedings, as ordered, if he tires before orally ingesting an adequate amount of formula or food.	7. Nasogastric feeding ensures that the child receives adequate nutrition.
8. Assess and record the child's fluid intake and output daily.	8. Too-rapid weight gain may indicate worsening CHF.
9. Restrict the child's fluid intake, as ordered.	9. Fluid restrictions may be ordered to decrease the circulatory volume associated with fluid retention.

Nursing diagnosis: *Potential for injury related to medication dosage or physiologic response to medication*

GOAL: The child will suffer no injuries from medication dosages or physiologic response to medication.

Interventions	**Rationales**
1. Monitor the child's heart rate and rhythm using a cardiac monitor.	1. Cardiac monitoring allows for observation of disturbances in the child's heart rate or rhythm related to medication use. For example, first-degree heart block or sinus bradycardia may indicate digoxin toxicity, and ventricular dysrhythmias may be caused by hypokalemia from diuretic use.
2. Monitor the child's electrolyte levels.	2. Monitoring electrolyte levels helps in detecting electrolyte imbalances caused by medication use. For example, diuretics can cause hypokalemia, which can potentiate the action of digoxin to toxic levels.
3. Double-check all dosage calculations for accuracy.	3. Verifying the accuracy of all dosages ensures that the child receives the correct medication in the exact amount necessary for therapeutic effectiveness.

Nursing diagnosis: *Anxiety (parent) related to the child's illness, hospitalization, and eventual home care*

GOAL: The parents will be less anxious as evidenced by asking appropriate questions about the child's condition.

Interventions	**Rationales**
1. Explain to the parents the nature of the child's illness and the reason for hospitalization. Also explain all procedures and treatments, advising them of discharge instructions from the start of the hospitalization.	1. Knowing this information should help the parents understand the child's condition and expected treatment and help ease their anxiety.

Interventions

2. Encourage the parents to participate in the child's care by helping to administer medications and by bathing, feeding, and monitoring the child.

3. Provide emotional support to the parents.

Rationales

2. By participating in the child's care, the parents will feel less anxious about the treatment and hospitalization. It also allows them to begin practicing home care instructions while under the nurse's supervision.

3. Providing emotional support helps relieve parental anxiety.

Nursing diagnosis: *Knowledge deficit related to the disease process and home care*

GOAL: The parents will verbalize an understanding of the disease process and home care instructions.

Interventions

1. Teach the parents the signs and symptoms of CHF, including, tachypnea, tachycardia, fatigue, poor feeding, restlessness, diaphoresis, rapid weight gain, dyspnea, cyanosis, wheezing, and peripheral edema.

2. Instruct the parents on the prescribed medication regimen, including details on dosages and potential adverse effects.

3. Instruct the parents on the purpose and use of home monitoring devices.

4. Explain to the parents the importance of feeding the child a high-calorie, low-sodium diet.

Rationales

1. Knowing the signs and symptoms of CHF should prompt the parents to seek medical advice and attention, when needed.

2. Explaining this information helps ensure correct medication administration and compliance with the overall treatment.

3. The child may require home monitoring to detect episodes of bradycardia, tachycardia, or apnea.

4. The child will need extra calories for growth and lowered sodium levels to prevent fluid retention and hypertension. Knowing this information should encourage compliance with the dietary regimen.

Documentation checklist

During the hospitalization, be sure to document the following:
___ the child's status and assessment findings upon admission
___ any changes in the child's status
___ pertinent laboratory and diagnostic findings
___ fluid intake and output
___ nutritional intake
___ the child's response to treatment
___ the child's and parents' reaction to the illness and hospitalization
___ patient and family teaching guidelines
___ discharge planning guidelines.

CARDIOVASCULAR SYSTEM
Dysrhythmias

Introduction

Any deviation in the normal heart rate or rhythm, dysrhythmias are directly related to disturbances in the conduction pathways of the heart. Generally classified according to their site of origin (ventricular or supraventricular), dysrhythmias may be congenital or may result from myocardial anoxia, infarction, or other causes. Their clinical significance depends on cardiac output, blood pressure, and site of origin.

Dysrhythmias, usually not common in children, often occur because of congenital reasons or in response to cardiac surgery. Treatment usually involves the use of antiarrhythmic medications, such as digitalis and verapamil.

Assessment
Cardiovascular
- abnormal heart rate for age
- irregular R-R intervals
- absence of P wave before each QRS complex
- long PR interval
- abnormally shaped P wave or QRS complex
- signs and symptoms of decreased cardiac output (decreased capillary refill time, peripheral edema, crackles, rhonchi, and tachycardia)

Nursing diagnosis: *Altered cardiac output: decreased related to cardiac dysrhythmia*

GOAL: The child will maintain effective cardiac output as evidenced by a capillary refill time of 3 to 5 seconds, pinkish mucous membranes, and increased energy levels.

Interventions

1. Monitor the child's cardiovascular status using a cardiac monitor.

2. Assess and record the child's apical heart rate, peripheral pulses, blood pressure, capillary refill time, intake and output, and skin characteristics (such as mottling, color, edema, temperature, and diaphoresis).

3. Administer cardiovascular medications, as ordered.

Rationales

1. Cardiac monitoring allows for immediate determination and documentation of deviations in the child's normal heart rate and rhythm.

2. Such assessment provides data on any changes from the child's baseline measurements, possibly indicating dysrhythmia.

3. Cardiovascular medications may be prescribed to help interrupt the electrical disturbances associated with the dysrhythmia.

Nursing diagnosis: *Potential for injury related to medication dosage or physiologic response to medication*

GOAL: The child will suffer no injuries from medication dosages or physiologic response to medication.

Interventions

1. After medication administration, monitor the child's heart rate and rhythm using a cardiac monitor.

2. Monitor the child's potassium and calcium levels.

3. Double-check the accuracy of all dosages before administration.

Rationales

1. Antiarrhythmic medications may produce dysrhythmias, which can be detected by cardiac monitoring.

2. The effectiveness of antiarrhythmic medications depends on proper adjustment of the intracellular electrolytes. Potassium imbalances can cause dysrhythmias; calcium imbalances can cause cardiac arrest.

3. Giving too much or too little of the medication can cause dysrhythmias.

Nursing diagnosis: *Potential for infection related to I.V. access site and use of cardiac electrodes*

GOAL: The child will have no sign of infection as evidenced by normal temperature and no change in vital signs.

Interventions	Rationales
1. Check the I.V. site hourly for signs of erythema or infiltration or for possible dislodgment of the I.V. line.	1. Assessing the I.V. site hourly helps to detect skin burns from chemical infiltration or the interruption of antiarrhythmic medications caused by dislodgment of the I.V. line—both possible sources of infection.
2. Change the I.V. tubing every 24 to 48 hours.	2. Changing the tubing on a regular basis helps prevent the growth of bacteria.
3. Check electrode sites every shift for signs of rash or erythema.	3. Electrode gel can cause skin irritation, possibly leading to infection. Removal of electrode adhesive pads can cause skin breakdown, creating a potential site for bacteria infiltration. Use of needle electrodes also provides a potential site for bacteria infiltration.

Nursing diagnosis: *Diversional activity deficit related to restricted activity from attachment to the cardiac monitor*

GOAL: The child will participate in child-life activities despite attachment to a cardiac monitor.

Interventions	Rationales
1. Consult a child-life worker (play therapist) regarding the child's condition.	1. A child-life worker can plan appropriate activities based on the child's developmental level and physical restrictions.
2. Encourage the child to interact with other children on the unit, providing the other children are free of respiratory infections.	2. Such contact with peers helps prevent feelings of isolation and encourages the child to participate in activities.
3. Provide toys, games, and books appropriate for the child's developmental level.	3. These activities help divert the child's attention from his condition and aid in decreasing boredom. They also provide stimulation to help the child grow developmentally.

Nursing diagnosis: *Knowledge deficit related to the child's illness, hospitalization, and eventual home care*

GOAL: The parents will verbalize an understanding of the child's illness, reason for hospitalization, and home care instructions.

Interventions	Rationales
1. Instruct the parents on the following:	1. Parents need to understand the nature and seriousness of the child's condition to comply with the treatment and monitor the child's progress.
• the cause of the child's dysrhythmias	• Understanding the cause of the child's illness helps parents to regain a sense of control over the situation.
• signs and symptoms of congestive heart failure, including tachypnea, tachycardia, diaphoresis, fatigue, difficulty feeding, peripheral edema, rapid weight gain, dyspnea, and cyanosis	• Recognizing the signs and symptoms of congestive heart failure should prompt them to seek medical advice and attention, when necessary, to help avert serious complications.

Interventions

• the action, administration, and potential adverse effects of antiarrhythmic medications.

2. Explain the purpose and use of the cardiac monitor to the parents and child (if age-appropriate). If the child requires home monitoring, explain how the system works, how to set the alarms, and the type of problems they may encounter when using the monitor at home.

3. Ensure that the parents attend a cardiopulmonary resuscitation (CPR) class before the child is discharged from the hospital.

Rationales

• Knowing the action, correct dosage, and administration of antiarrhythmic medications helps parents to comply with the child's treatment; recognizing the adverse effects should prompt them to seek medical attention, when necessary.

2. Such explanations are necessary to help alleviate parental fears and unnecessary preoccupation with the operation of the monitor, thereby allowing them to concentrate on other aspects of the child's care.

3. The parents need to know how to initiate CPR to sustain the child's circulation and respiration in the event of cardiac arrest related to the dysrhythmia.

Documentation checklist

During the hospitalization, be sure to document the following:
___ the child's status and assessment findings upon admission
___ any changes in the child's status
___ pertinent laboratory and diagnostic findings
___ fluid intake and output
___ nutritional intake
___ growth and development status
___ the child's response to treatment
___ the child's and parents' reaction to the illness and hospitalization
___ patient and family teaching guidelines
___ discharge planning guidelines.

NEUROLOGIC SYSTEM

Guillain-Barré Syndrome

Introduction

A neuromuscular condition of unknown causes, Guillain-Barré syndrome often follows a mild viral infection and is characterized by progressive muscle weakness. Onset usually is rapid, often beginning with a sore throat and progressing to paresthesia and paralysis. The condition may be mild or severe, sometimes requiring several months for complete recovery, depending on the degree of paralysis.

This condition occurs most often in children between ages 4 and 10 but may occur at any age. Treatment, which usually is symptomatic, may include ventilatory support and administration of corticosteroids.

Assessment

Neurologic
• sensory disturbances in the legs and feet
• dysphagia
• slurred speech
• pupillary dilation and constriction

Musculoskeletal
• acute ascending motor paralysis
• diminished or absent deep tendon reflexes

Respiratory
• history of a mild respiratory infection, such as influenza or infectious mononucleosis
• normal respirations that progress to shallow, irregular breathing and acute respiratory distress requiring mechanical ventilation

Cardiovascular
• vasoconstriction

Gastrointestinal
• constipation

Genitourinary
• urinary incontinence

Integumentary
• pallor
• flushing
• diaphoresis

Nursing diagnosis: *Ineffective breathing pattern related to ascending paralysis of disease process*

GOAL: The child will maintain adequate respiratory function as evidenced by equal and bilateral chest expansion with strong breath sounds and absence of cyanosis.

Interventions

1. Auscultate the child's breath sounds every 1 to 2 hours, noting depth and chest wall expansion.

2. Perform pulmonary function tests (such as testing the child's ability to exhale and the vital capacity and retained volume of air) three or four times each day during the initial phase of the illness.

3. Monitor the child's arterial blood gas (ABG) levels.

4. Place the child in a supine position with the head of the bed elevated.

5. Encourage the child to cough every 2 to 4 hours.

6. Provide ventilatory support, as ordered.

Rationales

1. Auscultating breath sounds helps in assessing paralysis of diaphragm and respiratory muscles.

2. Pulmonary function tests help assess the adequacy of the child's respirations.

3. Monitoring ABG levels helps assess the child's risk of respiratory failure and decreased cardiac output.

4. This position increases the child's lung expansion capacity.

5. Coughing helps clear mucus from the lungs and allows the nurse to assess the effectiveness of secretion management.

6. Because of decreasing respiratory function, the child may require oxygen therapy, intubation, or a tracheostomy.

Interventions	**Rationales**
7. Encourage the child to blow bubbles or to perform other respiratory exercises every 2 to 4 hours.	7. Such exercises facilitate lung expansion and gas exchange.

Nursing diagnosis: *Impaired physical mobility related to ascending paralysis*

GOAL: The child will maintain physical mobility as evidenced by joint mobility and lack of joint contractures.

Interventions	**Rationales**
1. Perform passive range-of-motion (ROM) exercises every 4 hours during the acute stage of illness, followed by active ROM exercises during the recovery phase.	1. ROM exercises help maintain joint mobility.
2. Place the child's feet on a foot board or in high-top sneakers. Remove the foot board or sneakers when performing ROM exercises.	2. High-top sneakers maintain the same joint angle as a foot board, which is used to prevent footdrop.
3. Maintain proper body alignment, and change the child's position every 2 hours.	3. Proper body alignment and position changes help prevent skin breakdown and contractures. Using hand or leg rolls and a proper back support should help prevent muscle strain.

Nursing diagnosis: *Ineffective thermoregulation related to autonomic instability*

GOAL: The child's temperature will remain between 98.6° and 100.4° F. (36° and 38° C.).

Interventions	**Rationales**
1. Monitor the child's temperature every 2 to 4 hours.	1. Temperature monitoring is essential to detect irregularities caused by autonomic instability.
2. Use a hyperthermia/hypothermia blanket to maintain normal body temperature if the child is unresponsive to other methods of temperature regulation, such as antipyretics or tepid sponge baths.	2. A hyperthermia/hypothermia blanket can be adjusted to maintain desired body temperature.
3. Administer antipyretics, as ordered.	3. Antipyretics aid in reducing high temperatures.
4. Assess for signs and symptoms of secondary infection, including elevated white blood cell count, greenish or yellowish sputum, and diarrhea.	4. Secondary infections may contribute to alterations in body temperature.
5. If the child's temperature is above 101° F. (38.4° C.), provide tepid sponge baths until the temperature begins falling or the child becomes chilled.	5. Cool, moist compresses help reduce temperature by evaporation and conduction.

Nursing diagnosis: *Altered cardiac output: decreased related to autonomic instability*

GOAL: The child will maintain an adequate cardiac output as evidenced by maintaining normal urine output and ABG and pH levels.

Interventions	**Rationales**
1. Monitor the child's vital signs every 1 to 2 hours for transient bradycardia, tachycardia, and blood pressure changes.	1. Monitoring is essential to detect abnormalities resulting from autonomic instability. Usually, no treatment is recommended for these abnormalities unless cardiac output decreases.

Interventions	Rationales
2. Carefully monitor the child's intake and output.	2. Urine output is an indication of cardiac output. Therefore, if urine output is decreased, cardiac output also is decreased.
3. Monitor the child's ABG and pH levels for signs of decreased cardiac output.	3. Monitoring these levels may reveal acidosis (pH level <7.35) or impending respiratory failure (PO_2 level <70 mm Hg).
4. Assess peripheral pulses every 4 hours.	4. Assessing peripheral pulses helps in determining the child's peripheral circulation and cardiac output.

Nursing diagnosis: *Altered nutrition: less than body requirements related to ascending paralysis*

GOAL: The child will exhibit no weight loss, proper wound healing, and good skin turgor.

Interventions	Rationales
1. Monitor the child's nutritional intake.	1. Such monitoring is essential to determine possible nutritional deficits, including insufficient calorie, protein, and vitamin intake.
2. Weigh the child daily.	2. Daily weight assessments provide a means of gauging whether the child is getting enough nutritional intake to prevent weight loss.
3. When serving meals, cut the child's food into small pieces.	3. Cutting the food into small pieces enables the child to manage food easily, thereby promoting increased intake.
4. Assess the child's food preferences, and try to incorporate favorite foods into his regular diet.	4. Children have specific food preferences. Serving the child's favorite foods helps ensure that he will consume more of each meal.
5. Assess the child's ability to chew and swallow.	5. Ascending paralysis may interfere with the child's ability to chew and swallow, necessitating the use of nasogastric or gastrostomy feedings.
6. Assess the child's skin integrity daily.	6. Skin breakdown and decreased wound healing may reflect nutritional deficits.

Nursing diagnosis: *Altered patterns of urinary elimination related to paralysis*

GOAL: The child will experience normal urinary elimination as evidenced by lack of urine retention.

Interventions	Rationales
1. Monitor the child's fluid intake and output.	1. Such monitoring provides a direct measure of the child's urine output.
2. Percuss and palpate the child's bladder every 2 to 4 hours.	2. Palpation and percussion may reveal bladder distention, a direct indication of urine retention.
3. Perform Credé's maneuver on the child's bladder as needed.	3. Performing Credé's maneuver helps stimulate the elimination process.
4. Monitor for signs of hematuria.	4. Hematuria may indicate the presence of renal stones caused by hypercalcemia resulting from the mobilization of calcium from the bone.

Nursing diagnosis: *Altered bowel elimination: constipation related to paralysis*

GOAL: The child will have no sign of constipation as evidenced by regular, frequent bowel movements.

Interventions	Rationales
1. Assess the child's bowel sounds, and monitor the frequency of bowel elimination.	1. Such assessment may reveal a tendency toward constipation related to the muscle paralysis and paralysis of the bowel.
2. Administer stool softeners, as ordered.	2. The child may require stool softeners to avoid fecal impaction, thereby reducing the risk of constipation.

Nursing diagnosis: *Potential for impaired skin integrity related to physical immobility*

GOAL: The child will maintain good skin integrity as evidenced by the lack of skin breakdown and decubiti.

Interventions	Rationales
1. Place the child on an eggcrate mattress or alternative bed, such as an air or a bead mattress.	1. Placing the child on such surfaces helps decrease or eliminate the risk of developing pressure sores.
2. Turn child every 2 hours.	2. Alternating positions helps relieve areas of pressure.
3. Assess the child's pressure points with every position change, noting areas of increased redness or shininess.	3. Redness or shininess of skin are indications of potential skin breakdown.
4. Massage the child's pressure points with every turning.	4. Massage increases circulation to the area and decreases the risk of skin breakdown.
5. Bathe the child daily.	5. Bathing increases circulation, thereby preventing skin breakdown.

Nursing diagnosis: *Potential for altered parenting related to the child's condition and hospitalization*

GOAL: The parents will maintain appropriate parental interaction as evidenced by visiting the child, responding to his needs, and providing support.

Interventions	Rationales
1. Assess the parents' knowledge of the child's condition and need for hospitalization.	1. Such assessment serves as a basis on which to begin teaching.
2. Explain all procedures and treatments to the parents.	2. Explaining the child's condition and expected treatment to the parents helps alleviate anxiety and fosters confidence in the child's care during hospitalization.
3. Encourage the parents to assist in the child's activities of daily living, such as bathing, serving meals, and performing ROM exercises.	3. Assisting in the child's care helps decrease anxiety and promotes parental-child attachments.
4. Provide support to the parents by listening to their feelings and concerns and referring them to auxiliary services, such as pastoral care or social services, if necessary.	4. Listening to the parents' feelings and concerns provides emotional support, reducing anxiety and stress. Referral to auxiliary services can provide additional support for areas of special concern.

Nursing diagnosis: *Disturbance in self-concept: personal identity (age-dependent) related to the disease process or rehabilitation process (or both)*

GOAL: The child will maintain a positive self-concept and age-dependent development despite his condition.

Interventions

1. Assess the child's knowledge of and feelings about his condition and expected recovery.

2. Allow the child to participate in his care, depending on his degree of paralysis.

3. Provide play stimulus according to the child's developmental level.

4. Explain all procedures to the child according to his developmental level.

Rationales

1. Such assessment reveals the child's current cognitive stage and emotional level.

2. This enables the child to assume some control over the situation.

3. Appropriate play allows the child to express various emotions and encourages developmental growth.

4. Explaining procedures helps decrease the child's anxiety and enables the child to assume a sense of control over his condition.

Nursing diagnosis: *Potential for infection related to immobility or invasive procedures (or both)*

GOAL: The child will exhibit no signs or symptoms of infection as evidenced by normal temperature and absence of purulent tracheal secretions and reddened areas at invasive sites.

Interventions

1. Monitor the child's vital signs every 2 to 4 hours.

2. Assess the child's breath sounds and respiratory secretions every 4 to 8 hours.

3. Assess I.V. sites and incisions every 8 hours for redness and tenderness.

Rationales

1. Monitoring vital signs provides ongoing assessment of changes in the child's status that may indicate infection.

2. Immobility increases the child's risk of developing pneumonia.

3. Invasive procedures increase the child's risk for infection.

Nursing diagnosis: *Anxiety (child) related to progressive muscle weakness*

GOAL: The child will have less anxiety as evidenced by decreased crying, restful periods, interaction with others, and less verbalization of fear and anxiety depending on degree of paralysis.

Interventions

1. Allow the parents to stay with the child unless the child is in the intensive care unit.

2. Explain all procedures and answer all the child's questions.

3. If possible, allow the child to make decisions regarding his daily routines, such as meals and bathing.

4. Use touch and talking to provide reassurance.

Rationales

1. Allowing the parents to stay with the child provides support, thereby decreasing the child's anxiety.

2. Explanations and honest answers decrease the fear of the unknown.

3. This enables the child to feel a sense of control over some of the aspects of his care, thereby reducing anxiety.

4. Touching and talking to the child may help to calm him and reduce anxiety.

Nursing diagnosis: *Knowledge deficit related to home care*

GOAL: The parents will verbalize an understanding of home care instructions.

Interventions

1. Teach the parents how to perform active ROM exercises.

2. Instruct the parents on the prescribed medication regimen, including details on administration and adverse effects.

3. Teach the parents necessary safety precautions, including gait training, having the child avoid stairs, never leaving the child unattended while bathing, avoiding the child's exposure to extreme heat or cold, and knowing how to perform cardiopulmonary resuscitation.

4. Teach the parents the importance of feeding the child a diet high in calories and protein.

Rationales

1. This enables the parents to provide exercises at home and ensures compliance with the prescribed physical therapy.

2. Providing the parents with detailed instructions on medication administration helps ensure compliance with the medication regimen. Knowing the potential adverse efffects should prompt them to seek medical advice and attention, when necessary.

3. Emphasizing safety precautions is necessary to reduce the risk of accidents caused by muscle weakness.

4. A high-calorie, high-protein diet is needed to replace weight and muscle mass lost during the illness.

Documentation checklist

During the hospitalization, be sure to document the following:
___ the child's status and assessment findings upon admission
___ any changes in the child's status
___ pertinent laboratory or diagnostic findings
___ fluid intake and output
___ nutritional intake
___ growth and development status
___ the child's response to treatment
___ the child's and parents' reaction to the illness and hospitalization
___ physical therapy guidelines
___ patient and family teaching guidelines
___ discharge planning guidelines.

NEUROLOGIC SYSTEM
Head Injury

Introduction

Head injury refers to any trauma to the scalp, skull, or brain, including concussion (most common), cerebral contusion or laceration, fracture, and vascular injuries (epidural or subdural hematoma). Types of skull fracture include linear (most common in children), depressed, compound (communication between lacerated scalp and brain), and basilar (involving either the base of the brain or the vault of the skull.)

Complications of head injury may include increased intracranial pressure (ICP), epidural or subdural hemorrhage, and cerebral edema. The prognosis depends on the severity of the injury and the length of time in a comatose state. Treatment includes the administration of I.V. fluids, anticonvulsants, and steroids.

Assessment

Because children do not always exhibit symptoms at the time of initial injury, they require close monitoring for 24 to 48 hours after any suspected head injury. Documentation of a fall or accident constitutes an important part of the assessment process. Because spinal injury may accompany head injury, children treated for head injuries should also be assessed and treated for spinal injury until spinal injury is ruled out.

CONCUSSION
Neurologic
- impaired consciousness for a variable period
- headache (postconcussion syndrome)
- vertigo
- depressed reflexes
- anxiety
- general malaise

Respiratory
- decreased respirations

Cardiovascular
- bradycardia
- hypotension

CEREBRAL CONTUSION
Note: The severity of the contusion will depend on the extent of cranial injury, the amount of cerebral edema, and the amount of bleeding.

Neurologic
- possible loss of consciousness
- mild motor or sensory weakness
- headache
- vertigo
- post-traumatic seizures (later sign)
- coma

- irritability
- restlessness

SKULL FRACTURE
Neurologic
- altered skull contour
- conjunctival hemorrhage (associated with fracture of the anterior fossa)
- cerebrospinal fluid (CSF) rhinorrhea
- periorbital ecchymosis (raccoon eyes)
- CSF otorrhea
- palsies of C1, C7, and C8 nerves
- post-traumatic seizures (later sign)
- coma

Cardiovascular
- hypovolemia (associated with fractures over the sagittal or lateral sinus)

Integumentary
- ecchymosis at the base of the neck (associated with basilar skull fracture and fractures over the mastoid process)

EPIDURAL HEMATOMA
Note: The following signs and symptoms of epidural hematoma occur after initial awakening and alertness.

Neurologic
- brief loss of consciousness
- sudden headache
- decreased level of consciousness
- signs of increased ICP (vomiting, headache, lethargy, decreased level of consciousness)
- unilateral pupillary dilation; bilateral pupillary dilation (if not decompressed)
- decerebrate posturing (later sign)
- hemiparesis

Respiratory
- respiratory depression
- apnea

Cardiovascular
- bradycardia

ACUTE SUBDURAL HEMATOMA
Note: Acute subdural hematoma usually presents with diffuse symptoms; however, signs and symptoms of cerebral laceration, contusion, or intracerebral hematoma also may be noted.

Neurologic
- headache
- loss of consciousness

- focal seizures
- unilateral pupillary dilation
- hemiparesis
- agitation
- drowsiness with confusion
- progressive slowness of thinking

CHRONIC SUBDURAL HEMATOMA
Neurologic
- headache
- progressive decrease in level of consciousness (may be over weeks or months resulting from a relatively minor injury)
- nuchal rigidity
- ipsilateral pupillary dilation

- hemiparesis
- tight or bulging fontanels (in infants)
- increased head circumference
- hyperactive reflexes
- irritability

Gastrointestinal
- anorexia
- vomiting

Eye, Ear, Nose, and Throat
- retinal hemorrhage

Integumentary
- low-grade fever

Nursing diagnosis: *Ineffective breathing pattern (with potential for respiratory failure) related to increased ICP*

GOAL: The child will maintain adequate respiratory effort and gas exchange as evidenced by normal respiratory patterns and arterial blood gas (ABG) levels and pink mucous membranes.

Interventions	Rationales
1. Establish an open airway by extending the child's neck after cervical vertebral fracture has been ruled out.	1. Extending the neck helps to decrease upper airway obstruction.
2. Insert an oral airway.	2. An oral airway helps prevent airway obstruction in a patient with a decreased level of consciousness.
3. Anticipate the need for endotracheal intubation.	3. Intubation may be necessary to provide mechanical ventilation to maintain adequate gas exchange.
4. Increase the head of the child's bed 30 degrees after spinal cord injury has been ruled out.	4. Increasing the head of bed helps to maximize diaphragmatic excursion, thereby assisting ventilatory effort.
5. Insert a nasogastric tube or an orogastric tube.	5. Insertion of either of these tubes decompresses the stomach, thereby decreasing the potential for vomiting and aspiration. For suspected basilar skull fracture, only an orogastric (not a nasogastric) tube should be used because of the risk of infection from an open pathway to the brain, especially if the child has a nasal CSF leak.
6. Provide suctioning, as needed.	6. Unnecessary suctioning is not recommended because of the potential for increased ICP. (*Note:* Nasal suctioning is contraindicated in suspected basilar skull fracture because of the risk of an open pathway to the brain.)
7. Monitor the child's respiratory effort for rate, depth, and pattern hourly until stable.	7. Abnormal breathing patterns may decrease breathing efficiency and adversely affect gas exchange.
8. Monitor ABG results for abnormal levels.	8. Partial pressure of carbon dioxide levels should be maintained at 25 to 30 mm Hg to induce vasoconstriction to lower the brain's blood volume, thereby decreasing increased ICP. (Levels less than 20 mm Hg may cause severe vasoconstriction, leading to lactic acidosis and secondary brain ischemia.) ABG levels may be normal if the physiologic response of hypoxia and hyperventilation is present.

Nursing diagnosis: *Altered tissue perfusion related to hypotension secondary to hypovolemic shock*

GOAL: The child will maintain adequate tissue perfusion as evidenced by strong peripheral pulses, warm extremities, lack of fever, a capillary refill time of 3 to 5 seconds, and normal blood pressure.

Interventions

1. Monitor the child's vital signs hourly, and check his extremities for warmth, brisk capillary refill, strong pulses, and pink nail beds.

2. Monitor central venous pressure and systemic arterial pressure hourly if the child is undergoing invasive monitoring.

3. Administer blood products, colloid solutions, or I.V. fluids, as ordered.

Rationales

1. An increase in rectal temperature and a decrease in skin temperature can indicate poor systemic perfusion, possibly a sign of hypovolemia. Fever may indicate an epidural hematoma. Cold stress increases oxygen consumption and produces peripheral vasoconstriction. Shock can result in hypotension, tachycardia followed by bradycardia, and increased respiratory rate.

2. Hypotension may cause brain injury secondary to cerebral ischemia. Central venous pressure and systemic arterial pressure decrease with hypertension.

3. Administering such fluids helps increase the circulating fluid volume. Hypotonic fluids usually are not administered since they can increase extracellular water uptake, causing cerebral edema. Hypovolemia may be secondary to intracranial hemorrhage or an associated traumatic injury.

Nursing diagnosis: *Potential for fluid volume deficit related to nausea and vomiting*

GOAL: The child will be adequately hydrated as evidenced by moist mucous membranes, good skin turgor, and electrolyte levels within normal limits.

Interventions

1. Monitor the child's fluid intake and output every 2 to 8 hours, depending on the outcome of specific gravity levels taken every 8 hours.

2. Weigh the child daily, and assess his skin turgor and mucous membranes every 8 hours.

Rationales

1. An increased urine concentration as noted by specific gravity may indicate a fluid deficit.

2. Weight loss, poor skin turgor (as evidenced by skin tenting), and dry mucous membranes indicate a fluid deficit.

Nursing diagnosis: *Altered cardiac output: decreased related to hemorrhage*

GOAL: The child will maintain adequate cardiac output as evidenced by normal heart rate, blood pressure, and hematocrit level.

Interventions

1. Monitor the child's vital signs hourly for the first 8 hours, then as ordered.

2. Assess the child initially and every 8 hours for physical evidence of hemorrhage, such as an alteration in the contour of the skull, bruising or external hematoma, or bleeding from the ear. Report these signs immediately to the doctor if they occur.

Rationales

1. The child may have tachycardia or hypotension, both of which are physiologic responses to hemorrhage.

2. Physical findings of potential hemorrhage may signify a decrease in circulatory volume.

Nursing diagnosis: *Potential for injury related to altered level of consciousness secondary to head injury or increased ICP (or both)*

GOAL: The child will have no signs of further injury.

Interventions

1. Assess the child's neurologic status hourly for the first 8 hours, then as ordered for the following:
• altered level of consciousness, such as lack of response to painful stimuli, altered pupillary response, decreased reflexes, and seizures
• unilaterally dilated, sluggish, or fixed pupils
• decreased motor activity.

2. Monitor the child's vital signs hourly (until stable) for signs of tachycardia, bradycardia, hypotension, widened pulse pressure, and decreased respiratory rate.

3. Ensure that the child maintains a cerebral perfusion pressure of >50 mm Hg by draining CSF fluid through the intracranial pressure line to reduce pressure.

4. Provide rest periods between nursing interventions or treatment.

5. Administer I.V. lidocaine or another analgesic, as ordered, before performing such noxious interventions as suctioning.

6. Administer diuretics, including mannitol and furosemide, as ordered.

Rationales

1. Altered level of consciousness may indicate increasing ICP. Unilaterally dilated, sluggish, or fixed pupils may precede an emergency, such as brain anoxia. Inappropriate motor responses, such as decreased reflexes, decreased reponse to stimuli, or seizures, may indicate brain damage.

2. These signs may indicate Cushing's syndrome (rare in children), which results from the use of steroids to treat cerebral edema.

3. Cerebral perfusion pressure, which measures the blood flow to the brain, must be maintained to prevent ischemia.

4. Adequate rest helps prevent a cumulative rise in ICP.

5. Administering an analgesic before suctioning or other noxious procedures reduces the risk of stimulating the child, which could lead to increased ICP.

6. These agents help reduce ICP by controlling the fluid volume in the cerebral spaces.
• Osmotic diuretics, such as mannitol, act to pull fluid from cerebral extracellular space into the bloodstream. However, a rebound effect may occur approximately 6 hours after the medication is stopped.
• Nonosmotic diuretics, such as furosemide, lower systemic blood flow through action on the kidneys, thereby decreasing cerebral fluid volume.

Nursing diagnosis: *Potential for injury secondary to seizure activity*

GOAL: The child will have no sign of further injury as evidenced by maintaining neurologic function despite seizure activity. (About 10% of children with cerebral contusions exhibit seizure activity beginning hours to years after the initial injury.)

Interventions

1. Take necessary seizure precautions, including keeping a tongue depressor, artificial airway, and suctioning equipment within easy reach and keeping side rails up and padded.

2. Administer anticonvulsant medications, as ordered.

Rationales

1. Because seizures can result in falls, head injuries, anoxia, choking, and possible death, these precautions are necessary to help prevent injury and the risk of further complications.

2. Anticonvulsant medications help control seizures.

Nursing diagnosis: *Altered comfort: pain related to head injury*

GOAL: The child will demonstrate minimal discomfort as evidenced by verbalizing reduced or lack of pain and maintaining vital signs within appropriate limits.

Interventions

1. Assess the child's complaints of pain, noting the pain's location, duration, and severity. Also assess vital signs for increased pulse rate, increased or decreased respiratory rate, and diaphoresis. To relieve pain, change the child's position, decrease stimulation, and administer pain medication.

2. Decrease the amount of light, noise, and other environmental stimuli in the child's room.

Rationales

1. Pain assessment is necessary, especially if the child is too young to verbalize his discomfort. Pain may result in increased ICP secondary to hypoventilation and Valsalva's maneuver. Increased pulse rate, increased or decreased respiratory rate, or diaphoresis may reflect discomfort.

2. Such stimuli may be disturbing to a head-injured child because stimulation increases neurologic irritability, which decreases his tolerance to pain. This also may lead to increased ICP.

Nursing diagnosis: *Anxiety (child and parent) related to traumatic head injury*

GOAL: The child and parents will demonstrate minimal anxiety as evidenced by exhibiting decreased agitation and asking appropriate questions about the illness and treatment.

Interventions

1. Explain to the child and parents the purpose of and procedure for all nursing measures.

2. Allow the parents to stay with the child, depending on the child's status.

Rationales

1. Knowing beforehand the reason and procedure for all nursing measures helps reduce the level of anxiety.

2. This allows the parents to provide the child with emotional support, thereby decreasing the child's anxiety. It also reduces parental anxiety by allowing the parents to see and participate in the child's care.

Nursing diagnosis: *Potential for infection related to injury*

GOAL: The child will have no signs or symptoms of infection as evidenced by normal body temperature, absence of drainage from the wound, and a normal white blood cell count.

Interventions

1. Assess the amount and character of any drainage from the child's nose, mouth, or auditory canal.

2. Monitor the child's temperature every 4 hours.

3. Assess for signs and symptoms of meningitis, including nuchal rigidity, irritability, headache, fever, vomiting, and seizures.

4. Change all wound dressings using sterile technique.

Rationales

1. Assessing such drainage may indicate a CSF leak, which suggests an open pathway to the brain. (Testing for CSF leakage may involve use of Tes-Tape to detect the amount of glucose present in CSF; decreased amounts may indicate infection.) An open pathway to the brain may increase the child's risk for infection.

2. Hyperthermia may signify an infectious process.

3. CSF leakage provides a medium for contracting meningitis because of the open pathway for infection.

4. Sterile technique aids in preventing the introduction of bacteria into the open wound, thereby decreasing the risk of infection.

Nursing diagnosis: *Potential for impaired skin integrity related to physical immobility*

GOAL: The child will have no have no signs of impaired skin integrity as evidenced by the lack of skin breakdown and decubitus ulcers.

Interventions

1. Provide passive range-of-motion (ROM) exercises every 4 hours.

2. Place the child's feet on a foot board or in high-top sneakers when not performing ROM exercises.

3. Maintain the child's proper body alignment, and change his position every 2 hours.

Rationales

1. Passive ROM exercises help maintain joint mobility, thereby decreasing the risk of skin breakdown.

2. Sneakers maintain the same joint angle as a foot board, preventing foot drop and skin breakdown.

3. Using hand and leg rolls and proper back support helps prevent muscle strain sometimes caused by proper alignment and improved positioning. Changing position aids in preventing skin breakdown.

Nursing diagnosis: *Knowledge deficit related to home care*

GOAL: The parents will verbalize an understanding of home care instructions.

Interventions

1. Instruct the parents on the nature and expected course of the child's head injury.

2. Instruct the parents on recognizing signs and symptoms of potential complications, including altered level of consciousness, changes in the child's gait, fever, and seizures.

3. Instruct the parents on the purpose and use of medications, including details on administration and potential adverse effects.

4. Teach the parents about seizure precautions, including keeping a padded tongue depressor available for emergency use, having the child wear a protective helmet, maintaining the child's airway during seizure episodes, and putting side rails on the child's bed.

5. Emphasize the importance of the child's performing activities of daily living, including daily or regular exercise, self-feeding, stimulation, and hygiene.

6. Provide safety-related information on the use of seat belts, car restraints, and safety helmets, and on driving while intoxicated.

Rationales

1. Such knowledge helps the parents to better understand the need for treatment and the possible long-term effects of the injury.

2. Knowing this information should prompt parents to seek medical advice and attention, when necessary.

3. Medications—whether for infection or seizures—must be given consistently to ensure therapeutic effectiveness. Knowing the potential adverse effects should prompt parents to seek immediate attention, when necessary.

4. Following these precautions helps prevent injury to the child during seizure episodes.

5. Because of the head injury, the child may have lost his ability to perform certain activities of daily living and may require retraining and continual encouragement.

6. Providing this information helps ensure that the parents and child follow necessary safety precautions to decrease the chance of another head injury.

Documentation checklist

During the hospitalization, be sure to document the following:

____ the child's status and assessment findings upon admission

____ any changes in the child's status

____ pertinent laboratory and diagnostic findings

____ the child's neurologic status

____ fluid intake and output

____ the child's repsonse to treatment

____ the child's and parents' reaction to illness and hospitalization

____ patient and family teaching guidelines

____ discharge planning guidelines.

NEUROLOGIC SYSTEM

Hydrocephalus

Introduction

Hydrocephalus, which is characterized by head enlargement, prominence of the forehead, brain atrophy, and mental deterioration, is caused by failure of circulating cerebrospinal fluid (CSF) to drain from cerebral ventricles. This results in increased fluid buildup and intracranial pressure (ICP), which, if unrelieved, may lead to brain damage and death.

Treatment involves surgery to relieve the ICP. Possible complications include infection, blockage, and subdural hematoma.

Assessment

The following assessment findings indicate shunt malfunction:

INFANTS
Neurologic
- split cranial sutures
- swelling along shunt tract
- high-pitched cry
- bulging fontanels
- irritability when awake

Gastrointestinal
- vomiting
- change in appetite

Musculoskeletal
- lethargy

TODDLERS
Neurologic
- headaches
- seizures
- swelling along the shunt tract
- irritability

Gastrointestinal
- vomiting

Musculoskeletal
- lethargy

SCHOOL-AGE CHILDREN
Neurologic
- headaches
- resplitting of cranial sutures
- seizures

Gastrointestinal
- vomiting

Musculoskeletal
- lethargy

Psychosocial
- decreased school performance
- change in attention span

ADOLESCENTS
Neurologic
- papilledema
- sunset eyes (setting-sun sign)
- prominent scalp veins
- seizures
- deterioration in level of consciousness
- Cushing's triad (bradycardia, widened pulse pressure, and apnea)
- pupil dilation

Respiratory
- Cheyne-Stokes respiration

The following assessment findings indicate shunt infection:

Neurologic
- swelling or redness along shunt tract
- signs and symptoms of shunt dysfunction (headaches, seizures, bulging fontanels, decreased level of consciousness)

Gastrointestinal
- poor appetite

Integumentary
- elevated temperature

Nursing diagnosis: *Altered thought processes related to increased intracranial pressure (ICP)*

GOAL: The child will maintain brain functioning and develop no further signs of ICP.

Interventions

1. Perform a neurologic assessment every 2 to 4 hours of the child's pupillary response, grip, grasp, pain response, interactive responses (smiling, talking, babbling), and disposition (pleasantness or irritability).

Rationales

1. Frequent assessments provide data for determining changes in the child's baseline neurologic status indicative of ICP. However, by the time clinical manifestations are present, the child already may have significant ICP.

Interventions	**Rationales**
2. Assess the child's vital signs every 2 to 4 hours, noting irregularities in respiration and heart rate and rhythm and widening of pulse pressures.	2. Frequent vital sign assessments help detect early signs of ICP (such as tachycardia, blood pressure fluctuation, and Cheyne-Stokes respiration) or later signs of advancing ICP (Cushing's triad: widened pulse pressure, bradycardia, and apnea).
3. Perform a cranial nerve assessment every 2 to 4 hours.	3. Changes in cranial nerve function are a direct reflection of ICP. Most commonly, C3 and C6 are affected as demonstrated by pupillary changes and extraocular eye movement. C7, C9, and C10 also may be affected as evidenced by asymmetrical facial movement, inability to speak and swallow, and stridor or crowing sounds on inspiration.
4. Elevate the head of the bed 30 degrees.	4. Elevating the head of the bed increases cerebral venous drainage by means of gravity, which aids in decreasing ICP.
5. Assess the child's fontanels every 4 hours for bulging. Be sure to perform the assessment during quiet periods, as the fontanels usually bulge during crying episodes.	5. Full and bulging fontanels directly reflect increased ICP.
6. If the child is under age 2, measure the head circumference daily.	6. Abnormal head enlargement in children under age 2, especially infants, indicates increased ICP. Normally, an infant's head grows an average of ¾" (2 cm) per month until age 3 months, then about ⅛" (0.2 cm) per month until age 1 year.
7. Assess for and report any swelling along the shunt tract every 8 hours.	7. Swelling along the shunt tract or around the shunt pump may indicate that the shunt is clogged.
8. Keep oxygen and suction equipment readily available at the child's bedside during periods of altered level of consciousness.	8. Oxygen and suction equipment are necessary in case seizures develop or the child becomes apneic.
9. Document the parents' recollection of the child's previous experiences with shunt malfunction.	9. Because each child experiences his own variation of the signs and symptoms of shunt malfunction, the parents' recollection of previous signs and symptoms helps the nursing and medical staff to determine whether the shunt is working properly.
10. Note the quality and pitch of the child's cry.	10. A high-pitched cry usually indicates increased ICP.
11. Perform shunt pumping only as ordered by the neurosurgeon.	11. Shunt pumping should only be done as ordered because pumping can pull tissue into the proximal end of the ventricular catheter tip, thereby clogging the tubing.
12. If the child is an infant, keep his body in proper alignment when holding him.	12. Because of his enlarged head, the infant may be difficult to hold; however, body alignment should be maintained to avoid putting a strain on his neck.

Nursing diagnosis: *Potential for infection related to surgical placement of shunt*

GOAL: The child will have no signs of infection related to shunt placement as evidenced by a normal or stable temperature and no signs of incisional swelling or drainage, irritability, lethargy, or loss of appetite.

Interventions	**Rationales**
1. Assess the child for temperature instability, decreased level of consciousness, loss of appetite, vomiting, increased white blood cell count, and swelling or redness along the shunt tract.	1. These signs and symptoms signal shunt infection, which usually occurs within the first month after shunt insertion.

Interventions	Rationales
2. Monitor the child's temperature every 4 hours.	2. Decreased temperature is an early sign of infection in a neonate, and elevated temperature is an early sign of infection in a child.
3. Position the child so that no weight is placed on the valve site for the first 24 to 48 hours postoperatively.	3. Positioning the head in this manner helps prevent skin breakdown on or around the shunt pump and thereby alleviates the risk of infection. Neonates are especially susceptible to shunt infection and may require special positioning for a longer period of time.
4. Assess the child's incision site every 4 hours for drainage or swelling. Note the amount and type of any drainage.	4. Swelling around the pump, shunt tract, or surgical incision—with or without drainage—may be an early sign of shunt infection.
5. Administer antibiotics, as ordered.	5. Prophylactic antibiotics usually are ordered at the time of surgery and continued for 1 to 2 days postoperatively to help prevent infection.

Nursing diagnosis: *Potential fluid volume deficit related to altered nutrition status in the preoperative and postoperative phases*

GOAL: The child will demonstrate no signs of dehydration as evidenced by stable weight, good skin turgor, stable electrolyte levels, adequate tearing, moist mucous membranes, and adequate fluid input and output.

Interventions	Rationales
1. Carefully monitor the child's fluid intake and output.	1. Careful monitoring is essential to detect fluid losses.
2. Weigh the child at the same time each day.	2. Monitoring weight gain or loss is vital in assessing hydration status.
3. Note the frequency of vomiting and the amount.	3. Vomiting, a common sign of increased ICP, may substantially affect the child's hydration status. Parenteral nutrition may be necessary to help correct fluid losses, especially in infants who cannot tolerate oral feedings.
4. Monitor the child's serum electrolyte levels daily if vomiting occurs. Pay particular attention to sodium and potassium levels.	4. Large amounts of sodium, potassium, and other electrolytes are lost through vomiting.
5. Initiate parenteral nutrition, as ordered, and monitor administration hourly.	5. Administration of parenteral fluids helps restore normal fluid and electrolyte balance.
6. If the child has undergone surgery for placement of a ventriculoperitoneal shunt, wait at least 24 hours after the return of active bowel sounds to begin giving clear liquids.	6. Waiting at least 24 hours after the return of bowel sounds ensures that the child does not have a paralytic ileus resulting from the surgery.

Nursing diagnosis: *Potential for injury related to onset of seizures*

GOAL: The child will suffer no injury resulting from seizures.

Interventions	Rationales
1. Determine whether the child has a history of seizures.	1. Seizures have been found to occur in up to 40% of children within 2 years after undergoing shunt placement.
2. Institute seizure precautions for a child with increasing ICP or shunt malfunction. Keep a padded tongue depressor and suction equipment on hand.	2. Seizures are a later sign of increased ICP. Seizure precautions are necessary to prevent injury to the child.

Interventions

3. During a seizure episode, take the following measures:

• Assist the child to his side, either on the bed or floor, and remove any obstacles from the area.

• Do not attempt to restrain the child, but remain at his side.

• Do not attempt to place anything in the child's mouth.

• Assess the child's respiratory status.

• Note any body movements and the duration of the seizure.

Rationales

3. Following these measures helps protect the child and aids in medical follow-up.

• Assisting the child to his side at the onset of a seizure prevents injuries incurred during a fall. Clearing the area of any obstacles helps reduce the possibility of the child suffering injury during convulsive or jerking seizure activity.

• Restraining or forcefully moving the child may cause trauma.

• Trying to force an object into the child's mouth may cause damage to teeth and gums.

• Respiratory resuscitation may be necessary if the child becomes apneic during or after a seizure.

• Seizures can be differentiated by characteristic movements and the duration of the event.

Nursing diagnosis: *Excess fluid volume related to placement of ventriculoatrial shunt*

GOAL: The child will develop no signs or symptoms of cardiac overload as evidenced by normal cardiac output and absence of respiratory distress.

Interventions

1. Assess the child's respiratory and cardiovascular status every 2 to 4 hours for signs and symptoms of decreased cardiac output and respiratory distress, including tachypnea, tachycardia, dyspnea, and cardiac dysrhythmias.

2. Weigh the child daily.

3. Monitor the child's fluid intake and output.

Rationales

1. During ventriculoatrial shunt placement, the distal end of the shunt is placed into the right atrium, where the CSF will flow. Because of the increased fluid volume in the right atrium, cardiac overload and respiratory distress may occur.

2. Weight gain may indicate fluid retention, which is associated with cardiac overload.

3. Such monitoring is essential to evaluate the child's fluid status.

Nursing diagnosis: *Anxiety (parent and child) related to lack of understanding about the child's condition and treatment*

GOAL: The parents and child (if appropriate) will verbalize an understanding of hydrocephalus, the necessity of shunt placement, and the usual operative routine.

Interventions

1. Explain to the parents and child (if appropriate) the definition of hydrocephalus, the anatomy of the ventricles, and the basic purpose of the shunt. Use diagrams and a sample shunt, if available, to help clarify your explanation. Also explain the purpose and procedure of any diagnostic tests ordered.

2. Describe the usual perioperative events, including:
• NPO status
• consent form signing
• establishment of an I.V. access
• transport of the child to the operating room
• waiting facilities for parents
• scheduled time of surgery
• expected length of surgery
• recovery room
• vital sign monitoring
• placement of incision
• dressings.

Rationales

1. Such explanations help decrease fear and anxiety and facilitate acceptance of the child's condition.

2. Explaining these events to the parents ensures that they are aware of what the child will undergo and helps encourage their participation in routine preoperative preparation, as allowed.

Interventions	**Rationales**
3. Allow time for the parents to ask questions and express their fears and concerns.	3. Parents need time to assimilate all the information so that they can formulate questions and express fears and concerns.
4. Provide an opportunity for child preparation, using a doll, actual hospital equipment, and diagrams and videos as appropriate for the child's developmental level.	4. Doll demonstration is extremely useful in helping a child deal with events that occur during hospitalization. Diagrams, videos, books, and honest explanations may be more appropriate for the older child.
5. Reinforce the surgeon's explanations.	5. Parents and children often receive large amounts of information in a short period of time. Repeated explanations help facilitate understanding of the child's condition.
6. Refer the parents to a social worker or other social services personnel, as needed.	6. A social worker can provide intense counseling to help parents cope with their child's condition and hospitalization and can assist the nurse in discharge planning and referral to community organizations.

Nursing diagnosis: *Knowledge deficit related to disease process and home care*

GOAL: The parents will verbalize an understanding of the disease process and home care instructions.

Interventions	**Rationales**
1. Assess the parents' understanding of the disease process and how the shunt functions.	1. Such assessment serves as a basis on which to begin teaching.
2. Instruct the parents on how to care for the shunt, including details on signs and symptoms of shunt malfunction (headache, irritability, vomiting, lethargy, decreased level of consciousness) and infection (fever, headache, neck rigidity) and on the specific care guidelines for the type of shunt in place (ventriculoperitoneal or ventriculoatrial).	2. The parents need to know how to care for the child's shunt and which signs and symptoms to report.
3. Emphasize the importance of continued neurologic follow-up examinations.	3. The child will require lifelong follow-up studies to assess shunt and tubing function and the child's general well-being. Typically, this involves regular assessments by means of computed tomography scans, ultrasonography, and skull and abdominal X-rays.
4. Allow time for the parents to ask questions and express concerns.	4. Asking questions and expressing concerns facilitates the parents' understanding of the discharge instructions.
5. Provide the parents with information on the availability of developmental programs for children with hydrocephalus. Assist them in completing the necessary paperwork for applying to the programs.	5. Children with hydrocephalus are at risk for various developmental delays because of the effects of the disease on brain functioning. Depending on the degree of brain dysfunction, such programs can help the child achieve a nearly normal developmental level.

Documentation checklist

During the hospitalization, be sure to document the following:
___ the child's status and assessment findings upon admission
___ any changes in the child's status
___ pertinent laboratory and diagnostic findings
___ fluid intake and output
___ shunt functioning
___ growth and development status
___ the child's and parents' reaction to the illness and hospitalization
___ patient and family teaching guidelines
___ discharge planning guidelines.

NEUROLOGIC SYSTEM

Intraventricular Hemorrhage

Introduction

Intraventricular hemorrhage (IVH) refers to bleeding into the ventricles of the cerebrum. This type of bleeding affects only premature infants; those of less than 34 weeks' gestation are at greatest risk for IVH. Physical signs and symptoms can range from acute to subtle to no observable signs.

Possible complications include intracranial pressure (ICP), brain anoxia and damage, developmental delays, and even death. Treatment usually is supportive and includes administration of anticonvulsants, vitamin E, and steroids and ventilatory support.

Assessment
ACUTE SIGNS AND SYMPTOMS
Neurologic
• seizures (generalized or focal)
• unresponsiveness to stimuli
• bulging or tautness of anterior fontanel

Respiratory
• apnea

Cardiovascular
• hypotension

Musculoskeletal
• hypotonicity

Integumentary
• ashen color
• temperature instability

SUBTLE SIGNS AND SYMPTOMS
Neurologic
• slight unresponsiveness to stimuli

Musculoskeletal
• slight hypotonicity

Integumentary
• pallor

Nursing diagnosis: *Potential for injury related to fragility of the capillary beds in the cerebrum*

GOAL: The infant will have no further signs of hemorrhage as evidenced by a stable hemodynamic status, normal intracranial pressure, and absence of seizures.

Interventions

1. Monitor and maintain the infant's PO_2, PCO_2, O_2Sat, and pH by maintaining a patent airway and using an oxygen-delivery device, such as an oxygen hood, continuous positive airway pressure, or a mechanical ventilator.

2. Monitor the infant's blood pressure every 4 hours.

3. Assess the infant's neurologic status every 2 to 4 hours, noting any seizure activity or increased tension in the fontanels. Document the anterior fontanel and head circumferences every 4 to 8 hours.

4. To decrease the risk of hypothermia or hyperthermia, avoid exposing the infant to drafts, keep him covered unless he is in an Isolette or on a warming table, and use a thermal sensor patch or probe to continuously monitor his body temperature.

5. If sodium bicarbonate is ordered to correct metabolic acidosis, administer a diluted 1:1 solution over 20 to 30 minutes.

Rationales

1. Maintaining the infant's blood gas levels is essential to prevent hypoxic episodes, which may lead to circulatory failure and increased cerebral perfusion. Increased cerebral perfusion causes increased pressure in vessels, which increases the likelihood of rupture.

2. Adequate cerebral blood flow depends on normal systemic blood pressure.

3. Seizure activity may decrease cerebral blood flow. The fontanels may bulge or become taut. Increased head circumference is an indication of IVH.

4. Extreme changes in temperature increase the stress on the infant's cardiovascular system, possibly leading to increased ICP.

5. Hyperosmolar solution may increase intravascular pressure, which may dilate cerebral vessels and cause hemorrhage.

Interventions

6. Monitor serial hemoglobin and hematocrit levels every 1 to 2 days.

7. Carefully monitor the infant's fluid intake and output.

8. Cluster nursing care measures to help minimize stressing the infant.

9. Elevate the head of the crib or Isolette 15 to 30 degrees.

10. Assist with ultrasonography or computed tomography scans, as necessary.

Rationales

6. Sudden, dramatic decreases in hemoglobin and hematocrit levels may indicate IVH.

7. Careful monitoring of fluid intake and output is necessary to prevent fluid overload or depletion, either of which could alter the infant's systemic pressure and cause hemorrhage.

8. Stressful stimuli may decrease the infant's PO_2 levels.

9. Elevating the head of the bed helps avoid increased blood flow and brain congestion.

10. These diagnostic tests help in assessing the infant's present condition.

Nursing diagnosis: *Knowledge deficit related to infant's condition and home care*

GOAL: The parents will verbalize an understanding of the infant's condition and home care instructions.

Interventions

1. Assess the parents' understanding of the infant's illness.

2. Provide explanations about the infant's medical condition, procedures, and required treatment.

3. Explain the purpose and use of prescribed medications, including details on dosages and potential adverse effects.

4. Instruct the parents to provide stimulation necessary for developmental growth, including bright colors, developmental toys, exercises for muscles, and talking to the infant.

5. Teach the parents seizure precautions and what to do in the event of a seizure, including positioning the infant on his side, maintaining respiratory status, protecting the infant from injury, and recording a description of the seizure activity.

Rationales

1. Such assessment serves as a basis on which to begin teaching.

2. Explaining this information to the parents helps clarify the disease process and need for hospitalization and helps decrease overall anxiety about the infant's well-being.

3. The parents need to know this information to correctly administer all medications prescribed for the infant's condition. Knowing the potential adverse effects should prompt them to seek medical advice and attention, when necessary.

4. Because IVH often causes developmental delays and potential brain damage, such stimulation is necessary to help the infant grow normally.

5. Parents need to know this information because infants with IVH are at high risk for seizures.

Documentation checklist

During the hospitalization, be sure to document the following:
___ the child's status and assessment findings upon admission
___ any changes in the child's status
___ pertinent laboratory and diagnostic findings
___ fluid intake and output
___ nutritional intake
___ growth and development status
___ ICP monitoring
___ ventilator settings
___ the parents' reaction to the illness and hospitalization
___ family teaching guidelines
___ discharge planning guidelines.

NEUROLOGIC SYSTEM
Reye's Syndrome

Introduction

A form of acute encephalopathy that follows a viral infection, Reye's syndrome usually affects children between ages 2 months and 18 years. Classic characteristics, which are stage-dependent, include rash, confusion, and vomiting with possible progression to coma. Researchers have identified a definite link between the development of Reye's syndrome, chicken pox, and aspirin use; however, the exact cause of the condition is still unknown.

Potential complications include seizures, coma, and even death (about 40% of all children die). Treatment includes administration of corticosteroids, dextrose 10% solution, mannitol, and urea. Additional measures include monitoring for intracranial pressure (ICP) and stabilizing respirations.

Assessment
GENERAL
Respiratory
• history of recent viral illness (such as influenza or chicken pox)

Gastrointestinal
• history of salicylate (aspirin) ingestion as treatment for viral illness

STAGE 1
Neurologic
• responsiveness to commands

Gastrointestinal
• vomiting

Musculoskeletal
• fatigue
• lethargy, sleepiness

STAGE 2
Neurologic
• disorientation
• delirium
• combativeness
• hyperactive reflexes
• responsiveness to noxious stimulus

Respiratory
• hyperventilation

Hepatic
• hepatic dysfunction

STAGE 3
Neurologic
• obtundation
• coma
• decorticate posturing
• preserved pupillary light reflexes
• possible dilated pupils
• intact oculovestibular and doll's eyes reflexes

Respiratory
• hyperventilation

STAGE 4
Neurologic
• deepening coma
• decerebrate posturing
• loss of oculocephalic reflexes
• large, fixed pupils
• dysconjugate eye movements

Nursing diagnosis: *Altered thought processes related to ICP*

GOAL: The child will remain oriented to person, place, and time.

Interventions

1. Perform a neurologic assessment every 2 to 4 hours or as needed.

2. Raise the head of the bed 30 to 45 degrees, and maintain the child's head in a neutral position (with the head and neck in complete alignment) to avoid neck flexion and rotation.

Rationales

1. Frequent assessments provide data for early detection of neurologic deterioration.

2. Positioning the child's head in this manner helps preserve cerebral blood flow and oxygenation.

Interventions	**Rationales**
3. Monitor the child's respiratory status every 2 to 4 hours for hyperventilation.	3. Hyperventilation may occur secondary to carbon dioxide retention and increased ICP.
4. Monitor the child hourly for decreased blood and pulse pressures and increased heart rate.	4. Such changes in vital signs signal ICP. However, the variations differ with each child and are therefore difficult to predict.

Nursing diagnosis: *Altered tissue perfusion: cerebral related to increased cerebral edema*

GOAL: The child will maintain adequate cerebral perfusion as evidenced by a cerebral perfusion pressure of above 50 mm Hg

Interventions	**Rationales**
1. Continuously monitor for ICP and increased cerebral perfusion pressure. Notify the doctor if the child's pressure is elevated.	1. Cerebral perfusion pressure measures the blood flow to the brain. Increased pressure may signify a worsening of the child's condition.
2. Hyperventilate the child to maintain ICP below 20 mm Hg or as ordered.	2. Hyperventilation will assist in decreasing ICP.
3. Monitor arterial blood gas (ABG) levels, as ordered.	3. ABG levels should be maintained at a constant level to prevent worsening of cerebral edema.
4. Administer diuretics, as ordered, and monitor the child's fluid intake and output.	4. Diuretics aid in decreasing fluid retention. Monitoring fluid intake and output helps in determining the effectiveness of diuretic therapy.
5. Monitor the child's vital signs and perform neurologic assessments every 2 hours.	5. Careful monitoring is essential because vital signs and neurologic status alter with ICP.

Nursing diagnosis: *Potential for injury (hypoglycemia) related to decreased calorie intake or possible metabolic dysfunction (or both)*

GOAL: The child will have no sign of injury as evidenced by maintaining a serum glucose level of 100 to 200 mg/dl.

Interventions	**Rationales**
1. To ensure I.V. patency, infuse the child with a dextrose solution.	1. Maintaining a patent I.V. access facilitates delivery of adequate amounts of glucose.
2. Monitor the child's blood glucose level every 2 to 4 hours or as ordered.	2. Such monitoring is essential to prevent hypoglycemic brain damage.

Nursing diagnosis: *Altered tissue perfusion: renal, cerebral, cardiopulmonary, gastrointestinal, peripheral (specify) related to increased ICP*

GOAL: The child will maintain adequate circulatory volume as evidenced by a normal central venous pressure, hematocrit level, and urine output.

Interventions	**Rationales**
1. Monitor the child's vital signs (pulse rate, blood pressure, peripheral pulses, temperature) and central venous pressure every 1 to 2 hours.	1. Such monitoring provides data to assess changes in the child's perfusion status. Temperature often is increased related to malfunctioning of the central nervous system.

Interventions

2. Monitor fluid and electrolyte levels, as ordered.

3. Carefully monitor the child's fluid intake and output (including nasogastric feedings).

Rationales

2. Electrolyte imbalances may be caused by the disease process (such as phosphaturia or hypoglycemia) or treatment (such as diuretic therapy). Hyponatremia and hyposmolarity may occur with inappropriate secretion of antidiuretic hormone.

3. Careful monitoring ensures accurate replacement of any fluid loss and decreases the risk of dehydration or cerebral edema.

Nursing diagnosis: *Ineffective breathing pattern (with the potential for respiratory failure) related to cerebral edema*

GOAL: The child will maintain adequate gas exchange as evidenced by normal PaO_2 and $PaCO_2$ levels.

Interventions

1. Auscultate the child's breath sounds every 2 to 4 hours or as needed.

2. Monitor the child's ABG levels for adequate gas exchange.

3. If the child requires endotracheal intubation, perform the following nursing measures:

• After intubation, monitor the ventilator readings for fraction of inspired air (FIO_2) and respiratory rate hourly.
• Provide chest physiotherapy, as needed. Hyperventilate and sedate the child 4 hours before performing chest physiotherapy.

• Administer muscle relaxants, as ordered, to maintain ventilatory control.
• Use soft restraints, as needed, to prevent the child from removing the tube. Check circulation hourly.

Rationales

1. Auscultation provides data for assessment of respiratory function.

2. Decreasing PaO_2 and increasing $PaCO_2$ levels indicate poor gas exchange.

3. Endotracheal intubation may be ordered to control respiratory effort and hyperoxygenation if the child has increased cerebral edema.
• Monitoring the FIO_2 and respiratory rate is essential to prevent respiratory failure.

• Chest physiotherapy helps clear the airway and improve gas exchange. However, because the suctioning performed in physiotherapy may cause dangerous increases in ICP, hyperventilation and sedation are necessary beforehand.
• Muscle relaxants may be needed to reduce agitation and ensure that the child does not fight the ventilator.
• Soft restraints help limit the child's movement, preventing access to the mouth and nose.

Nursing diagnosis: *Potential for impaired skin integrity related to physical immobility*

GOAL: The child will maintain good skin integrity as evidenced by the lack of skin breakdown and decubitus ulcers.

Interventions

1. Move and position the child carefully, as ordered, depending on his degree of ICP.

2. Place the child on an eggcrate mattress or alternative bed (air or bead mattress).

3. Turn and reposition the child every 2 hours.

4. Assess pressure points with every position change, noting areas of increased redness or shininess.

Rationales

1. Movement may cause increased ICP.

2. This type of bedding helps reduce or eliminate the risk of pressure sores.

3. Turning and repositioning help relieve pressure areas. However, because movement may cause an increase in ICP, turning and repositioning will depend on the child's current degree of ICP.

4. Increased redness or shininess indicate increased pressure, possibly leading to skin breakdown.

Interventions	**Rationales**
5. Massage pressure points with every turning.	5. Massage increases circulation to the area and decreases the risk of skin breakdown.
6. Bathe the child daily.	6. Bathing helps increase circulation, thereby preventing skin breakdown.

Nursing diagnosis: *Anxiety (child) related to hospitalization*

GOAL: The child will show minimal fear and anxiety as evidenced by blood pressure, pulse rate, and ICP within normal ranges.

Interventions	**Rationales**
1. Administer sedatives, as ordered, in conjunction with the child's drug-induced coma. However, do not give if the child has bradycardia, hypotension, or decreased respirations.	1. The child may be placed in a drug-induced coma with a paralytic or other agent to decrease metabolic needs on the body. However, because paralytic drugs have no effect on pain, sedatives also may be necessary. Sedatives help reduce anxiety and can help to prevent ICP.
2. Encourage the parents to bring in some of the child's objects from home, such as a stuffed animal, blanket, or a recording of familiar voices.	2. Familiar objects help reduce anxiety. Tape recordings are particularly helpful to adolescents; besides reducing anxiety, they also help decrease environmental noises when used with earphones.
3. Encourage the parents to visit the child regularly.	3. Regular visits promote continuity of the parent-child relationship.

Nursing diagnosis: *Disturbance in self-concept (age-dependent) related to the disease process or rehabilitation process (or both)*

GOAL: The child will maintain a positive self-concept and maintain age-dependent development.

Interventions	**Rationales**
1. Assess child's knowledge of the disease process and his feelings about the situation.	1. Such assessment helps determine the child's current cognitive stage and emotional level (fear, anger, shame).
2. Allow the child to participate in his care.	2. This gives the child a sense of control over his condition.
3. Provide play stimulus according to the child's developmental level.	3. Play allows the child to unconsciously express various emotions.
4. Explain to the child all procedures and treatments according to his developmental level.	4. Such explanations help decrease anxiety.

Nursing diagnosis: *Potential for altered parenting related to the child's hospitalization or lack of knowledge about the child's condition*

GOAL: Parents will maintain appropriate parental interaction as evidenced by visiting the child, responding to his needs, and providing support.

Interventions	**Rationales**
1. Assess the parents' knowledge about the child's condition.	1. Such assessment serves as a basis on which to begin teaching.

Interventions

2. Explain all procedures and nursing care measures to the parents.

3. Encourage the family to assist in activities of daily living, such as daily baths, meals, and range-of-motion exercises.

4. Provide support to the parents by listening to their fears and concerns and referring them to auxiliary services, such as pastoral care or social services, if necessary.

Rationales

2. Knowing this information eases anxiety and helps the parents to feel confident in the child's care during recovery.

3. Such encouragement helps decrease the parents' anxiety by allowing them to participate in their child's care.

4. Listening to the parents' fears and concerns helps decrease anxiety and stress. Auxiliary services can provide support for areas of special concern.

Nursing diagnosis: *Knowledge deficit related to home care*

GOAL: The parents will verbalize an understanding of home care instructions.

Interventions

1. Explain to the parents the child's need for physical therapy.

2. Explain the importance of feeding the child a diet high in calories and protein.

Rationales

1. Physical therapy is necessary to help develop wasted muscles.

2. A high-calorie, high-protein diet is essential to help repair injured tissues.

Documentation checklist

During the hospitalization, be sure to document the following:
___ the child's status and assessment findings upon admission
___ any changes in the child's status
___ pertinent laboratory and diagnostic findings
___ fluid intake and output
___ nutritional intake
___ growth and development status
___ the child's neurologic status
___ the child's response to treatment
___ the child's and parents' reaction to the illness and hospitalization
___ patient and family teaching guidelines
___ discharge planning guidelines.

NEUROLOGIC SYSTEM

Spina Bifida (Meningomyelocele)

Introduction

Meningomyelocele, the most common form of spina bifida, is characterized by incomplete formation of the spinal column in which a thin sac protrudes on the back and contains a portion of the spinal cord, meninges, and spinal fluid. The defect, which occurs in about 1 in 1,000 live births, can be detected by alpha-fetoprotein levels in amniotic fluid. The location of the defect determines the severity of the symptoms.

Potential complications include paralysis, joint deformities, meningitis, and lack of bladder or bowel control. Treatment involves surgery, antibiotic administration, physical therapy, and bladder and bowel retraining. Many children are able to walk with the use of crutches or braces.

Assessment

Neurologic
• decreased level of consciousness
• increased head circumference
• bulging fontanels
• lethargy
• irritability

Respiratory
• apnea

Gastrointestinal
• vomiting
• poor sucking reflex

Genitourinary
• dysuria
• urine retention
• dribbling

Integumentary
• leakage of cerebrospinal fluid (CSF) from the sac
• temperature instability
• skin breakdown

Nursing diagnosis: *Impaired skin integrity related to presence of sac and surgical procedure*

GOAL: The infant will have no signs of postoperative infection as evidenced by lack of fever, normal white blood cell count, and no purulent drainage.

Interventions

1. During the preoperative and early postoperative periods, maintain the infant in a prone position with the buttocks elevated higher than head.

2. Use blanket rolls or sandbags, if necessary, to keep the infant from moving from side to side.

3. During the preoperative period, cover the sac with a sterile dressing soaked in normal saline solution. Reinforce the site frequently with new dressings; however, avoid removing any adherent dressing from the lesion.

4. Notify the doctor immediately if any leakage of CSF occurs from sac.

5. During the postoperative period, place a transparent occlusive (Op-Site) dressing over the infant's buttocks distal to the sac.

6. Every 4 hours, assess the infant for signs and symptoms of infection (including fever, increased white blood cell count, and purulent drainage from the sac) or seizure.

7. Emphasize the importance of good hand-washing technique to all visitors.

Rationales

1. Maintaining the infant in a prone position minimizes pressure on the sac, thereby preventing the risk of rupture.

2. This helps ensure that the infant remains in a prone position.

3. Maintaining a moist covering over the sac prevents drying of the membrane which could otherwise cause tearing or rupture of the sac, leading to leakage of CSF.

4. Leakage of CSF places the child at higher risk for developing meningitis.

5. The plastic covering helps prevent contamination of the sac or surgical incision.

6. Frequent assessments allow for early detection and treatment of infection.

7. Good hand-washing technique minimizes the risk for infection.

Nursing diagnosis: *Hypothermia related to presence of sac*

GOAL: The infant will maintain a normal temperature.

Interventions

1. During the initial preoperative and early postoperative periods, place the infant in an Isolette or a radiant warmer.

2. Monitor the infant's temperature every 4 hours for instability.

Rationales

1. Because of the sac protrusion, the infant has an increased amount of skin surface area exposed. An Isolette or radiant warmer minimizes heat loss from convection and evaporation from the skin surface.

2. Temperature instability may be a sign of a central dysfunction or an early sign of infection, such as sepsis or meningitis.

Nursing diagnosis: *Altered tissue perfusion: cerebral related to hydrocephalus and increased intracranial pressure (ICP)*

GOAL: The infant will develop no signs of increased ICP.

Interventions

1. Assess the infant's neurologic status every 2 to 4 hours, noting any signs of lethargy, bulging fontanels, pupillary changes, or seizures.

2. Measure the infant's head circumference daily.

3. Assess the infant's anterior fontanel every 4 to 8 hours.

4. Report any swelling around or leakage of clear fluid from the infant's back incision.

5. Assess the infant's respiratory rate and rhythm every 2 to 4 hours for signs of apnea, stridor, or an ineffective or weak sucking reflex.

Rationales

1. Frequent neurologic assessments provide a baseline for identification of early changes signifying the development of hydrocephalus. About 70% to 90% of all infants with meningomyelocele develop hydrocephalus either in utero or during the neonatal period.

2. Increasing head circumference beyond the normal limits is a sign of developing or progressive hydrocephalus.

3. Normally, the anterior fontanel closes around age 12 to 15 months. Until then, any bulging at the site may indicate increased ICP.

4. Swelling or leakage of fluid may indicate progressive hydrocephalus or surgical infection (or both).

5. Such signs and symptoms indicate Arnold-Chiari syndrome, a malformation of the hindbrain. All infants with meningomyelocele have Arnold-Chiari syndrome; however, only about 10% of these infants become symptomatic. Hydrocephalus aggravates this problem. (See Arnold-Chiari syndrome.)

ARNOLD-CHIARI SYNDROME

Arnold-Chiari syndrome, an elongation or tonguelike downward projection of the cerebellum and medulla through the foramen magnum into the spinal canal, occurs in all infants with the meningomyelocele form of spina bifida. Hydrocephalus often accompanies the defect, resulting from impaired drainage of cerebrospinal fluid.

Besides the signs and symptoms of hydrocephalus, other indications of Arnold-Chiari syndrome include nuchal rigidity, noisy respirations, irritability, vomiting, weak sucking reflex, and hyperextension of the neck.

Treatment requires surgical placement of a shunt like that used in hydrocephalus. Surgical decompression of the cerebellar tonsils at the foramen magnum sometimes is indicated.

Nursing diagnosis: *Altered patterns of urinary elimination related to the level of spinal cord involvement with defect*

GOAL: The infant will develop no signs of urinary tract infection.

Interventions

1. Carefully note frequency and amount of the infant's urine.

2. Monitor and record the infant's fluid intake and output carefully.

3. Maintain or implement intermittent catheterization every 4 hours. Teach the parents how to perform catheterization using clean technique.

4. Perform post-void catheterization.

5. Weigh the infant daily.

6. Encourage increased fluid intake.

7. Observe, report, and record any signs or symptoms of urinary tract infection, including foul-smelling urine, elevated temperature, and cloudy urine

Rationales

1. Neurogenic bladder and sphincter commonly occur in children with meningomyelocele. Function depends on the integrity of the sacral nerve roots. Often, voiding occurs by overflow of urine in the bladder.

2. Such monitoring ensures early detection of inadequate voiding, which can lead to urinary tract infection.

3. Intermittent catheterization ensures complete emptying of the bladder, thereby decreasing the risk of urinary tract infection.

4. Post-void catheterization helps in determining how well the infant is emptying the bladder on his own. Overdistention of the bladder causes ischemia to the bladder wall and weakens its resistance to infection. Also, residual urine provides a medium for bacterial growth in the bladder.

5. Weight changes can reflect hydration status.

6. Increased fluid intake increases renal blood flow and helps flush bacteria from the urinary tract.

7. Children with meningomyelocele are at increased risk for urinary tract infections. Early recognition of signs and symptoms facilitates early treatment.

Nursing diagnosis: *Altered bowel elimination: constipation related to level of spinal cord involvement with defect*

GOAL: The infant will maintain normal, regular bowel movements as evidenced by no sign of constipation.

Interventions

1. Observe, report, and record characteristics of the infant's anal opening and stool pattern.

2. Assess for abdominal distention, vomiting, and difficulty feeding.

3. Feed the infant a formula containing corn oil.

Rationales

1. Anal sphincter assessments may reveal the presence of the anal reflex, anal "wink," indicating abnormal bowel function. Assessment of the infant's stooling pattern ensures early recognition of constipation and lack of sphincter control.

2. These may be indications of constipation.

3. Corn oil facilitates the passage of regular bowel movements.

Nursing diagnosis: *Potential for impaired skin integrity (perineal region) related to altered pattern of elimination*

GOAL: The infant will develop no signs of skin breakdown or excoriation in the perineal region.

Interventions	Rationales
1. Clean the infant's perineum as soon as possible after each soiling; then pat, not rub, the area dry.	1. Cleansing the perineum helps prevent irritation from urine and feces. Patting the area dry is recommended, as rubbing may cause further irritation.
2. Apply an appropriate ointment or cream, such as A & D Ointment or Sween Cream, around the perineal region.	2. Ointments and creams serve as a protective barrier to the skin.
3. Leave excoriated areas open to air as much as possible.	3. This keeps the area dry and promotes healing.

Nursing diagnosis: *Potential for impaired skin integrity related to altered mobility*

GOAL: The infant will develop no signs of pressure sores, contractures, or hip dislocation.

Interventions	Rationales
1. Place the infant on a sheepskin surface, waterbed pad, or eggcrate mattress.	1. Placing the infant on one of these surfaces helps prevent pressure sores.
2. Keep bed linens clean and dry at all times. Place a soft nonirritating pad or cloth under the infant's face.	2. Clean, dry linens and a soft, nonirritating pad help minimize irritation to the infant's skin.
3. Change the infant's position at least every 2 hours.	3. Immobilization or maintaining the same position for prolonged periods can lead to skin breakdown.
4. Massage the infant's pressure points with lotion every 2 hours.	4. Massage increases blood flow to tissues, thereby preventing skin breakdown.
5. Lift the infant by the buttocks rather than the feet when changing diapers after the acute postoperative period.	5. Lifting the infant in this manner helps prevent hip dislocation.
6. Use sandbags or small blanket rolls to provide appropriate alignment of extremities when positioning the infant.	6. Because of the defect and level of spinal cord involvement, the infant may have contractures, which impair muscle movement and proper body alignment. Proper positioning helps maintain alignment to prevent further deterioration of contractures.
7. Perform range-of-motion (ROM) exercises on the infant's legs and arms as instructed by the physical therapist.	7. ROM exercises help prevent contractures and stretches those which the infant already has. The physical therapist works with the doctor to carefully evaluate alignment, movement, and integrity of the infant's extremities, joints, and muscle groups. Based on this evaluation, an individualized exercise plan is created. Because of potential injury to the infant, the nurse should never independently initiate ROM exercises without first consulting the physical therapist.
8. Assess for altered sensation by pricking the skin on the infant's arms and legs with a pin every 2 hours. Use a clean pin and be careful not to scratch or puncture the skin.	8. Because response to stimuli often parallels the level of motor functioning, testing for altered sensation should indicate the infant's neuromuscular status. Altered sensation places the child at risk for skin breakdown because of his inability to detect pain.

Interventions	**Rationales**
9. Protect the infant from exposure to excessive heat or cold.	9. Because of the defect, the infant may be unable to sense extremes in temperature, possibly resulting in skin damage.
10. Assess for signs of swelling, erythema, or skin breakdown.	10. Early recognition and treatment help prevent the development pressure sores and infection.

Nursing diagnosis: *Altered nutrition: less than body requirements related to surgery*

GOAL: The infant will receive adequate nutrition intake to meet caloric requirements as evidenced by weight gain.

Interventions	**Rationales**
1. Maintain the infant on an I.V. dextrose solution during the preoperative and early postoperative phase.	1. Maintaining the infant on an I.V. infusion ensures that he receives adequate nutrition during periods when he cannot receive anything by mouth.
2. Advance the infant to formula within 24 to 48 hours after surgery, by either bottle-feeding or gavage.	2. As long as infant has no respiratory difficulties, he should be able to tolerate formula within 24 to 48 hours after surgery, thereby ensuring adequate nutritional intake.
3. If the infant must be maintained in a prone position postoperatively, turn his head and elevate his chin slightly to feed him with a bottle.	3. This position ensures adequate nutritional intake and promotes his use of the sucking reflex.
4. Assess the infant's sucking capabilities.	4. Poor sucking reflexes may be related to increased intracranial pressure.
5. If the infant is to be breast-fed, take the following measures: • If the mother is available for breast-feeding, position the infant on the mother's lap on at least two pillows.	5. In most cases, an infant with meningomyelocele may be breast-fed despite his medical condition. • Positioning the infant in this manner minimizes pressure on the back incision and brings the baby's head to the level of the breast, thus facilitating improved intake.
• If the mother is unavailable for feedings, make sure that breast milk is stored properly in the refrigerator or freezer. Instruct the parents on pumping methods and transportation of milk.	• Proper storing and transportation of breast milk is essential to preserving the milk's nutritional value.

Nursing diagnosis: *Altered parenting related to separation from the infant and hospitalization at birth*

GOAL: The parents will establish patterns of attachment before discharge as evidenced by stroking, touching, and talking to the infant and by taking over some of the routine caregiving activities.

Interventions	**Rationales**
1. Explain to the parents the nature of the defect and what they may expect during the hospitalization, using diagrams and written information as appropriate.	1. The parents need a basic understanding during the initial hospitalization to facilitate their progress through the stages of grieving and to establish a foundation for home care instruction.
2. Help the father or significant other to schedule his activities to allow for more time to spend with the infant and mother.	2. In most cases, the father or significant other is the nurse's first contact while the mother is recovering from recent delivery. Helping him to schedule activities helps promote parental bonding.

Interventions

3. Model attachment behaviors for the parents by moving from simple to complex tasks, such as touching and stroking the infant to performing such caregiving tasks as changing diapers, bathing, and clothing the infant.

4. Teach home care instructions after the parents begin demonstrating attachment behaviors.

Rationales

3. Parents normally begin the attachment process through touching, stroking, and talking to the infant immediately after birth. This often is disrupted because of the urgency of the situation at the time of delivery. Therefore, the nurse may need to serve as a role model to demonstrate to parents that touching and stroking are desirable behaviors that will not hurt the infant. Helping parents progress to more complex caregiving tasks reinforces parental-infant bonds.

4. Home care instructions are better retained after parents successfully progress through the grieving process and begin demonstrating attachment behaviors.

Nursing diagnosis: *Altered growth and development related to hospitalization*

GOAL: The infant will develop at an appropriate rate despite the hospitalization.

Interventions

1. Provide the infant with auditory, tactile, and sensory stimulation (such as touching, stroking, and talking with the infant; hanging a black and white mobile over the crib; playing soft music or a recording of the mother's voice; and changing the infant's position) during nursing care procedures.

2. Provide a referral to an appropriate developmental program after the infant is discharged from the hospital.

3. Instruct the parents on normal infant development and the importance of infant stimulation.

Rationales

1. Such stimulation enhances the infant's physical, emotional, and mental development.

2. Infants with meningomyelocele and hydrocephalus are at risk for developmental delay.

3. Knowing the stages of normal infant development helps parents to provide the infant with appropriate developmental activities, thereby maximizing potential intellectual achievemnt.

Nursing diagnosis: *Knowledge deficit related to home care*

GOAL: The parents will verbalize an understanding of the infant's condition, treatment, follow-up appointments, and home care instructions.

Interventions

1. Assess the parents' stage in the grieving process and their understanding of the infant's defect and treatment.

2. Provide several short teaching sessions on the following topics, allowing the parents to practice necessary caregiving skills:
• catheterization
• feeding
• medication administration
• skin care
• recognizing the signs and symptoms of increased intracranial pressure.

3. Provide appropriate education materials on caregiving skills, including booklets, videotapes, and diagrams.

Rationales

1. Such an assessment helps determine the parents' readiness to learn complex caregiving tasks.

2. Short teaching sessions facilitate comprehension by focusing the parents' attention for limited periods of time. Allowing the parents to practice necessary skills reinforces their understanding of what was learned during the teaching sessions.

3. These materials allow the parents to review at their own convenience what was discussed in the teaching sessions and offer other perspectives on caregiving skills.

Interventions

4. Help the parents to organize community service assistance for the infant's follow-up after discharge from the hospital. Areas of special concern may include:
• support groups, such as a spina bifida association or parent support group
• babysitting for other children
• financial assistance
• home health care
• durable medical equipment
• occupational and physical therapy.

Rationales

4. Comprehensive follow-up will be necessary throughout the infant's life. By age 10, the child will have had an average of 11 other surgeries, causing a financial and emotional drain on the family unit.

Documentation checklist

During the hospitalization, be sure to document the following:
___ the child's status and assessment findings upon admission
___ any changes in the child's status
___ pertinent laboratory and diagnostic findings
___ fluid intake and output
___ nutritional intake
___ the child's preoperative and postoperative status
___ the child's neurologic status
___ the child's response to treatment
___ the parents' reaction to the illness and hospitalization
___ growth and development status
___ patient and family teaching guidelines
___ discharge planning guidelines.

Spinal Cord Injury

Introduction

Spinal cord injury—damage that occurs to any level of the spinal cord—can be classified according to one of three major categories: traumatic injuries, tumors, or congenital defects (most common). Such injuries impair nerve impulse transmission, leading to varying degrees of dysfunction depending on the cause, the degree of transection (complete or incomplete), the location of the lesion (lower or upper motor neuron), and the level of spinal cord injury (C1 to S4). Generally, the higher the level of spinal cord damage, the more extreme the damage.

Treatment includes preventing further trauma to the spinal cord by use of stabilization or traction. Other measures include corticosteroid administration to help decrease edema and surgery, if necessary.

This care plan focuses on the acute phase of the illness and does not fully address the rehabilitative process.

Assessment

The following assessment findings indicate spinal cord injury, depending on the specific type of injury involved:

Neurologic
• absent voluntary motor activity
• absence of asymmetry in sensory evaluation
• areflexia

Respiratory
• dyspnea
• ineffective cough

Cardiovascular
• bradycardia
• hypotension

Musculoskeletal
• stiff neck
• muscle spasms

Integumentary
• warm, dry skin

Nursing diagnosis: *Impaired gas exchange related to loss of use of the phrenic nerve, intercostal muscles, or abdominal muscles secondary to the spinal injury*

GOAL: The child will exhibit adequate ventilatory effort as evidenced by good air exchange and normal respiratory rate and arterial blood gas (ABG) levels.

Interventions

1. Assess the child's respiratory status every 1 to 2 hours for breath sounds, chest expansion, respiratory rate, tidal volume (if on a ventilator), and use of accessory muscles.

2. Assess the child's ability to cough every 1 to 2 hours.

Rationales

1. Although deterioration in respiratory function is expected, it may not develop for several days depending on the amount of edema to the cord. Injuries above C4 are associated with partial or complete inability to breathe from loss of use of the phrenic nerve. The loss of use of intercostal muscles in low cervical or high thoracic injuries may result in the inability to breathe deeply.

2. An ineffective cough increases the risk for aspiration, infection, and atelectasis, possibly leading to respiratory failure.

Interventions	**Rationales**
3. Encourage the child to breathe deeply every 2 hours.	3. Deep breathing helps to maintain rib cage flexibility.
4. Provide gentle tracheal suctioning if the child's cough is ineffective.	4. Suctioning helps to keep the airway clear.
5. Reposition the child every 2 hours.	5. Changing position prevents the pooling of secretions.
6. Maintain ABG levels within normal ranges by adjusting oxygen flow rates or ventilator settings.	6. Hypoxia may contribute to further degeneration of the cord injury.
7. Administer bronchodilators or mucolytic agents, as ordered.	7. Bronchodilators and mucolytic agents help increase the diameter of the bronchioles, which facilitates breathing.
8. Monitor the child's temperature every 2 hours until stable.	8. Because of the interruption of the sympathetic pathways to the hypothalamus, the child may become poikilothermic, exhibiting fluctuations in body temperature based on environment temperatures. (For each increase of 1.8° F. [1° C.], the brain demands about 7% more oxygen to meet metabolic demands.)

Nursing diagnosis: *Altered cardiac output related to autonomic dysfunction and immobility*

GOAL: The child will maintain adequate cardiac output as evidenced by a normal heart rate and blood pressure.

Interventions	**Rationales**
1. Monitor the child's heart rate, blood pressure, skin color and temperature, and capillary refill time hourly until stable.	1. Bradycardia, hypotension, and warm, dry skin are classic signs of spinal shock as a result of the loss of sympathetic control. The higher the lesion to the spinal cord, the more severe the spinal shock will be.
2. Assess for the following signs and symptoms of hemorrhage from associated trauma (keeping in mind, however, that internal hemorrhage may not be detectable): • weak, rapid, thready pulse • tachypnea • pallor • tachycardia	2. Such changes in vital signs result from changes in circulatory status brought on by hemorrhage.
3. Apply antiembolism stockings or elastic bandages from the child's toes to his groin.	3. Massive vasodilatation may occur below the injury, causing pooling of venous blood in the child's abdomen, legs, and feet.
4. Monitor the child's central venous and arterial pressures if invasive lines are in place.	4. Such monitoring helps detect fluid overload, which may lead to pulmonary edema and respiratory failure.
5. Administer vasopressor agents, as ordered.	5. Low-dose vasopressors may be used to maintain adequate cerebral and renal perfusion.
6. Avoid moving the child or tilting (elevating the head of the bed) him while he has spinal shock.	6. Position changes may precipitate hypotensive episodes because of loss of compensatory mechanisms with autonomic dysfunction.
7. Assess the child's extremities every 8 hours for signs and symptoms of venous thrombosis, including Homans' sign, redness in the calf or thigh, and warmth.	7. Venous stasis or thrombosis may result from decreased blood flow and flaccid paralysis.

Nursing diagnosis: *Impaired physical mobility related to medical treatment or spinal cord injury*

GOAL: The child will exhibit no further injury related to impaired mobility as evidenced by good skin integrity, muscle tone, and joint mobility.

Interventions

1. Maintain spinal alignment, as ordered, using cervical traction, a special bed, or hyperextension of the child's regular bed.

2. Reposition the child every 2 hours, and evaluate pressure points. During the acute stage, carefully position the extremities as follows:
• arms and legs extended and slightly abducted
• ankles dorsiflexed (may use high-top sneakers)
• wrist extended with metaphalangeal joints flexed about 60 to 70 degrees and interphalangeal joints flexed 35 degrees.

3. Provide passive range-of-motion exercises every 4 hours.

4. Maintain traction devices, as ordered, following the manufacturer's recommendations.

5. Assess the child for presence or absence of voluntary motor activity in each major muscle group during each shift.

6. Assess the child's sensory level, noting deficits and lack of symmetry. Use a clean pin for pin prick, being careful not to scratch or puncture the skin. Record the sensory level by describing its location in reference to anatomic landmarks.

Rationales

1. Maintaining spinal alignment promotes healing of the lesion and prevents further injury to the spine.

2. Changing position decreases venous pooling (especially over bony prominences), which can lead to skin breakdown. Proper positioning promotes healing without producing flexor spasms or contractures.

3. Range-of-motion exercises help prevent spasms and joint contractures and maintain muscle tone.

4. Improper use of traction devices may increase the risk of improper healing.

5. Such assessment helps determine the extent of spinal cord injury and possible improvement.

6. The sensory examination will provide data to determine the level of the spinal lesion and possible changes in neurologic status.

Nursing diagnosis: *Altered patterns of urinary elimination related to interruption of neural innervation*

GOAL: The child will maintain adequate urine output for his age.

Interventions

1. Monitor the child's urine output hourly during the acute stage. Clamp the urinary catheter periodically, initially for 1 hour, then 2 hours, then gradually increasing the time.

2. After removal of the urinary catheter, assess the child's urinary function. If necessary, assist the child's to empty his bladder by performing Credé's maneuver or by providing intermittent catheterization every 4 to 6 hours, then every 6 to 8 hours.

3. Start the child on a bladder training program focused toward home care. Begin with clamping the catheter for periods of time, then using Credé's maneuver or intermittent catheterization every 4 hours.

Rationales

1. Monitoring urine output helps evaluate fluid balance and renal function. Periodic clamping of the urinary catheter promotes development of micturition reflexes and may prevent contractions caused by either an empty bladder or prolonged distention.

2. The child may require assistance to empty the bladder fully after removal of the urinary catheter. Credé's maneuver and intermittent catheterization help prevent bladder distention and urinary tract infection.

3. Bladder training helps improve the bladder's muscle control and tone. Bladder control enables the child to maintain some control over his bodily functions.

Nursing diagnosis: *Potential for infection related to catheterization*

GOAL: The child will remain free of urinary tract infection.

Interventions

1. Monitor urinalysis results and urine culture and sensitivity tests for abnormal values.

2. Provide catheter care every 8 hours.

Rationales

1. Urinalysis and urine culture and sensitivity testing are used to determine the presence of infection and to help identify the causative organism.

2. Routine cleansing around the catheterized area helps decrease the risk of infection.

Nursing diagnosis: *Altered bowel elimination: constipation related to loss of bowel control*

GOAL: The child will have adequate, regular bowel movements as evidenced by lack of diarrhea, constipation, or fecal impaction.

Interventions

1. Inspect the child's abdomen for distention, and insert a nasogastric tube for intermittent suctioning of gastric contents.

2. Monitor the child's fluid intake, and start him on a diet with increased fiber after the ileus clears.

3. Develop a bowel training program that incorporates a digital examination at a routine time, preferably 30 minutes to 1 hour after a designated meal.

4. Administer stool softeners, as ordered.

Rationales

1. During the spinal shock stage, the child's gastrointestinal system becomes atonic, possibly resulting in overdistention that may lead to vomiting and aspiration. Insertion of a nasogastric tube ensures the elimination of gastric contents by suctioning, thereby preventing overdistention and improper bowel elimination.

2. Adequate fluid intake and increased fiber in the diet encourage the ease of bowel elimination.

3. Digital examination encourages the use of the anal sphincter. Scheduling this after a designated meal enables the child to rely on normal bowel peristalsis along with digital stimulation to produce a bowel movement.

4. Stool softeners help to eliminate hard, impacted stools.

Nursing diagnosis: *Altered nutrition: less than body requirements related to acute injury*

GOAL: The child will demonstrate an improved nutritional status as evidenced by minimal weight loss and no sign of skin breakdown.

Interventions

1. Administer I.V. fluids and electrolytes, as ordered, during the initial shock phase.

2. Progress from clear liquids to a normal diet, depending on the child's ability to swallow after the acute phase.

3. Carefully monitor the child's dietary intake. Increase his protein intake to one to two times the normal amount.

Rationales

1. I.V. fluids and electrolytes are necessary to ensure adequate nutrition during the initial shock phase, as paralytic ileus or endotracheal intubation may prohibit oral or nasogastric feedings.

2. Because spinal cord injury sometimes interferes with swallowing during the acute phase, frequent assessments are necessary to determine the child's ability to tolerate a normal diet.

3. Monitoring the child's caloric and protein intake is necessary to maintain proper nitrogen balance, which is necessary for skin healing.

Nursing diagnosis: *Disturbance in self-concept: body image related to physical disability*

GOAL: The child will demonstrate a healthy self-image as evidenced by verbalizing an acceptance of the physical disabilities imposed by his condition.

Interventions	Rationales
1. Encourage the child and parents to express their feelings about the injury.	1. Allowing the child and parents to express feelings helps them to overcome some of the grief brought on by the child's illness and resulting physical disabilities.
2. Provide honest explanations about the child's expected future functioning and possible dependence.	2. Honest explanations help the child and parents to face the reality of the disabilities and allow them to plan for the future.
3. Encourage the child and parents to seek counseling, if appropriate.	3. Individual or family counseling may be necessary to help the child and parents work through the grieving process. Peer discussions may be especially helpful, depending on the child's age.

Nursing diagnosis: *Knowledge deficit related to home care*

GOAL: The parents will verbalize an understanding of home care instructions.

Interventions	Rationales
1. Assess the parents' understanding of the child's condition and prescribed treatment.	1. Such assessment serves as a basis on which to begin teaching.
2. Explain to the parents the necessity and importance of all treatments, procedures, and equipment related to home care.	2. Knowing this information helps lessen the parents' anxiety and emphasizes the importance of complying with the prescribed regimen.
3. Teach the parents the importance of encouraging the child to drink plenty of fluids.	3. Adequate fluids are necessary to dilute the child's urine concentration, to help prevent the buildup of bacteria.
4. Teach the parents the signs and symptoms of urinary tract infection, including cloudy, foul-smelling urine, fever, and burning and urgency upon urination.	4. Early recognition of the signs and symptoms of urinary tract infection help prevent extensive infection caused by urinary stasis or catheterizations.
5. Refer the parents to a physical therapist for ongoing treatment after discharge.	5. Such a referral is necessary because the child will require extensive physical therapy to achieve his maximum level of wellness.

Documentation checklist

During the hospitalization, be sure to document the following:
___ the child's status and assessment findings upon admission
___ any changes in the child's status
___ pertinent laboratory and diagnostic findings
___ fluid intake and output
___ nutritional intake
___ the child's neurologic status
___ the child's response to treatment
___ the child's and parents' reaction to the illness and hospitalization
___ patient and family teaching guidelines
___ discharge planning guidelines.

GASTROINTESTINAL AND HEPATOBILIARY SYSTEMS

Biliary Atresia

Introduction

A congenital defect, biliary atresia is caused by the absence or obstruction of one or more of the extrahepatic or intrahepatic bile ducts, which results in the improper drainage of bile.

Biliary atresia usually is surgically corrected using the Kasai procedure in which the nonfunctioning extrahepatic ducts are removed and a substitute duct (usually the jejunum) is anastomosed to the liver. Liver transplantation, a possible alternative, is sometimes successful in correcting the atresia; however, it is associated with several complications, including the risk of hemorrhage, organ rejection, and possible death.

Assessment

Gastrointestinal
• clay-colored stools
• distended abdomen with hepatomegaly

• feeding problems (such as slowness in feeding, occasional disinterest in feeding)

Genitourinary
• dark-colored urine

Musculoskeletal
• lethargy

EENT
• scleral jaundice at age 2 to 3 weeks

Hematologic
• bleeding tendencies

Integumentary
• jaundice

Nursing diagnosis: *Fluid volume deficit related to poor absorption of nutrients*

GOAL: The infant will maintain fluid and electrolyte balance as evidenced by a capillary refill time of 3 to 5 seconds, good skin turgor, adequate urine output (1 to 2 ml/kg/hour), and no sign of lethargy, dysrhythmias, or tachycardia.

Interventions

1. Monitor the infant's intake and output hourly. When measuring intake, be sure to note I.V. fluids, total parenteral nutrition, and any nasogastric or oral feedings. When measuring output, weigh diapers for urine and stool content. If input exceeds output, administer increased fluids, as ordered.

2. Weigh the infant at the same time each day, using the same scale to obtain accurate measurements.

3. Check the pH level of the infant's stools with Tes-Tape.

4. Measure the infant's abdominal girth, as ordered, using a consistent point of reference for accurate measurements.

5. Observe for clinical signs of dehydration (oliguria, dry skin, poor skin turgor, and sunken fontanels and eyes) or overhydration (bulging fontanels, decreased urine specific gravity, and possible signs of congestive heart failure including tachycardia and crackles).

6. Monitor the infant's total peripheral resistance and blood pressure, as ordered.

Rationales

1. Such monitoring provides objective data to evaluate the infant's fluid balance and the need for further intervention.

2. Daily weight is used to assess the infant's fluid balance.

3. Knowing the pH level of stools helps in determining the infant's nutritional absorption of fat and carbohydrates.

4. Measuring the abdominal girth helps in detecting ascites, the effusion and accumulation of serous fluid in the abdominal cavity.

5. Signs of dehydration or overhydration should alert the nurse to the need for prompt and appropriate intervention to correct the child's fluid deficit or excess.

6. Monitoring the total peripheral resistance and blood pressure helps in evaluating fluid and electrolyte balance. Imbalances can be corrected by administering total parenteral nutrition or I.V. fluids or by altering the child's diet. Uncorrected, such imbalances can lead to tachycardia, bradycardia, dysrhythmias, or hypotension.

Interventions

7. Monitor the infant's electrolyte, total protein, albumin, blood urea nitrogen, and creatinine levels as well as the complete blood count (see Appendix B: Normal Vital Sign Measurements). Report any abnormalities immediately to the doctor.

Rationales

7. Such monitoring helps in evaluating fluid and electrolyte balance. Abnormal findings may indicate liver rejection or malfunctioning and should be reported immediately.

Nursing diagnosis: *Altered growth and development related to chronic illness*

GOAL: The infant will develop normally as evidenced by achievement of age-appropriate developmental milestones.

Interventions

1. Institute an infant stimulation program that emphasizes the achievement of gross motor skills. Be sure to include range-of-motion exercises and positioning (sitting the infant upright) in the program. Also provide objects the infant can reach for as well as an open space for crawling.

2. Counsel the parents regarding the infant's developmental achievement as compared to that of other, healthy infants. Encourage them to attend parent support group sessions or to meet with other parents of infants with biliary atresia.

Rationales

1. A planned stimulation program helps to promote the infant's optimal abilities in meeting developmental milestones. It also provides a means for parents to effectively bond with the infant.

2. Parents of chronically ill infants often need special counseling concerning the infant's expected developmental progression. Support groups and discussions with other parents facing similar problems can help alleviate some of the stress and fears associated with the infant's chronic illness and can provide important information on exercises to help stimulate development.

Nursing diagnosis: *Knowledge deficit related to home care*

GOAL: The parents will verbalize an understanding of home care instructions.

Interventions

1. Instruct the parents on the purpose and use of all prescribed medications, including details on administration, dosages, and potential adverse effects.

2. Instruct the parents on the importance of providing the infant with appropriate auditory, visual, and tactile stimulation.

3. Explain the importance of monitoring the infant for nausea and vomiting, muscle cramps, diarrhea, and irregular heart rate. Tell them to report such signs and symptoms immediately to the doctor.

Rationales

1. Parents need to know how and when to give medications so that they can comply with the treatment regimen. Knowing the potential adverse effects should prompt them to seek medical advice and attention, when necessary.

2. Such stimulation is essential to help the infant achieve developmental milestones.

3. These are signs and symptoms of fluid and electrolyte imbalances and possible indications of liver rejection or malfunctioning.

Documentation checklist

During the hospitalization, be sure to document the following:
___ the infant's status and assessment findings upon admission
___ any changes in the infant's status
___ pertinent laboratory and diagnostic findings
___ fluid intake and output
___ nutritional intake
___ growth and development status
___ the infant's response to treatment
___ the parents' reaction to the illness and hospitalization
___ family teaching guidelines
___ discharge planning guidelines.

GASTROINTESTINAL AND HEPATOBILIARY SYSTEMS

Hepatitis

Introduction

Hepatitis, a leading cause of illness and death in childhood, is marked by inflammation of the liver usually resulting from a viral infection. Hepatitis A usually is transmitted by the fecal or oral route; hepatitis B, by a parenteral route.

Usual treatment includes isolation, bed rest, and a high-carbohydrate, low-fat diet. Although the prognosis is generally favorable, hepatitis may lead to potentially serious complications, including permanent liver damage.

Assessment

Gastrointestinal
• gastrointestinal upset (nausea, vomiting, diarrhea)
• anorexia
• light-colored stools
• right upper quadrant pain (more common in hepatitis B)

Hepatic
• enlarged liver

Genitourinary
• dark-colored urine

Musculoskeletal
• lethargy

Integumentary
• elevated temperature
• jaundice with pruritus
• arthralgia and rash (occasionally seen early in course of hepatitis B)
• papular acrodermatitis (seen in young infants with hepatitis B)

Nursing diagnosis: *Potential for fluid volume deficit related to vomiting, diarrhea, and bleeding*

GOAL: The child will maintain adequate fluid volume as evidenced by moist mucous membranes, adequate skin turgor, normal electrolyte levels, normal urine output, and absence of bleeding.

Interventions

1. Weigh the child daily, and carefully monitor his intake and output, including the amount and color of urine and stools. Report any output abnormalities (such as decreased urine output or diarrhea) immediately to the doctor.

2. Assess the child's skin turgor and mucous membranes each shift. Notify the doctor immediately of any significant changes in the child's status.

3. Monitor the child for third-space fluid shifting by:
• measuring the abdominal girth at the largest area daily and as needed
• assessing for orthostatic hypotension every 4 hours
• assessing for changes in heart rate every 4 hours.

4. Monitor the child for decreased sodium levels (<138 mEq/liter), decreased potassium levels (<3.4 mEq/liter), and increased albumin levels. Report any abnormalities immediately to the doctor.

5. Monitor the child for signs and symptoms of bleeding, including bloody stools, bleeding from venipuncture sites, hematuria, and ecchymoses.

Rationales

1. Daily monitoring of weight and intake and output are direct measurements of the child's current hydration status. Children with hepatitis often have dark-colored urine from the passage of bilirubin and urobilinogen, and light-colored stools from the lack of pigment. Decreased urine output may indicate renal problems; diarrhea can lead to dehydration.

2. Poor skin turgor and dry mucous membranes indicate dehydration for which the doctor might order increased fluid intake.

3. Third-space fluid shifting reflects impaired liver function. This shifting results from edema caused by decreased albumin levels in plasma, which causes an increased flow of water from the capillaries to intracellular compartments.

4. Abnormal electrolyte and albumin levels indicate fluid imbalances that require prompt treatment.

5. Because of liver disease associated with hepatitis, the child's prothrombin time will be elevated, placing him at risk for increased bleeding. Bleeding can lead to decreased circulatory volume and fluid imbalances.

Interventions	Rationales
6. Maintain a patent I.V. access.	6. Because of anorexia and vomiting, the child may require rehydration with I.V. fluids to maintain fluid balance.

Nursing diagnosis: *Altered comfort: pain related to inflammation of the liver*

GOAL: The child will demonstrate increased comfort as evidenced by vital signs within the normal limits for his age, verbalization of decreased pain and itching, and relaxed body movements.

Interventions	Rationales
1. Administer antipyretics, analgesics, and antihistamines, as ordered.	1. Analgesics may be ordered to relieve pain. Antihistamines inhibit the action of histamines on body tissues, thereby reducing pruritus. Antipyretics help reduce fever.
2. Monitor the child's vital signs every 4 hours, as needed.	2. Changes in vital signs can indicate the child's current comfort level. For example, increased blood pressure, heart rate, and respiratory rate may signify increased discomfort.
3. Encourage the use of distraction (such as toys, games, television, and books) to help decrease the child's pain. However, keep in mind that children with hepatitis should not share objects, such as toys, because of the risk of spreading infection.	3. Distraction helps to decrease pain and discomfort by allowing the child to focus his attention and concentration on objects and activities rather than on his immediate pain.
4. Encourage the child to take frequent rest periods and naps.	4. Frequent resting and napping are important because fatigue can reduce the child's tolerance to pain.
5. If the child has a fever, give sponge baths with tepid water to reduce his temperature.	5. Using tepid water can help decrease the child's temperature by allowing increased evaporation of heat without causing chilling and shivering.
6. Administer cool, medicated baths (such as oatmeal, baking soda, or cornstarch baths), as desired, to decrease pruritus.	6. Cool compresses and vasoconstriction effectively decrease pruritus. Medicated baths also have been found useful in decreasing pruritus in some children.
7. Each shift, assess and document the child's pain and itching along with his response to supportive measures.	7. Such documentation provides data for assessing the effectiveness of nursing interventions.

Nursing diagnosis: *Altered nutrition: less than body requirements related to gastrointestinal disturbances (anorexia, diarrhea, nausea, or vomiting)*

GOAL: The child will have improved nutritional intake as evidenced by stable weight and adequate caloric intake as monitored by a dietitian.

Interventions	Rationales
1. Weigh the child daily, and carefully monitor his intake and output.	1. Daily weight and monitoring of intake and output are necessary to help determine the child's current nutritional status.
2. Consult the hospital dietitian regarding the child's dietary requirements.	2. Because of anorexia, the child requires careful dietary planning to ensure that he receives adequate nutrition.

Interventions	**Rationales**
3. Serve the child small, frequent meals that are high in carbohydrates. Make sure that the largest meal is served early in the day.	3. Serving small, frequent meals helps ensure that the child eats most of each meal. A high-carbohydrate diet is thought to protect liver cells. Serving the largest meal in the early part of the day is recommended because, at this time, children usually are hungry and less tired.
4. Administer vitamins, as ordered.	4. Vitamin supplements help replenish nutrients that are diminished as a result of liver disease. Increasing the child's nutritional state helps the damaged liver to heal.

Nursing diagnosis: *Potential for activity intolerance related to increased fatigue and bed rest*

GOAL: The child's activity level will return to normal, prehospital levels without recurrence of illness.

Interventions	**Rationales**
1. Encourage the child to remain in bed during the acute phase of the illness.	1. Bed rest helps to decrease work load on the liver and thereby prevent liver damage.
2. Provide a quiet environment by decreasing the number of visitors and unnecessary interruptions by hospital staff.	2. Decreasing stimuli helps to promote rest and enhance healing.
3. After the acute phase, encourage the child to slowly increase his activities, as tolerated.	3. Increasing activity, as tolerated, helps to prevent long-term bed rest complications (such as muscle weakness, contractures, and bed sores) and assists in recovery.
4. Monitor the child's vital signs and transaminase levels (serum glutamic-oxaloacetic transaminase, serum glutamic-pyruvic transaminase).	4. Changes in vital signs can indicate changes in activity tolerance. For example, increased heart and respiratory rates along with signs of respiratory distress indicate that the child's activity levels need to be limited. Monitoring transaminase levels is important because rapidly increased activity may increase enzyme levels, thereby causing recurrence of the illness.

Nursing diagnosis: *Potential for impaired skin integrity related to pruritus, frequent diarrhea, and prolonged bed rest*

GOAL: The child will maintain skin integrity as evidenced by no signs of increased redness, irritation, or abrasions.

Interventions	**Rationales**
1. Keep the child's skin clean and dry at all times.	1. Keeping the skin clean and dry is important because moisture or debris can lead to skin breakdown.
2. Assess the child's skin each shift for signs and symptoms of breakdown, including redness, chapping, and tenderness. If the child has any evidence of skin breakdown, change his position every 2 hours and use padding or an eggcrate mattress for extra support.	2. Frequent assessments ensure the early detection and prompt treatment of skin breakdown.
3. Administer cool, medicated baths (such as oatmeal, baking soda, or cornstarch baths) and antihistamines, as ordered, to help decrease pruritus.	3. Cool compresses and vasoconstriction effectively decrease pruritus, thereby decreasing the risk of skin breakdown from itching. Antihistamines are used to reduce histamine-induced pruritus.
4. Keep the child's fingernails clean and short.	4. Clean, short fingernails help prevent skin damage and infection from scratching.

Nursing diagnosis: *Potential for infection related to spread of hepatitis virus through contact with visitors and staff*

GOAL: Visitors and staff will remain free of infection as evidenced by maintaining strict isolation procedures.

Interventions

1. Instruct all visitors and staff to use good hand-washing technique (involves thoroughly scrubbing the hands with an antimicrobial soap).

2. Maintain strict blood and body fluid isolation procedures by:
• using liners for trash receptacles, according to hospital protocol
• wearing, then disposing of gloves, as indicated, when touching soiled materials or obtaining blood samples
• disposing of needles in appropriate containers after use
• wearing, then disposing of gloves when measuring or obtaining body fluids, such as urine or stool samples
• using disposable dishes and utensils.

Rationales

1. Good hand-washing technique is necessary to help reduce the risk of spreading infection.

2. Strict blood and body fluid isolation procedures are necessary to ensure the containment of any potentially contaminated specimens, needles, or containers to prevent the risk of cross-contamination and spread of infection.

Nursing diagnosis: *Impaired social interaction related to isolation status (if the child has hepatitis B)*

GOAL: The child will maintain social interaction with parents and significant others despite being placed in isolation.

Interventions

1. Explain to the child and parents the purpose of instituting isolation precautions in cases of hepatitis B (usual protocol includes the wearing of gowns and gloves when in contact with infected blood or body fluids).

2. Encourage the child to maintain contact with his parents and significant others, even if by phone.

3. Encourage the child to express his feelings regarding changes in life-style and body perceptions resulting from isolation.

4. Encourage the parents to participate in the child's care.

5. Offer the child toys, games, books, television, and other age-appropriate materials (such as newspapers and magazines) to divert his attention from illness and isolation.

Rationales

1. Such explanations should increase compliance with the isolation regimen and decrease the child's anxiety about being alone.

2. Continual contact helps to decrease feelings of isolation.

3. Allowing the child to ventilate feelings helps in assessing the child's understanding of his isolation status and encourages him to verbalize any problems he may have concerning lack of social interaction.

4. Parental involvement in the child's care helps preserve some semblance of family unity and enables the child to interact socially with others.

5. Diversional activities help decrease the trauma of isolation. Newspapers and magazines allow the child to keep current on timely events, thereby lessening his feelings of social isolation.

Nursing diagnosis: *Knowledge deficit related to home care, disease process, and prevention of recurrence of hepatitis*

GOAL: The child and parents will verbalize an understanding of home care instructions, disease process, and instructions for preventing the recurrence of hepatitis.

Interventions

1. Assess the child's and parents' understanding of hepatitis, including its signs and symptoms (epigastric pain, pruritus, and jaundice) and the usual route of transmission (fecal or oral route).

2. Instruct the child and parents on appropriate hygiene for preventing the spread of infection, including:
• washing hands after toileting and before eating
• cleaning eating utensils with hot water and detergent
• keeping the child's toothbrush, eating utensils, cups, and other personal items separate from those of other family members.

3. Involve the hospital dietitian in teaching sessions on food preparation and storage if improper storage or preparation is found to be the source of contamination.

4. If appropriate, emphasize the importance of the child's avoiding alcoholic beverages while recuperating from hepatitis.

5. Instruct the parents to contact the doctor regarding the use of such over-the-counter medications as acetaminophen, cold preparations, and aspirin.

6. Instruct the parents to monitor the child's activity level for signs and symptoms of the illness' recurrence, including jaundice, pruritus, and epigastric pain.

7. Instruct family members and the child's sexual contacts (if appropriate) exposed to the virus to contact their doctor for evaluation and instruction on preventive measures.

8. Instruct the child and parents on the importance of keeping follow-up appointments.

Rationales

1. Such assessment provides a basis on which to begin teaching.

2. Maintaining proper hygiene practices helps prevent the spread of virus.

3. The dietitian can provide detailed information on proper storage and preparation techniques to ensure that the virus is not transmitted through food.

4. Because alcohol has a direct toxic effect on the liver, consumption of alcoholic beverages might impair the liver's healing process during the recuperative phase.

5. Many over-the-counter medications are metabolized by the liver and may cause further hepatic damage.

6. Rapid increases in activity level may induce a relapse or recurrence of illness.

7. Such evaluation and instruction helps prevent transmission of the disease.

8. Follow-up is necessary to evaluate the clinical progress of the disease and to prevent permanent liver damage.

Documentation checklist

During the hospitalization, be sure to document the following:
___ the child's status and assessment findings upon admission
___ any changes in the child's status
___ pertinent laboratory and diagnostic findings
___ nutritional intake
___ growth and development status
___ the child's response to treatment
___ the child's and parents' reaction to the illness and hospitalization
___ patient and family teaching guidelines
___ discharge planning guidelines.

GASTROINTESTINAL AND HEPATOBILIARY SYSTEMS

Hirschsprung's Disease

Introduction

Hirschsprung's disease, also known as aganglionic megacolon, is a congenital disease marked by the absence of parasympathetic ganglion cells in a portion of the colon (and occasionally the ileum). This aganglionosis results in lack of peristalsis in the affected bowel, which usually leads to obstruction and difficulty or inability to pass stool.

Hirschsprung's disease, which occurs more commonly in males, usually is diagnosed in infancy although occasionally the diagnosis is made later in life. Treatment usually includes a temporary colostomy or ileostomy proximal to the affected bowel until the corrective surgery is performed. Surgery may include resection of the affected bowel and closure of the colostomy or ileostomy.

Potential complications of this disease include bowel obstruction and dehydration. The prognosis depends on the extent of aganglionosis.

Assessment
NEONATES
Gastrointestinal
• abdominal distention
• bilious vomitus
• no passage of meconium during the first 48 hours of life, especially if followed by diarrhea
• lack of interest in feedings

Integumentary
• unexplained fever

OLDER CHILDREN
Gastrointestinal
• constipation
• vomiting
• abdominal distention
• signs of malnutrition (weight loss, physical underdevelopment)
• ribbonlike stools

Nursing diagnosis: *Altered bowel elimination: constipation related to aganglionosis*

GOAL: The child will have normal, regular bowel movements as evidenced by decreased abdominal distention, decreased discomfort, and clear return of enemas or rectal irrigations.

Interventions
1. Administer enemas or rectal irrigations, as ordered.

2. Assess the child's bowel sounds and abdomen every 4 hours. Report decreased or absent bowel sounds immediately to the doctor.

Rationales
1. Bowel evacuation increases the child's comfort level and decreases the risk of bowel perforation from obstruction.

2. Such assessment is necessary to ensure proper bowel functioning and appropriate treatment when necessary.

Nursing diagnosis: *Potential for fluid volume deficit related to decreased intake, nausea, vomiting, diarrhea, or increased absorptive surface of distended bowel*

GOAL: The child will maintain fluid balance within normal limits as evidenced by normal urine output, brisk capillary refill time, good skin turgor, and moist mucous membranes.

Interventions
1. Weigh the child daily, and carefully monitor his fluid intake and output.

Rationales
1. Daily weights and careful monitoring of intake and output are indicative of the child's current fluid status.

Interventions	**Rationales**
2. Administer I.V. fluids, as ordered.	2. I.V. fluids may be necessary if the child becomes dehydrated or is at risk for dehydration.
3. Use saline or antibiotic solutions rather than tap water when administering enemas or rectal irrigations.	3. Tap water should be avoided because water intoxication can result from the increased absorptive surface associated with bowel distention.

Nursing diagnosis: *Anxiety (parent) related to lack of knowledge about the disease process and prescribed treatment*

GOAL: The parents will be less anxious as evidenced by verbalizing an understanding of the disease process and prescribed treatment.

Interventions	**Rationales**
1. Explain to the parents, in simple terms, the anatomy and physiology of the normal gastrointestinal tract and the disease process involved in the child's illness. Supplement your explanation with written information and diagrams or illustrations (if available).	1. Understanding the normal functioning of the gastrointestinal system helps the parents to understand the seriousness of the child's condition and the need for treatment. Increased awareness of the situation should help to ease parental anxiety.
2. Provide the parents with an outlined plan for scheduled diagnostic studies.	2. Knowledge of scheduled events should help decrease the parents' anxieties and fears.
3. Provide the parents with preoperative and postoperative information regarding interventions for colostomy or ileostomy surgery. Provide details on dressings, the appearance and function of the colostomy, ambulation, I.V. fluids, postoperative breathing exercises, and pain control.	3. Such information helps decrease parental anxiety and allows for increased parental involvement in health plan objectives.
4. Explain to the parents the expected activities and events during the postoperative period (such as the need for I.V. fluids, nothing-by-mouth status, laboratory tests, X-rays, administration of pain medications, dressing changes, and nasogastric suctioning). Use visual aids, such as sample equipment, if available.	4. Explaining the expected postoperative events helps alleviate the parents' anxiety by preparing them beforehand for their child's condition after surgery. Such explanations also reinforce the importance of surgical intervention and the need for parental cooperation and involvement in postoperative care.

Nursing diagnosis: *Impaired skin integrity related to exposure to stool secondary to colostomy or ileostomy*

GOAL: The child will have no sign of skin breakdown as evidenced by intact skin around the colostomy or ileostomy site.

Interventions	**Rationales**
1. Use a wire-fitted ostomy bag with an effective skin barrier (Hollihesive, Stomahesive, Comfed) to protect the skin from coming in contact with stool.	1. A properly fitting appliance and skin barrier protects the periostomal area from the caustic effects of stool. Diapering without a bag usually results in skin breakdown.
2. Change the ostomy bag whenever leaking occurs or is suspected. Check the bag every 2 hours.	2. Leaking causes stool to come in contact with skin, thereby increasing the risk of skin breakdown.
3. Empty the ostomy bag whenever it is one-fourth to one-third full.	3. Allowing the bag to fill up increases the risk of leaking, as the weight of stool can pull the seal away from the skin.

Interventions	Rationales
4. Change the ostomy bag at least once every 24 hours until the periostomal site is healed.	4. Changing the ostomy bag daily allows for frequent monitoring of the periostomal area and ensures prompt treatment in case of improper healing (the periostomal site usually heals within 1 to 3 days).
5. If skin breakdown occurs, administer wound treatment as ordered by the doctor, enterostomal therapist, or ostomy nurse.	5. Depending on the degree of skin breakdown, various treatments (flotation or eggcrate mattress, donut pads, skin preparations, karaya rings) may be required.

Nursing diagnosis: *Potential for infection (postoperative incisional wound) related to contamination from stool*

GOAL: The child's incision will heal normally, without infection, as evidenced by no signs or symptoms of erythema, induration, drainage, or fever.

Interventions	Rationales
1. Change the ostomy bag immediately if leaking occurs or is suspected. This is especially important if the skin barrier or ostomy bag partially or completely covers the incision.	1. Changing the ostomy bag ensures that prolonged contact between the incision and stool, and thus skin breakdown, does not occur.
2. If the incision is covered by an ostomy bag, change the ostomy bag daily until the incision is healed. Note any signs or symptoms of infection, including redness, purulent drainage, or swelling.	2. Changing the ostomy bag daily allows for early detection of contamination and signs of infection, thereby allowing for prompt treatment.

Nursing diagnosis: *Disturbance in self-concept: body image related to colostomy or ileostomy*

GOAL: The child will have an improved self-concept as evidenced by verbalization about the colostomy and ostomy bag and showing interest in self-care.

Interventions	Rationales
1. Promote and encourage such self-care activities as daily hygiene, grooming, feeding, and dressing.	1. Self-care activities enable the child to continue caring about himself and his appearance despite his altered body image, thereby improving his self-esteem.
2. Encourage the child to verbalize his feelings about the colostomy or ileostomy.	2. Such verbalization allows the child to deal with his feelings without fear of rejection and helps to improve his self-image.
3. Refer the child and parents to a local Hirschsprung's disease support group or ostomy support group, as appropriate.	3. Group support can help the child to feel better about himself by introducing him to others in similar situations who have learned to cope with altered body images.

Nursing diagnosis: *Knowledge deficit related to home care*

GOAL: The parents will verbalize an understanding of home care instructions.

Interventions	Rationales
1. Instruct the parents on the importance of feeding the child a high-calorie, high-fiber diet.	1. A high-calorie, high-fiber diet is important to replace lost calories and to prevent constipation.
2. Instruct the parents on how to care for the child's colostomy (see the "Colostomy, Ileostomy" care plan, page 250).	2. The parents need to know how to properly care for the colostomy to ensure healing and to prevent skin breakdown and other potential complications.

Documentation checklist

During the hospitalization, be sure to document the following:

___ the infant's status and assessment findings upon admission

___ any changes in the infant's status

___ pertinent laboratory and diagnostic findings

___ fluid intake and output

___ nutritional intake

___ the child's response to treatment

___ the child's and parents' reaction to the illness and hospitalization

___ patient and family teaching guidelines

___ discharge planning guidelines.

GASTROINTESTINAL AND HEPATOBILIARY SYSTEMS

Inflammatory Bowel Disease

Introduction

Inflammatory bowel disease—a combination of ulcerative colitis and Crohn's disease—is marked by chronic inflammation of the colon. In ulcerative colitis, the mucosa and submucosa of the colon are affected. In Crohn's disease, the entire alimentary tract is involved.

Usual treatment for inflammatory bowel disease includes the administration of a high-protein, high-calorie, low-fat, low-fiber diet and anti-inflammatory medication. Prognosis for this incurable disease is unfavorable. Often, children have lifelong bowel problems and an increased incidence of colon cancer.

Assessment
Gastrointestinal
• abdominal pain and cramping
• weight loss
• abdominal distention
• anorexia
• diarrhea
• steatorrhea
• vomiting
• bloody stools

Musculoskeletal
• fatigue
• arthralgia
• arthritis

Hematologic
• anemia

Nursing diagnosis: Anxiety (child and parent) related to lack of knowledge about the disease process, diagnostic testing, and expected treatment

GOAL: The child and parents will be less anxious as evidenced by verbalizing an understanding of the disease process, diagnostic studies, and expected treatment.

Interventions

1. Explain to the parents and child (as appropriate) the basic anatomy and physiology of the upper and lower GI tracts. Also explain the normal process of food passage through the GI system, paying particular attention to the nutritional aspects and functions of the small and large intestines. Use visual aids, if available, during explanations.

2. Provide the parents and child with an outline of scheduled diagnostic studies, such as an upper GI series with a small-bowel follow-through, a barium enema, an upper and lower endoscopy, and biopsies.

3. Instruct the parents and child about each scheduled diagnostic test, including information on the preparation, length of testing, and postprocedural care.

4. Instruct the parents on the importance of maintaining the child on a high-protein, high-calorie, low-fat, low-fiber diet to promote maximum nutritional adsorption.

5. Explain to the parents and child the purpose, use, correct dosage, and potential adverse effects of anti-inflammatory agents (sulfasalazine, corticosteroids).

Rationales

1. Understanding the normal functioning of the GI system enables the parents and child to better understand the abnormal functioning that occurs in inflammatory bowel disease. Using visual aids helps increase retention of information.

2. Knowing when to anticipate events helps decrease anxiety and fear.

3. Understanding the purpose and procedure of each ordered test helps reduce anxiety and increases the child's cooperation, as well as the parents' support and involvement, in the preparation, actual testing, and postprocedural care.

4. Maintaining the child on such a diet ensures that he receives adequate nutrition during periods of acute illness as well as remission. A diet high in calories and protein and low in fat replaces the nutrients and blood lost through frequent diarrhea and anorexia. A diet low in fiber reduces stress on the bowel, allowing it to heal.

5. Anti-inflammatory agents may be ordered to help reduce inflammation, which allows the bowel to rest. Teaching the parents and child about the medication regimen helps to improve compliance with therapy and with monitoring of potential complications.

Interventions

6. As indicated, provide information about the need for surgery and placement of a colostomy bag. Explain that surgery is necessary to remove the inflamed area and to create a colostomy for normal elimination. Also explain the purpose and appearance of the colostomy as well as details on the use of dressings, I.V. fluids, and pain-control medications.

7. Encourage the child and parents to express their feelings regarding the need for a colostomy. Refer the parents and child, as appropriate, to a local ostomy support group, or arrange for them to meet with other parents and children undergoing the same problem.

8. Encourage the parents and child to ask questions about the disease process, diagnostic tests, or expected treatment during teaching sessions and to write down any further questions as they arise.

Rationales

6. Providing the parents and child with this information helps them to understand and better anticipate the potential course of the disease, thereby lessening their anxiety.

7. Because colostomy often has an effect on body image, the child and parents may have difficulty dealing with their feelings. A support group or meeting with others sharing the same problem may help to reduce anxiety.

8. Asking questions during teaching sessions allows for immediate responses. Writing down questions as they occur ensures that the nurse will clarify pertinent information at a later date.

Nursing diagnosis: *Altered nutrition: less than body requirements related to impaired nutritional adsorption*

GOAL: The child will have improved nutritional intake as evidenced by increased intake and weight gain.

Interventions

1. Maintain the child on a a high-protein, high-calorie, low-fat, low-fiber diet.

2. Administer nutrition through alternate methods (such as a high-protein, high-carbohydrate, high-vitamin liquid diet; short-term peripheral total parenteral nutrition [TPN] for 1 to 2 weeks; or long-term central line TPN therapy) during periods of exacerbation.

3. Monitor the child for changes in stool consistency, melena, abdominal pain, bloating, nausea and vomiting, or fever. Monitor biochemical results (complete blood count and electrolyte, blood urea nitrogen, and glucose levels), reporting any alterations immediately to the doctor.

4. Consult the hospital dietitian when planning the child's meals, and serve the child some of his favorite foods as allowed.

Rationales

1. Extra protein and calories help replace protein and blood lost from the ulcerated bowel and restore calories lost through diarrhea and weight loss. A low-fat, low-fiber diet decreases bowel irritation by controlling the amount of stool that could lead to diarrhea.

2. During acute periods, the child may require additional measures to ensure he is receiving adequate nutrition. An oral liquid diet replaces lost nutrients; short-term TPN replaces lost nutrients while the child's oral intake is restricted. Long-term TPN may be necessary if chronic diarrhea, fluid loss, or nutritional malabsorption occurs.

3. These changes may signal infection, GI disturbance, or electrolyte imbalances related to nutritional imbalances.

4. Consulting the dietitian ensures that the child receives adequately balanced meals. Serving some of the child's favorite foods helps ensure that he eats most of each meal.

Nursing diagnosis: *Disturbance in self-concept: body image related to the disease, medication use, and the need for a colostomy*

GOAL: The child will exhibit a positive body image as evidenced by demonstrating self-care, such as hygiene and personal grooming, and verbalizing an understanding of the need for his colostomy.

Interventions

1. Instruct the child and parents to report adverse effects of corticosteroid therapy, such as acne and rapid weight gain, immediately to the doctor.

2. Prepare the child for the possibility of colectomy surgery and need for a colostomy. Refer the child and parents to a local ostomy support group for ongoing counseling, if appropriate.

3. Encourage the child to participate regularly in an exercise program, sport, or hobby with other children in his age-group. Also encourage active participation in school, church, and community activities.

Rationales

1. Acne and weight gain can be devastating to a child, especially an adolescent. Reporting these adverse effects to the doctor allows for prompt treatment, thereby decreasing their physical and emotional impact.

2. Because the need for a colostomy often has devastating psychological effects, parents and children require education, patience, support, and time to accept the condition. Local ostomy groups offer support and first-hand knowledge on ways to deal with the effects of an altered body image.

3. Promoting such activities helps to distract the child's attention from the disease, thereby decreasing his negative feelings of an altered body image. Interest and participation in activities with other children helps the child to maintain a healthy self-image and life-style.

Nursing diagnosis: *Knowledge deficit related to home care*

GOAL: The parents and child will verbalize an understanding of home care instructions.

Interventions

1. Instruct the parents and child in the purpose and importance of proper colostomy care, including maintaining and cleaning colostomy bags, using irrigation solutions, and maintaining skin care (see the "Colostomy, Ileostomy" care plan, page 250).

2. Explain the importance of maintaining the child on a high-protein, high-calorie, low-fat, and low-fiber diet.

Rationales

1. The parents and child must know how to provide proper care of the colostomy to prevent skin breakdown and infection and to ensure the proper bowel functioning.

2. Extra calories and protein help to supplement those lost through the GI tract. Decreased levels of fat and fiber in the diet help to control the flow of stool that could lead to diarrhea.

Documentation checklist

During the hospitalization, be sure to document the following:
___ the child's status and assessment findings upon admission
___ any changes in the child's status
___ pertinent laboratory and diagnostic findings
___ nutritional intake
___ growth and development status
___ the child's response to treatment
___ the child's and parents' reaction to the illness and hospitalization
___ patient and family teaching guidelines
___ discharge planning guidelines.

GASTROINTESTINAL AND HEPATOBILIARY SYSTEMS
Liver Transplant

Introduction

Liver transplantation involves the surgical replacement of a nonfunctioning liver with a liver donated from a "living" donor (a brain-dead donor sustained by life support), not a cadaver. Typically, this procedure is indicated for children suffering from a congenital defect, such as biliary atresia. Each hospital requires that the surgery candidate meet certain criteria before being accepted for transplantation, including such compatibility factors as organ size and blood and tissue type matching.

Recovery from transplant surgery varies, depending on the number of complications. Potential complications include hemorrhage, infection, organ rejection, and death. The procedure carries a success rate of 50% to 75%.

Assessment

Hepatic
• slight to moderate jaundice

Gastrointestinal
• abdominal distention with large abdominal incision
• malnourishment
• poor weight gain

Respiratory
• coarse bilateral breath sounds
• pink, moist mucous membranes

Cardiovascular
• pink nail beds with a capillary refill time of <3 seconds

Psychosocial
• developmental delays

Nursing diagnosis: *Potential for infection related to incision and immunosuppression*

GOAL: The child will have no sign of infection as evidenced by normal temperature and lack of purulent drainage from the incision.

Interventions

1. Observe good hand-washing technique before caring for the child.

2. Keep the child in a private room.

3. Monitor the child's temperature every 4 hours, every 2 hours when elevated; notify the doctor of any elevation.

4. Monitor the child's vital signs every 4 hours.

5. Assess the incision for redness, edema, and drainage. Report any of these signs immediately to the doctor.

6. Use sterile technique for such invasive procedures as central line care or wound care.

7. Monitor the child's contact with other patients and visitors. Institute reverse isolation precautions, as ordered (see *Reverse isolation*).

Rationales

1. Good hand-washing technique helps prevent the risk of nosocomial infection.

2. Keeping the child in a private room decreases the risk of exposure to other patients with potentially contagious diseases.

3. A temperature of >100.4° F. (38° C.) may indicate infection.

4. Changes in vital signs, such as elevated temperature and increased pulse rate, may indicate early infection.

5. Redness, edema, and purulent drainage are signs of wound infection.

6. Sterile technique decreases the risk of nosocomial infection.

7. Screening other patients and visitors for contagious diseases before they enter the child's room helps prevent infection. Reverse isolation further protects the child because of the required hospital gowns and masks and other safeguards against infection.

Interventions

8. Administer antibiotics, as ordered.

9. Monitor the child's complete blood count daily.

10. Obtain specimens for blood and urine cultures and a chest X-ray if the child's temperature is >100.4° F. (38° C.).

Rationales

8. Antibiotics are given prophylactically to prevent postoperative infection.

9. An increased or decreased white blood cell count indicates infection. Shifts in the differential may also indicate infection.

10. These tests are used to rule out the possibility of infection and to identify the source of fever.

Nursing diagnosis: *Altered tissue perfusion: cardiopulmonary related to blood loss, alterations in the renin-angiotensin system, and recovering liver function*

GOAL: The child will maintain normal tissue perfusion as evidenced by maintaining stable vital signs, a capillary refill time of <3 seconds, and a normal CBC and by having no sign of active bleeding.

Interventions

1. Assess the child's blood pressure every 4 hours. Take corrective measures, as ordered, if the pressure is increased or decreased.

2. Assess the child's capillary refill time, peripheral pulses, and color of skin and mucous membranes every 4 hours.

3. Assess the child for signs of active bleeding, such as bloody vomitus and tarry stools, and for color and volume of drainage output. Notify the doctor immediately of any abnormal findings, and perform a type and cross matching for blood replacement.

4. Administer antihypertensive agents (propranolol, hydralazine) or antihypotensive agents (packed red blood cells, fresh frozen plasma, or platelets), as ordered, depending on the child's blood pressure.

Rationales

1. Decreased blood pressure may indicate active bleeding. Increased blood pressure may result from alterations in the renin-angiotensin system produced by steroid and immunosuppressant therapy.

2. A capillary refill time of >3 seconds, diminished peripheral pulses, and cyanosis indicate poor peripheral perfusion and impending shock.

3. Active bleeding may indicate coagulopathies related to previous liver disease and the grafting recovery period.

4. These agents help to maintain blood pressure and hematologic values within normal limits.

REVERSE ISOLATION

Because immunosuppression increases the child's risk for infection, reverse (protective) isolation often is required postoperatively. Below is a list of general precautionary measures used in many hospitals:

• After locating the child in a private room, explain isolation procedures to him to help ease anxiety and promote cooperation.
• Make sure the room is cleaned and has new or scrupulously clean equipment. Because the child does not have a contagious disease, articles leaving the room require no special precautions after the child is discharged.
• Keep supplies, such as gowns, gloves, masks, caps, and plastic bags, in a clean, enclosed cart or in an anteroom outside the child's room. Also stock linens and head and shoe coverings for the child if he is especially susceptible to infection. Keep additional supplies, such as a thermometer, stethoscope, and blood pressure cuff, in the room to minimize trips in and out and to prevent contaminating the child with equipment used on other patients.
• Keep the door to the room closed. Post reverse isolation cards on the door.

• Put on a clean gown, mask, cap, and gloves each time you enter the child's room.
• Wash your hands with an antiseptic agent before putting on gloves to prevent bacterial growth on gloved skin; wash the gloves with an antiseptic if they become contaminated during procedures or other care; wash your hands after leaving the room.
• Instruct the housekeeping staff to put on gowns, gloves, caps, and masks before entering the room; advise them not to enter the room if they are ill or infected.
• Do not allow visits by anyone known to be infected or ill. Show visitors how to put on gowns, gloves, caps, and masks, and instruct them to remove them only after they leave the room.
• Do not perform invasive procedures, such as urethral catheterization, unless absolutely necessary because of the risk of infection.
• Avoid transporting the child out of the room; if he must be moved, put a gown and mask on him first.

Nursing diagnosis: *Potential for fluid volume deficit related to high-dose steroid therapy and fluid loss*

GOAL: The child will maintain fluid and electrolyte balance as evidenced by normal serum electrolyte levels and normal urine output.

Interventions	Rationales
1. Carefully monitor the child's intake and output, including parenteral intake, oral fluid intake (after the child can tolerate fluids), and urine and drainage output.	1. Accurate monitoring is essential to determine the child's fluid requirements. Decreased urine output may indicate hypovolemia or acute renal failure.
2. Weigh the child daily each morning using the same scale.	2. A weight fluctuation of ± 9 oz (250 g) in a 24-hour period indicates fluid imbalance.
3. Assess for edema, weight gain, hypertension, increased ascites, gallop rhythms, and coarse breath sounds.	3. These signs of hypervolemia indicate the need for immediate treatment, such as decreased fluid intake and diuretic therapy.
4. Monitor the child's serum electrolyte levels.	4. Increased sodium levels indicate hypovolemia (usually treated with fluid volume expanders); decreased sodium levels indicate hypervolemia (usually treated with decreased fluid intake and diuretic therapy).
5. Administer diuretics, as ordered.	5. Diuretics are ordered in cases of hypervolemia to increase the excretion of excess fluids.
6. Maintain the child on a low-sodium diet.	6. This is to prevent high sodium intake, which leads to fluid retention.
7. When preparing I.V. medications, be sure to use the minimum amount of fluid necessary for dilution.	7. Using minimal fluids is especially important in small children and infants to prevent fluid overload.

Nursing diagnosis: *Ineffective breathing pattern related to prolonged general anesthesia and a large abdominal incision*

GOAL: The child will maintain an adequate respiratory status as evidenced by a pinkish skin color, a normal respiratory rate, clear breath sounds, and effective air movement.

Interventions	Rationales
1. Instruct the child or help him to cough, turn, and breathe deeply every 2 hours.	1. Coughing helps clear mucus from the lungs; turning helps loosen secretions; deep breathing facilitates oxygenation.
2. Perform chest physiotherapy every 4 hours (see *Performing chest physiotherapy,* page 4).	2. Chest physiotherapy helps loosens and remove secretions, thereby allowing the child to breathe easier.
3. Suction the child, as needed.	3. Suctioning helps to clear mucus from the airway.
4. Assess for increased respiratory rate, decreased air movements, coarse breath sounds, and changes in the color or consistency of sputum.	4. These signs of respiratory infection usually indicate the need for antibiotic administration.

Nursing diagnosis: *Altered comfort: pain related to surgery*

GOAL: The child will have decreased pain.

Interventions	Rationales
1. Administer pain medication, such as meperidine hydrochloride, as ordered.	1. Meperidine has sedative properties that help to decrease the child's pain.

Interventions	Rationales
2. Change the child's position every 2 hours.	2. Position changes help relieve pressure on bony prominences and prevent stiffness.
3. Provide diversional activities, such as toys, books, television, or games.	3. Such activities help to divert the child's attention from his pain.

Nursing diagnosis: *Altered nutrition: less than body requirements related to chronic illness, initial postoperative nothing-by-mouth status, and anorexia*

GOAL: The child will maintain adequate nutritional status as evidenced by adequate caloric intake and weight gain.

Interventions	Rationales
1. Carefully monitor the child's intake and output.	1. Accurate monitoring of intake and output is necessary to assess the child's caloric requirements.
2. Weigh the child daily.	2. Slow, steady weight gain indicates adequate nutritional intake.
3. When planning the child's meals, consult the hospital dietitian and consider anthropometric findings.	3. Adequate nutrition is necessary for wound healing. Anthropometric findings help to determine the child's current nutritional status and caloric requirements.
4. Administer nasogastric feedings or total parenteral nutrition, as ordered.	4. Supplemental forms of nutrition may be necessary when the child's oral intake does not meet caloric requirements.
5. Serve the child some of his favorite foods, if they are within dietary limits.	5. Offering some of the child's favorite foods helps to ensure that he will eat more of each meal.

Nursing diagnosis: *Anxiety (child and parent) related to extended hospitalization and chronic illness*

GOAL: The child and parents will be less anxious as evidenced by verbalizing their fears and demonstrating a realistic problem-solving approach to coping with those fears.

Interventions	Rationales
1. Assume the role of the primary nurse to establish a trusting relationship with the child and parents.	1. Generally, the primary nurse establishes consistent nursing care and serves as advocate for the patient and family, which helps ease anxiety.
2. Explain all procedures to the child and parents in appropriate terms.	2. Such explanations help to reduce anxiety by preparing the child and parents for upcoming events.
3. Answer all questions honestly, consulting appropriate resources as needed.	3. Answering all questions enhances knowledge and understanding, thereby decreasing anxiety.
4. Allow the child and parents to express their fears and frustrations.	4. Expression of feelings promotes trust and open communication, thereby helping to decrease anxiety.
5. Allow the child and parents to make choices concerning the child's care (such as bathing, feeding, and performing other activities), when possible.	5. This helps to ease anxiety by fostering a sense of control and allowing for active participation in the child's care.
6. Integrate the services of a social worker, child-life worker, and spiritual counselor, as needed, in the child's care.	6. Offering ancillary support helps to ease anxiety during particularly stressful times.

Nursing diagnosis: *Altered growth and development related to chronic illness and long-term hospitalization.*

GOAL: The child will achieve his appropriate developmental level as evidenced by demonstrating age-appropriate developmental tasks.

Interventions

1. Provide the child with age-appropriate toys and activities.

2. Use the Denver Developmental Screening Test (DDST) to assess the child's current developmental level.

3. Develop a daily schedule of all activities and treatments for the staff and family to use.

4. Provide for routine psychological evaluation of the child's coping skills and support systems.

Rationales

1. Providing such toys and activities encourages normal development.

2. The DDST is widely accepted as a measure of a child's current developmental level.

3. A daily schedule provides consistency and improved organization of care.

4. Such evaluation provides information on the child's developmental progress and ability to cope with the illness.

Nursing diagnosis: *Altered parenting related to chronic life-threatening disease*

GOAL: The parents will interact appropriately with the child as evidenced by visiting regularly, talking with the child, and providing support.

Interventions

1. Encourage the parents to visit or stay with child (if permitted).

2. Explain all treatments and procedures to the parents.

3. Encourage the parents to attend support group meetings.

Rationales

1. Regular visits or rooming-in allows for continued parent-child contact.

2. Such explanations help to decrease fear and anxiety, which can lead to stress and alterations in the parent-child relationship.

3. Attending support group meetings allows the parents to interact with other parents of children with chronic illnesses, which encourages improved parenting skills.

Nursing diagnosis: *Knowledge deficit related to home care*

GOAL: The parents will verbalize an understanding of home care instructions.

Interventions

1. Instruct the parents on the following:
• the signs and symptoms of infection, such as elevated temperature and purulent drainage from the incision
• the signs and symptoms of organ rejection, such as elevated temperature, pain at the graft site, swelling and tenderness, jaundice, and decreased hemoglobin and hematocrit levels.

2. Instruct the parents on the purpose and use of each ordered medication, including details on proper administration and potential adverse effects.

Rationales

1. Knowing the signs and symptoms of infection and organ rejection should prompt them to seek medical advice and attention, when necessary.

2. Such instruction helps to ensure accurate administration and compliance with the medication regimen. Knowing the potential adverse effects should prompt parents to seek medical advice and attention, when necessary.

Interventions

3. Explain to the parents the child's immunosuppressed state and the need for certain precautions, such as avoiding persons with known infection and avoiding large crowds, to protect the child from infection.

4. Instruct the parents to monitor the child's temperature twice daily.

5. Explain the importance of keeping regular laboratory appointments when the child is receiving cyclosporine therapy.

Rationales

3. Because of the child's immunosuppressed state, he is at risk for infection, which may have life-threatening implications.

4. Frequent monitoring ensures early recognition of rejection or infection and allows for prompt treatment.

5. Regular laboratory visits ensure accurate blood level measurements and help to determine when medication adjustments are necessary.

Documentation checklist

During the hospitalization, be sure to document the following:

___ the child's status and assessment findings upon admission
___ any changes in the child's status
___ pertinent laboratory and diagnostic findings
___ fluid intake and output
___ nutritional intake
___ growth and development status
___ the child's response to treatment
___ the child's and parents' reaction to the illness and hospitalization
___ patient and family teaching guidelines
___ discharge planning guidelines.

Necrotizing Enterocolitis

Introduction

Most common in preterm infants, necrotizing enterocolitis (NEC) is characterized by necrosis of the intestinal wall. Although the exact cause of this serious, life-threatening condition has not been determined, formula feeding may be involved. The severity of the problem depends on the amount of intestinal necrosis.

Usual treatment for NEC includes nasogastric suctioning, the administration of antibiotics, and possible bowel resectioning. Potential complications include permanent ostomy, short gut syndrome, bowel obstruction, peritonitis, and death. The prognosis usually depends on the extent of bowel necrosis and sepsis.

Assessment

Gastrointestinal
- increased residual gastric contents
- abdominal distention
- absent bowel sounds
- grossly bloody stools (guaiac-positive)
- bilious or bloody vomitus
- reddening or shininess of the abdominal wall

Cardiovascular
- sudden vascular collapse

Neurologic
- coma (if metabolic acidosis is severe)

Nursing diagnosis: *Altered nutrition: less than body requirements related to necrotic bowel*

GOAL: The child will have no signs of decreased gastric intestinal function as evidenced by normal bowel sounds and lack of residual gastric contents.

Interventions

1. Use breast milk, if available, for enteric feedings.

2. Measure the amount of gastric residuals before each nasogastric feeding.

3. Assess for abdominal distention. If distention is noted, measure the infant's abdominal girth before each feeding and as needed.

4. Test the infant's stools using a guaiac reagent.

5. Assess for bowel sounds every shift and as needed.

6. Assess the infant's abdomen for redness or shininess.

Rationales

1. Hyperosmolar formula feedings may have a synergistic effect in contributing to NEC. Breast milk is preferred because it provides the infant with passive immunity, macrophages, and lysozymes.

2. Increased gastric residuals, one of the first indications of NEC, suggest that the infant is not absorbing the formula or breast milk.

3. Abdominal distention indicates carbohydrate malabsorption.

4. Guaiac-positive or grossly bloody stools indicate that the intestinal wall is becoming hemorrhagic. Feeding at this time may result in perforation of the bowel.

5. Absence of bowel sounds indicates paralytic ileus and the need for immediate treatment.

6. Redness or shininess of the abdominal wall indicates that the skin is being stretched because of peritonitis, a serious complication of NEC.

Nursing diagnosis: *Altered tissue perfusion: gastrointestinal related to intestinal infarction and inflammation*

GOAL: The infant will demonstrate normal perfusion as evidenced by the ability to tolerate full-strength feedings and by having minimal pregastric aspiration, no abdominal distention, and guaiac-negative stools.

Interventions

1. Monitor the infant's vital signs every 2 to 4 hours. When taking the temperature, use the axillary, not rectal, route.

2. Place the infant in a supine or side-lying position in an Isolette or radiant heat warmer on an open diaper.

3. Handle the infant gently and as minimally as possible.

4. Remove soiled diapers and meticulously cleanse the perineal area as soon as possible after the infant defecates. Assess the infant's skin integrity, noting any redness or breaks in the skin.

5. Insert a nasogastric tube for intermittent suctioning.

6. Administer enteric and systemic antibiotics, as ordered.

7. Reinstitute and monitor enteric feedings, as ordered (usually after 1 to 2 weeks of the child's being given nothing by mouth [NPO status]). Begin with glucose-electrolyte solutions, and follow with diluted formula until the infant can tolerate the formula full strength.

8. If the infant requires surgery, provide the same nursing care as for any infant who has undergone abdominal surgery, including intestinal ostomy care.

Rationales

1. Such monitoring may reveal impending sepsis or cardiovascular shock, which indicates extensive involvement. The rectal route should be avoided for temperature measurement because of the risk of rectal perforation.

2. Placing the infant in this position avoids putting pressure on the distended abdomen, allows easy access to the abdominal area for assessment, and does not impede tissue perfusion.

3. Handling the infant in this manner helps to prevent trauma to the abdominal area.

4. Infants with NEC often have diarrhea and are at risk for skin breakdown around the perineal area.

5. Suctioning facilitates the removal of gastric contents.

6. Studies indicate that bacterial infection is involved in NEC. Broad-spectrum antibiotics often are ordered until the pathogen is identified by culture or culture results are negative.

7. Introducing enteric feedings too soon or too quickly can result in exacerbation of NEC.

8. The child may require removal of the diseased bowel, resulting in the creation of a temporary or permanent ostomy.

Nursing diagnosis: *Altered parenting related to infant's acute illness*

GOAL: The parents will remain attentive and caring as evidenced by verbalizing an understanding of the infant's illness and treatment and by touching and talking to the infant.

Interventions

1. Provide parents with a simple, honest explanation of the infant's condition and treatment regimen. Answer all questions with patience and empathy.

2. Encourage parental participation in the infant's daily care, including stroking and talking to the infant, taking axillary temperatures, and cleansing the perineal area.

Rationales

1. Such explanations help the parents to prepare for the disease's possible consequences and allows them to begin developing a means for coping. Answering questions with patience and empathy fosters a feeling of support.

2. Parents often feel that they must relinquish their parental roles when their child is hospitalized, especially if the child is a neonate who requires minimal handling and placement on NPO status. Encouraging parental participation promotes continued parent-child contact.

Nursing diagnosis: *Knowledge deficit related to home care*

GOAL: The parents will verbalize an understanding of home care instructions.

Interventions

1. Explain to the parents the anatomy and physiology of the normal GI system as well as the pathology involved in NEC.

2. Explain the signs and symptoms of obstruction or perforation, including intestinal obstruction and pain, abdominal distention, decreased bowel sounds, and decreased or absent stools.

3. Instruct the parents on how to care for a colostomy, if appropriate (see the "Colostomy, Ileostomy" care plan, page 250).

Rationales

1. Such explanations increase the parents' understanding of the infant's disease and aid in compliance with the treatment regimen.

2. Knowing these signs and symptoms should prompt the parents to seek medical advice and attention, when needed.

3. Parents need to know how to perform such care, as they will be the primary caregivers when the infant is discharged from the hospital.

Documentation checklist

During the hospitalization, be sure to document the following:
___ the infant's status and assessment findings upon admission
___ any changes in the infant's status
___ pertinent laboratory and diagnostic findings
___ nutritional intake
___ growth and development status
___ the parents' reaction to the illness and hospitalization
___ family teaching guidelines
___ dischage planning guidelines.

Pyloric Stenosis

Introduction

Pyloric stenosis—a blockage of the pyloric sphincter caused by a narrowing of the pylorus that leads from the stomach to the small intestine—is characterized by hypertrophy of the pylorus muscle. Apparent soon after birth (usually within 6 weeks), this disorder is marked by severe projectile vomiting and dehydration.

The prognosis for pyloric stenosis is favorable. Usual treatment includes pyloroplasty and rehydration. Potential complications include aspiration pneumonia and infection.

Assessment

Gastrointestinal

- projectile vomiting
- weight loss
- palpable mass in the upper abdomen
- visible peristaltic waves

Integumentary

- signs and symptoms of dehydration (lethargy, weakness, dry skin, and poor skin turgor)

Nursing diagnosis: Anxiety (parent) related to lack of understanding about the disease, diagnostic studies, and treatment

GOAL: The parents will be less anxious as evidenced by verbalizing an understanding of the disorder and the need for diagnostic testing and treatment.

Interventions

1. Explain to the parents the basic anatomy and physiology of the normal upper GI tract and the process of food passage through this section of the GI system. Use visual aids, if available, in your explanations.

2. Provide the parents with a schedule of the ordered diagnostic tests.

3. Provide preprocedural instruction on each ordered diagnostic test (upper GI series, ultrasonography, and laboratory testing), including details on the preparation, length of testing, and postprocedural care.

4. Provide the parents with information on the preoperative and postoperative events surrounding the surgery. Include details on withholding oral feedings, laboratory workups, X-rays, pain medication, feeding plan, how to hold the infant, and nasogastric intubation. Use sample equipment and demonstrations, as appropriate.

5. Encourage the parents to write down any questions they have concerning the child's care as they arise. Answer their questions simply and honestly.

Rationales

1. Understanding the normal functioning of the GI system helps parents to better understand the abnormal functioning associated with the disorder and the need for testing and treatment.

2. Providing the parents with a schedule of diagnostic tests helps them to anticipate upcoming events, thereby helping to decrease anxiety and fear.

3. Knowing this information should help to decrease anxiety and increase cooperation, support, and parental involvement in diagnostic testing and postprocedural care.

4. Knowing the surgical preparation and postoperative care measures helps decrease anxiety and fear and allows for increased parental involvement in health plan objectives.

5. Parents often have additional questions regarding their child's care after meeting with the nurse. Encouraging them to write down questions for further discussion can be reassuring and helps to lessen anxiety.

Nursing diagnosis: Altered nutrition: less than body requirements related to frequent projectile vomiting

GOAL: The infant will maintain an adequate nutrition status as evidenced by retained feedings and decreased vomiting.

Interventions

1. Feed the infant in upright position, burping him after every ½ to 1 oz. Maintain a quiet, relaxed environment.

Rationales

1. Feeding and burping the infant in this manner prevents aerophagia and ensures optimal retention of feeding.

Interventions

2. Offer small, frequent feedings every 2 to 3 hours. Refeed after each vomiting episode.

3. Offer oral feedings of an electrolyte solution (such as Pedialyte) during diagnostic workups.

4. Assess the infant for signs and symptoms of worsening dehydration, including decreased urine output, dry skin, poor skin turgor, and sunken fontanels and eyes. Report these signs immediately to the doctor.

5. Position the infant upright after each feeding.

Rationales

2. Small, frequent feedings decrease the total fluid volume in the stomach at one time, thereby decreasing the risk for vomiting and providing optimal hydration until I.V. therapy is initiated.

3. Electrolyte solutions replace electrolytes lost through alkalosis, hypokalemia, and hypochloremia, which may occur with repeated vomiting.

4. The doctor may order I.V. fluids to provide appropriate fluid replacement and prevent shock.

5. Positioning the infant in this manner helps prevent aspiration.

Nursing diagnosis: *Fluid volume deficit related to dehydration or shock (or both)*

GOAL: The infant will maintain normal fluid and electrolyte balance as evidenced by normal output (11 to 18 ml/hour for neonates; 17 to 25 ml/hour for infants), a capillary refill time of <3 seconds, good skin turgor, normal potassium levels, and normal vital signs.

Interventions

1. Rehydrate the infant, as indicated, with an oral electrolyte solution or I.V. fluids.

2. Monitor laboratory test results for complete blood count, specific gravity, and electrolyte, blood urea nitrogen, and arterial blood gas levels.

3. Monitor the infant every 2 to 4 hours for signs and symptoms of shock, including increased heart and respiratory rates, decreased blood pressure, and pallor.

4. Assess the infant's skin for signs and symptoms of dehydration, including grayish color, dryness, poor turgor, and depressed fontanels.

5. Weigh the infant daily, and monitor his intake and output hourly, including the amount of I.V. and oral intake, vomitus, nasogastric drainage, urine, and stool. Be sure to weigh diapers to obtain accurate urine and stool measurements.

Rationales

1. Oral electrolyte solutions and I.V. fluids replace fluids and electrolytes lost through vomiting and dehydration.

2. Dehydration causes increases in the hemoglobin and hematocrit levels. Vomiting causes decreased potassium and sodium levels, increased specific gravity, increased PCO_2 levels, and decreased pH.

3. Frequent monitoring allows for early detection and treatment of shock, which can occur with vomiting and postoperative hypervolemia. Treatment may include the administration of fluids and electrolytes (sodium and potassium) or a plasma volume expander (albumin).

4. Dehydration indicates the need for increased fluid intake.

5. Daily weights and frequent monitoring of intake and output ensure continual assessment of the infant's fluid status.

Nursing diagnosis: *Potential for infection related to surgery*

GOAL: The infant's surgical incision will remain free of infection postoperatively as evidenced by decreased swelling and redness around the incision site and a lack of foul-smelling odor and purulent discharge.

Interventions

1. Monitor the incisional dressing and site for signs of infection (erythema, purulent drainage, edema, increased tenderness and wound dehiscence, elevated core temperature) every 2 hours. Report any evidence of infection immediately and administer antibiotics, as ordered.

Rationales

1. Frequent monitoring allows for early detection and prompt treatment of infection.

Interventions

2. Use clean and sterile technique when in contact with the incision site until the healing process is complete. For example, wash hands before any skin contact, keep dressings sterile, and cleanse the wound thoroughly.

Rationales

2. Clean and sterile technique provides optimal protection to prevent bacterial infection.

Nursing diagnosis: *Altered comfort: pain related to surgical incision*

GOAL: The infant will have minimal pain as evidenced by decreased irritability, fussing, and crying.

Interventions

1. Administer analgesics on a regular basis during the first 24 hours postoperatively. Document the medication's effectiveness.

2. Change the infant's position (from side to back to abdomen) every 2 hours, when possible.

3. Demonstrate to the parents the proper holding technique while encouraging them to hold and cuddle the infant.

4. Monitor the infant for abdominal distention, peristaltic waves, absent or decreased bowel sounds, and signs and symptoms of obstruction (such as bilious vomitus) every 4 hours. Notify the doctor immediately if the infant has any of these abnormalities.

Rationales

1. Analgesics are usually ordered postoperatively to provide pain relief. Documenting the medications' effectiveness helps in determining the infant's current comfort level.

2. Position changes promote increased mobility, comfort, and muscle relaxation and decreased guarding of the incisional site.

3. Holding promotes parent-child interaction, thereby increasing the infant's sense of security, love, and support. Demonstrating the proper technique ensures that the parents will not cause the infant any discomfort.

4. Such abnormalities are signs of postoperative complications, such as bowel obstruction or paralytic ileus, and require prompt treatment.

Nursing diagnosis: *Knowledge deficit related to home care*

GOAL: The parents will verbalize an understanding of home care instructions.

Interventions

1. Instruct the parents on the infant's feeding, including details on specific formulas, preparation methods, feeding volume, and feeding technique.

2. Instruct the parents on proper wound care, including details on dressing changes, cleansing techniques, and signs and symptoms of infection.

3. Instruct the parents on the purpose and use of medications (such as bethanechol chloride), including details on the administration, dosages, and potential adverse effects.

Rationales

1. Knowing this information should promote compliance with the feeding regimen and ensure that the infant receives adequate nutrition.

2. Such instruction should help the parents to provide adequate care and careful monitoring for signs and symptoms of infection.

3. Such instruction promotes compliance with the medication regimen. Knowing the signs and symptoms of potential adverse effects should prompt parents to seek medical advice and attention, when necessary.

Documentation checklist

During the hospitalization, be sure to document the following:
___ the infant's status and assessment findings upon admission
___ any changes in the infant's status
___ pertinent laboratory and diagnostic findings
___ fluid intake and output
___ nutritional intake
___ growth and development status
___ the infant's response to treatment
___ the parents' reaction to the illness and hospitalization
___ family teaching guidelines
___ discharge planning guidelines.

GASTROINTESTINAL AND HEPATOBILIARY SYSTEMS

Tracheoesophageal Fistula

Introduction

A congenital malformation of the trachea and esophagus, tracheoesophageal fistula is characterized by failure of the trachea and esophagus to develop as a continuous passage from the throat to the stomach. The abnormality, which commonly results in obstruction of the infant's normal swallowing route, may occur as a blind pouch that terminates at the proximal end of the esophagus and connects to a fistula extending from the trachea at the distal end; as a fistula between the trachea and esophagus; or as some other abnormality.

Usual treatment includes reanastomosis of the esophagus and closure of the fistula. Potential complications include aspiration pneumonia and bowel obstruction. The prognosis usually is favorable.

Assessment

Gastrointestinal
- excessive mucus around the mouth
- frothy saliva around the mouth and nose

Respiratory
- triad of choking, coughing, and cyanosis with first feeding

Nursing diagnosis: *Ineffective breathing pattern related to choking, coughing, and cyanosis during feeding*

GOAL: The infant will have decreased respiratory distress as evidenced by quiet, relaxed breathing during feedings.

Interventions

1. Observe the infant's behavior before, during, and after feedings. Notify the doctor immediately if the infant shows signs of choking, increased respiratory rate, vomiting, and cyanosis.

2. Carefully suction the infant's oropharynx.

3. Prepare the infant for diagnostic X-ray studies, according to hospital protocol.

4. Keep the head of the infant's crib elevated 45 degrees until the defect is corrected.

Rationales

1. Observing the infant's behavior ensures early detection and prompt treatment of complications.

2. Careful suctioning helps decrease the risk for aspiration. Suctioning past the pharynx should be avoided to prevent accidental perforation of the esophagus.

3. Diagnostic X-rays are necessary to identify the specific abnormality and further define the appropriate medical or surgical intervention.

4. Elevating the head of the crib helps prevent aspiration of secretions.

Nursing diagnosis: *Anxiety (parent) related to lack of knowledge about the disorder, diagnostic testing, and treatment*

GOAL: The parents will be less anxious as evidenced by verbalizing an understanding of the disorder and the need for diagnostic testing and treatment.

Interventions

1. Explain to the parents the basic anatomy and physiology of the normal upper GI tract and the process of food passage through this section of the gastrointestinal system. Use visual aids, if available, in your explanation.

Rationales

1. Understanding the normal functioning of the GI system enables parents to better understand the abnormal functioning associated with the disorder and the need for diagnostic testing and treatment.

Interventions	Rationales
2. Provide the parents with a schedule of the ordered diagnostic tests.	2. Providing the parents with a schedule of the ordered diagnostic tests helps them to anticipate upcoming events, thereby helping to reduce anxiety and fear.
3. Explain to the parents that the infant may require a gastrostomy tube until he is mature enough to undergo temporary or permanent repair of the abnormality.	3. A gastrostomy tube may be necessary to provide feedings.
4. Provide the parents with information about the pre-operative and postoperative events surrounding surgery. Include details on withholding oral fluids, I.V. lines, laboratory workups, X-rays, pain medication, feeding plans (gastrostomy or total parenteral nutrition), and how to hold the infant. Include sample equipment and tours of the intensive care unit, when possible.	4. Knowing the surgical preparation and postoperative events helps decrease anxiety and allows for increased parental involvement in the health plan objectives.
5. Encourage the parents to write down any additional questions they may have concerning the infant's care as they arise. Answer their questions honestly and simply.	5. Parents often have many questions concerning their child's care after meeting with the nurse. Encouraging them to write down questions for further discussion can be reassuring and helps to lessen anxiety.

Nursing diagnosis: *Ineffective breathing pattern related to aspiration of secretions or feedings (or both)*

GOAL: The infant will have an improved respiratory status as evidenced by stable respirations and no signs of respiratory distress.

Interventions	Rationales
1. Take the following measures to maintain the infant's respiratory status and prevent pneumonia:	1. Taking these measures ensures that the infant receives adequate oxygenation at all times.
• Maintain positioning of the nasal catheter in the esophageal pouch when providing gentle suctioning.	• Maintaining the catheter in this position facilitates the draining of secretions and helps prevent aspiration.
• Maintain the infant's head and thorax at a 20-degree elevation.	• Maintaining the infant in this position helps prevent aspiration.
• Suction the infant, as needed.	• Suctioning helps clear secretions, thereby clearing the airway.
• Maintain a patent airway.	• Maintaining airway patency allows for adequate oxygenation.
2. Administer antibiotics, as ordered.	2. Antibiotics may be ordered to treat aspiration pneumonia.

Nursing diagnosis: *Delayed growth and development related to hospitalization and deprivation of normal parent-child interactions and environmental stimulation*

GOAL: The infant will grow and develop normally as evidenced by achieving optimal growth and developmental milestones.

Interventions	Rationales
1. Use appropriate auditory, visual, and tactile stimulation (such as music, bright colors, mirrors, and different shaped objects) when caring for the infant. Instruct the parents and other staff to use the same stimulation when in contact with the infant.	1. Consistent auditory, visual, and tactile stimulation is essential to help the infant achieve optimal growth and developmental skills.

Interventions

2. Demonstrate to the parents the proper way to hold the infant, and encourage frequent holding and cuddling.

3. Help the parents to understand and distinguish the infant's behavioral cues, such as crying, grimacing, and fussing.

4. Instruct the parents to perform range-of-motion exercises or to use appropriate play when the infant is not confined by I.V. setups or dialysis, such as during his bath and diaper changes.

5. Encourage the parents to talk to and establish eye contact with the infant.

Rationales

2. Frequent holding and cuddling help promote infant-parent bonding, which is essential to normal growth and development.

3. Parents of infants who require emergency care often have difficulty understanding and distinguishing their infant's needs. Helping them to differentiate behavioral cues allows them to respond promptly and appropriately to the infant's needs, thereby promoting normal growth and development.

4. Range-of-motion exercises and play techniques allow for increased infant stimulation and parental bonding, which promote normal growth and development.

5. Verbal and visual communication increase parental bonding and help to stimulate the infant, thereby promoting normal growth and development.

Nursing diagnosis: *Knowledge deficit related to home care*

GOAL: The parents will verbalize understanding of home care instructions.

Interventions

1. Instruct the parents on recognizing the signs and symptoms of aspiration, including respiratory distress, vomiting of bright red blood, elevated temperature, and choking. Make sure they receive proper training in cardiopulmonary resuscitation and the Heimlich maneuver before the infant is discharged from the hospital.

2. Instruct the parents to keep the infant's head elevated during feedings and to place the infant on his side after feedings.

3. Explain the need for follow-up care, including surgery.

Rationales

1. Parents need to know the signs and symptoms of aspiration so that they can provide emergency treatment, when necessary.

2. These positions help prevent the aspiration of food.

3. The infant may require surgery at a later date if he was too unstable to undergo corrective surgery during the initial hospitalization.

Documentation checklist

During the hospitalization, be sure to document the following:
___ the infant's status and assessment findings upon admission
___ any changes in the infant's status
___ pertinent laboratory and diagnostic findings
___ nutritional status
___ growth and development status
___ the infant's response to treatment
___ the parents' reaction to the illness and hospitalization
___ family teaching guidelines
___ discharge planning guidelines.

Acute Glomerulonephritis

Introduction

The most common noninfectious renal disease of childhood, acute glomerulonephritis affects the glomeruli and filtration rate of the kidneys, resulting in water and sodium retention and hypertension. Usually caused by a reaction to streptococcal infection, this disease seldom has any long-term effects on the renal system.

Acute glomerulonephritis affects boys more than girls, usually occurring at about age 6. Treatment typically includes the administration of antibiotics, antihypertensives, and diuretics as well as dietary restrictions. Potential complications include hypertension, congestive heart failure, and end-stage renal disease.

Assessment

Genitourinary
- cloudy, smoky brown urine
- proteinuria
- elevated urine specific gravity
- decreased urine output

Cardiovascular
- mild hypertension

Neurologic
- lethargy
- irritability

Gastrointestinal
- anorexia
- vomiting
- diarrhea

EENT
- moderate periorbital edema

Hematologic
- transient anemia

Integumentary
- pallor
- generalized edema

Nursing diagnosis: *Altered tissue perfusion: cerebral related to water retention and hypernatremia*

GOAL: The child will have normal tissue perfusion as evidenced by normal blood pressure, reduced water retention, and no signs of hypernatremia.

Interventions

1. Monitor and document the child's blood pressure every 2 to 4 hours during the acute phase.

2. Institute the following seizure precautions:
- Keep a padded tongue depressor, oral airway, and suction equipment at the child's bedside.
- Post signs above the child's bed and on his door alerting health care personnel to the child's seizure status.

3. Administer an antihypertensive agent, such as hydralazine hydroxide (the drug of choice), as ordered. Monitor the child for potential adverse reactions.

4. Monitor the child's fluid volume status closely.

5. Assess the child's neurologic status (level of consciousness, reflexes, and pupillary response) every 8 hours. Notify the doctor immediately of any significant changes in the child's status.

6. Administer diuretics, such as hydrochlorothiazide or furosemide, as ordered.

Rationales

1. Frequent monitoring allows for early detection and prompt treatment of changes in the child's blood pressure, such as hypertension.

2. Instituting seizure precautions helps prevent injury during a seizure episode. Although uncommon, seizures can occur as a result of lack of oxygen perfusion to the brain.

3. Antihypertensives may be ordered because uncontrolled hypertension may lead to kidney damage. Although the exact reason for hypertension is unknown, it may be related to fluid overload in the circulatory system.

4. Monitoring is essential because volume expansion further increases blood pressure.

5. Frequent assessments allow for early detection and prompt treatment of any changes in the child's neurologic status.

6. Diuretics helps in the excretion of the retained fluid.

Nursing diagnosis: *Fluid volume excess related to oliguria*

GOAL: The child will maintain normal fluid volume as evidenced by maintaining a urine output of approximately 1 to 2 ml/kg/hr.

Interventions

1. Weigh the child daily, and monitor his urine output every 4 hours.

2. Assess the child for edema and measure his abdominal girth every 8 hours.

3. Monitor the child closely for adverse reactions to diuretic therapy, specifically when using hydrochlorothiazide or furosemide.

4. Monitor and record the child's intake.

5. Assess the color, consistency, and specific gravity of the child's urine.

6. Monitor the results of all ordered laboratory tests.

Rationales

1. Daily weight monitoring and frequent monitoring of intake and output allow for early detection and prompt treatment of changes in the child's fluid status. Rapid weight gain indicates fluid retention. Decreased urine output may indicate impending renal failure.

2. Frequent assessments and measurements allow for early detection and prompt treatment of any changes in the child's condition. An increase in abdominal girth usually indicates ascites.

3. These diuretics can cause hypokalemia, which requires the administration of I.V. potassium supplements.

4. Intake often is restricted because of the child's fluid retention and lowered filtration rate of the kidneys. Sodium and fluid restrictions may be required.

5. Frothy urine indicates increased protein depletion, signifying impaired kidney functioning.

6. Elevated blood urea nitrogen and creatinine levels may indicate impaired kidney functioning.

Nursing diagnosis: *Altered nutrition: less than body requirements related to anorexia*

GOAL: The child will have improved nutritional intake as evidenced by eating 80% of each meal.

Interventions

1. Provide a high-carbohydrate diet.

2. Serve small, frequent meals that include some of the child's favorite foods.

3. Restrict the child's sodium and protein intake, as ordered.

Rationales

1. A high-carbohydrate diet, usually more palatable to a child, provides essential calories for improved intake.

2. Serving smaller quantities of food at one meal seems less overwhelming to a child and enables him to eat more at each sitting. Serving some the child's favorite foods helps ensure that he eats more of each meal.

3. Sodium causes fluid retention and often is restricted in children with this disorder. Protein restrictions may be necessary in severe cases because of the kidneys' inability to metabolize protein.

Nursing diagnosis: *Activity intolerance related to fatigue*

GOAL: The child will have increased activity tolerance as evidenced by the ability to play for increasingly longer periods of time.

Interventions

1. Schedule rest periods to follow each activity.

Rationales

1. Frequent resting conserves energy and decreases the production of waste in the body, which can further stress the kidney.

Interventions	**Rationales**
2. Provide quiet, challenging age-appropriate games.	2. These types of games conserve energy yet keep the child mentally stimulated.
3. Schedule the child's nursing care to allow for periods of uninterrupted sleep at night.	3. Scheduling care enables the child to obtain needed sleep.

Nursing diagnosis: *Potential for impaired skin integrity related to immobility and edema*

GOAL: The child will maintain normal skin integrity as evidenced by maintaining a pinkish skin color and having no signs of redness, edema, or skin breakdown.

Interventions	**Rationales**
1. Provide an eggcrate mattress for the child's bed.	1. An eggcrate mattress provides padding to reduce pressure on body prominences, thereby decreasing the risk of skin breakdown.
2. Assist child to change position every 2 hours.	2. Frequent position changes reduce pressure on the capillary beds and improve circulation, thereby decreasing the risk of skin breakdown.
3. Bathe the child daily using a soap with a high fat content.	3. Deodorant and perfumed soaps dry the skin, contributing to skin breakdown.
4. Support and elevate edematous extremities.	4. Supporting and elevating extremities promotes venous return and helps decrease swelling.

Nursing diagnosis: *Anxiety (parent) related to the child's hospitalization*

GOAL: The parents will be less anxious as evidenced by verbalizing their fears and understanding the child's need for hospitalization.

Interventions	**Rationales**
1. Listen to the parents' concerns.	1. Listening provides support during the stress of hospitalization.
2. Explain all procedures to the parents and involve them in discussions about the child's care.	2. Keeping the parents informed and involving them in discussions on the child's care helps to decrease anxiety by fostering a sense of control.
3. Refer the parent to appropriate support groups, if needed.	3. Support groups provide parents with an alternative outlet for expressing their feelings and concerns.

Nursing diagnosis: *Knowledge deficit related to home care*

GOAL: The parents will verbalize an understanding of home care instructions.

Interventions	**Rationales**
1. Explain to the parents the pathophysiology of the disease.	1. Explaining this information increases the parents' understanding of the disease and aids in compliance with the treatment regimen.
2. Reassure the parents that usually no long-term effects are associated with the disease.	2. Parents often are worried about the effects of the disease, especially if the child has been on dialysis to help filter impurities from the body until the kidneys resume normal functioning.

Interventions

3. Explain to the parents the need to maintain the child on a sodium-restricted diet until his edema subsides and the kidneys resume normal functioning.

4. Instruct the parents to limit the child's activity level until otherwise specified by the doctor.

5. Teach the parents the signs and symptoms of upper respiratory infection leading to a streptococcal infection, including elevated temperature, sore throat, and cough.

6. Advise the parents of the importance of keeping all follow-up appointments.

Rationales

3. This type of diet is necessary because excessive sodium intake limits water excretion.

4. Limited activity is necessary to prevent stress on the kidneys, which could cause a relapse of the disease.

5. Knowing the signs and symptoms of recurring infection should prompt parents to seek medical advice and treatment, when necessary.

6. Follow-up visits are essential to determine resolution of disease and any further complications.

Documentation checklist

During the hospitalization, be sure to document the following:
___ the child's status and assessment findings upon admission
___ any changes in the child's status
___ pertinent laboratory and diagnostic findings
___ fluid intake and output
___ nutritional intake
___ the child's response to treatment
___ the child's and parents' reaction to the illness and hospitalization
___ patient and family teaching guidelines
___ discharge planning guidelines.

GENITOURINARY SYSTEM

Hypospadias, Epispadias

Introduction

Congenital defects that are detectable at or shortly after birth, hypospadias and epispadias involve abnormalities of the male urethral opening. In hypospadias, the more common defect, the urethral opening usually appears behind the penis or somewhere along the ventral side of the penile shaft. Often, although not always, the defect is associated with a chordee, a downward bowing of the penis. In epispadias, the urethral opening appears on the dorsal side of the penis.

Treatment for hypospadias or epispadias involves surgery to repair the cosmetic appearance and normal functioning of the penis. Surgery usually is not scheduled until age 1 to 2, when the penis is of a more operable size. Potential complications include infection and urethral obstruction.

Assessment
PREOPERATIVE
Genitourinary
• absence of ventral foreskin
• dimple or groove at tip of penis
• spade-shaped glans penis
• possible chordee with or without an erection
• urethral opening on the ventral (hypospadias) or dorsal (epispadias) side of penis

POSTOPERATIVE
Genitourinary
• penile swelling
• bleeding at surgical site
• dysuria

Neurologic
• irritability
• restlessness

Nursing diagnosis: *Anxiety (child and parent) related to surgical procedure (urethroplasty)*

GOAL: The child and parents will be less anxious as evidenced by verbalizing an understanding of the surgical procedure.

Interventions

1. Explain to the child and parents, in appropriate terms, the surgical procedure and expected postoperative care. Use pictures and dolls when explaining procedures to the child. Explain that surgery involves correcting the placement of the urethral opening. Also explain that an indwelling (Foley) catheter will be in place and that restraints may be necessary to prevent the child from disturbing the catheter. Advise them that the child may be discharged with the catheter in place.

2. Allow the child to act out fears and fantasies with puppets and dolls.

Rationales

1. Explaining the surgery and postoperative care helps alleviate anxiety and fear by allowing the child and parents to anticipate and prepare for the upcoming events. Using pictures and dolls to explain procedures to the child enables the child to understand complicated concepts through demonstrations.

2. Acting out allows the child to ventilate his fear and enables the nurse to better assess the child's cognitive level concerning the condition and need for hospitalization.

Nursing diagnosis: *Potential for infection (urinary tract) related to placement of indwelling catheter*

GOAL: The child will remain free of infection as evidenced by normal urinalysis results on removal of the catheter.

Interventions

1. Keep the catheter drainage bag below the child's bladder level, making sure the tubing is free of kinks and loops.

Rationales

1. Maintaining the drainage bag in this postion prevents infection by keeping nonsterile urine from flowing back into the bladder.

Interventions

2. Use aseptic technique when emptying the catheter bag.

3. Monitor the child's urine for cloudiness or sedimentation. Also monitor surgical dressings for foul odor or purulent drainage every 4 hours.

4. Encourage the child to drink 2 to 3 oz (60 to 90 ml) or more per hour.

5. Administer prophylactic antibiotics, as ordered, to help prevent infection. Monitor the child for therapeutic or adverse effects.

Rationales

2. Aseptic technique prevents contaminants from entering the urinary tract system.

3. These signs may indicate infection and should be reported promptly to the doctor.

4. Increased fluid intake promotes dilution of urine and encourages voiding.

5. Such monitoring provides a means for determining the efficacy of and the child's tolerance to antibiotics.

Nursing diagnosis: *Altered comfort: pain related to surgery*

GOAL: The child will have decreased amounts of pain during hospitalization as evidenced by decreased crying, restlessness, and verbalization of pain.

Interventions

1. Administer analgesics, as ordered.

2. Make sure the child's catheter is correctly positioned and free of kinks, which could cause pressure and pain.

Rationales

1. Analgesics may be ordered to provide pain relief.

2. Improper catheter positioning may cause pain from inadequate drainage or friction resulting from pulling against the inflated balloon.

Nursing diagnosis: *Potential for injury related to dislodged catheter or catheter removal (suprapubic or Foley)*

GOAL: The child will remain free of injury as evidenced by maintaining correct catheter placement until removal by the nurse or doctor.

Interventions

1. Secure the catheter to the child's penis with bandages and tape.

2. Place restraints on the child's arms when he is unsupervised or asleep.

3. Use a bed cradle to keep linens from contacting the catheter and penis.

4. Restrict the child from straddling a bicycle or rocking horse.

Rationales

1. A secure dressing helps decrease the chance of accidental removal.

2. Restraints prevent the child from pulling out or dislodging the catheter.

3. Keeping bed linens from contact with the catheter and penis is necessary to prevent accidental dislodgment.

4. Such restrictions are necessary to prevent catheter dislodgment and damage to the operative site.

Nursing diagnosis: *Anxiety (parent) related to the physical imperfection of the child's penis after surgery*

GOAL: The parents will be less anxious as evidenced by verbalizing their feelings regarding the child's defect.

Interventions

1. Encourage the parents to express their feelings and concerns about the child's imperfection.

2. Assist the parents through the normal grieving process.

3. Refer the parents to an appropriate support group, if needed.

Rationales

1. Allowing the parents to express feelings and concerns provides support and understanding, thereby helping to reduce their anxiety.

2. Grieving allows the parents an alternate mechanism for working through their anxiety and distress.

3. Support groups provide an alternative method for the parents to cope with the child's imperfection.

Nursing diagnosis: *Knowledge deficit related to home care*

GOAL The parents will verbalize an understanding of home care instructions.

Interventions

1. Instruct the parents on the signs and symptoms of urinary tract or incisional infection, including increased temperature, cloudy urine, and purulent drainage from the incisional site.

2. Instruct the parents on how to care for the catheter and penis, including cleaning around the catheter, emptying the drainage bag, and securing the catheter, and on the need for monitoring the color and clarity of urine.

3. Instruct the parents on the purpose and use of antibiotics and medication for bladder spasms (meperidine hydrochloride, acetaminophen, B & O Supprettes), including details on administration, dosages, and potential adverse effects.

Rationales

1. Knowing the signs and symptoms of infection should prompt parents to seek medical advice and attention, when needed.

2. Such information helps promote increased compliance with the medical regimen and helps prevent the risk of catheter dislodgment and infection.

3. Analgesics help to control pain. Bladder spasms may occur from bladder irritation. Knowing the potential adverse effects should prompt parents to seek medical advice and attention, when needed.

Documentation checklist

During the hospitalization, be sure to document the following:
___ the child's status and assessment findings upon admission
___ any changes in the child's status
___ pertinent laboratory and diagnostic findings
___ fluid intake and output
___ nutritional intake
___ the child's response to treatment
___ the child's and parents' reaction to the illness and hospitalization
___ family teaching guidelines
___ discharge planning guidelines.

Kidney Transplant

Introduction

Kidney transplantation may be indicated for children whose kidneys are no longer functioning because of infection, end-stage renal disease, or cancer. The procedure involves the replacement of the nonfunctioning kidney with a fully functioning kidney taken from a living donor or a cadaver. Children awaiting kidney transplants must meet certain hospital criteria before being put on a waiting list.

Potential complications include hemorrhage, infection, organ rejection, and death. The survival rate usually is above 50%.

Assessment

The following assessment findings are indicative of postoperative complications:

Genitourinary
• increased urine output

Cardiovascular
• hypertension

Neurologic
• restlessness
• irritability

Gastrointestinal
• increased appetite
• gastric distress

EENT
• periorbital edema

TRANSPLANT REJECTION
Genitourinary
• tenderness and swelling at graft site
• decreased urine creatinine levels
• proteinuria
• hematuria

Hematologic
• increased white blood cell count
• increased serum creatinine levels

Musculoskeletal
• general malaise

Integumentary
• fever

Nursing diagnosis: *Potential fluid volume excess related to function of transplanted kidney*

GOAL: Child will maintain appropriate fluid volume status as evidenced by good skin turgor, moist mucous membranes and lack of periorbital edema.

Interventions

1. Weigh the child at same time each day, with the child in the same clothes, using the same scale.

2. Monitor the child's fluid intake and output hourly for the first 48 to 72 hours, then every 4 hours until stable, and then every 8 hours.

3. Monitor the child's blood pressure hourly until stable, then every 4 hours.

4. Monitor the child for hematuria, which should clear within 2 to 4 days after surgery.

5. Assess the child's skin turgor and mucous membranes every 8 hours.

6. Closely monitor serum electrolyte and creatinine levels.

Rationales

1. Daily weights help determine whether the child has fluid retention or depletion.

2. Frequent monitoring provides information on the child's fluid status and kidney functioning.

3. Monitoring is essential because blood pressure changes with fluid shifts and degree of shock after surgery.

4. Increased bleeding may signal transplant rejection or hemorrhage after surgery.

5. Poor skin turgor and dry mucous membranes indicate dehydration.

6. Electrolyte and creatinine levels should return to normal with normal kidney function.

Interventions	Rationales
7. Maintain the child on a sodium-restricted diet.	7. Maintaining the child on a sodium-restricted diet helps decrease fluid retention.

Nursing diagnosis: *Potential for infection related to lowered resistance secondary to immunosuppression*

GOAL: The child will remain free of infection as evidenced by maintaining a temperature between 97.5° and 99° F. (36.5° and 37.2° C.), clear lungs, and normal urinalysis results.

Interventions	Rationales
1. Monitor the child for increased temperature and for swelling, redness, warmth, or drainage around the surgical site.	1. These signs indicate possible infection and the need for appropriate nursing measures, such as the administration of antibiotics.
2. Assess the child's pulmonary status (respiratory rate, depth, and rhythm) every 4 hours. Notify the doctor immediately of any significant changes in the child's status.	2. Such assessment is necessary for the early detection and prompt treatment of infection.
3. Have the child turn, cough, and deep-breathe every 2 hours. Be sure to splint the surgical site before having the child cough.	3. Turning, coughing, and deep breathing help to mobilize secretions, thereby preventing infection. Splinting provides support to the incision during coughing.
4. Assess the child's urine for cloudiness or increased sedimentation.	4. These signs indicate possible infection and should be treated promptly with antibiotics.
5. Use sterile technique during all dressing changes.	5. Sterile technique helps prevent the introduction of bacteria into the wound.
6. Cleanse the wound with hydrogen peroxide or sterile saline solution.	6. Proper cleansing decreases crusting and bacterial buildup.
7. Provide proper catheter care, such as cleaning around the catheter and urinary meatus with an antimicrobial agent.	7. Keeping the catheter clean decreases bacterial exposure of the urinary tract.

Nursing diagnosis: *Altered nutrition: potential for more than body requirements related to increased appetite secondary to use of immunosuppressant agents and limitations on potassium and sodium*

GOAL: The child will maintain appropriate nutritional balance as evidenced by ingesting a balanced diet.

Interventions	Rationales
1. Monitor the child's daily weight and dietary intake.	1. Such monitoring allows for continual assessment of the child's current nutritional status and ensures early detection of changes and prompt intervention, when needed.
2. Discuss dietary modifications, such as sodium and potassium restrictions, with the child and parents.	2. Understanding the reasons for dietary modifications should promote compliance with the dietary regimen. Sodium increases fluid retention; potassium is supplemented in medications.
3. Inform the child and parents that the child's appetite should decrease in 2 to 4 months, when the immunosuppressant drug (prednisone) dosage is decreased.	3. Immunosuppressant agents cause increased appetite. Knowing this should prompt the child and parents to comply with the dietary regimen.
4. Incorporate some of the child's favorite foods, as allowed, into the dietary regimen.	4. Serving some of the child's favorite foods helps the child to comply with the dietary regimen by increasing his sense of control over the situation.

Nursing diagnosis: *Altered comfort: pain related to frequent invasive procedures and surgery*

GOAL: The child will be more comfortable and in less pain as evidenced by relaxed features, active involvement in play, and verbalization of comfort.

Interventions

1. Before any invasive procedure, explain to the child and parents what will occur.

2. Assess the child for the severity and location of any pain or discomfort, using pediatric pain assessment tools (such as a face interval or number line pain-rating scale).

3. Maintain the child in a comfortable position while maintaining proper body alignment and supporting pressure points.

4. Allow the child to have familiar objects, such as toys and blankets, from home.

5. Administer an analgesic, as ordered.

6. Provide diversional activities, such as toys, games, television, or books.

Rationales

1. Such explanations help to decrease anxiety, fear, and feelings of loss of control.

2. Knowing the severity and location of the child's pain helps in determining appropriate nursing measures used to control pain. Such measures might include the use of medications, positioning, diversion, imagery, relaxation, and breathing techniques.

3. Positioning the child in this manner decreases pressure being placed on one part of the body for extended periods of time.

4. Familiar objects help increase feelings of security and decrease anxiety, which can affect the child's comfort level.

5. Analgesics provide pain relief, thereby increasing the child's comfort level.

6. Diversional activities refocus the child's attention and concentration from his pain.

Nursing diagnosis: *Ineffective individual coping related to sensory overload*

GOAL: The child will demonstrate effective coping skills as evidenced by responses and behavior appropriate for his developmental level.

Interventions

1. Allow the child to make small decisions about his care, especially concerning his daily bath and mealtimes. Allow him limited flexibility regarding medications and treatments. For example, ask him if he wants his medication now or in 10 minutes.

2. Set limits for the child regarding acceptable and nonacceptable behavior. Encourage the parents to maintain discipline as they would at home.

3. Take the child to a treatment room for any invasive procedure.

4. Schedule periods of quiet time for the child.

Rationales

1. Allowing the child some control over simple routines helps him to better cope with his situation by increasing feelings of self-control.

2. Establishing reasonable behavioral limits and providing consistent discipline increase feelings of security and normalcy, thereby enabling the child to cope with his current situation.

3. Using a treatment room for invasive procedures allows the child to feel secure in his room, fostering a sense of normalcy necessary for effective coping.

4. Quiet time allows the child to block out sensory stimuli that may be hindering his ability to cope.

Nursing diagnosis: *Disturbance in self-concept: body image related to adverse effects of steroid therapy*

GOAL: The child will have an improved self-concept as evidenced by verbalizing acceptance of his altered body image.

Interventions

1. Listen attentively to the child's feelings and concerns about his altered body image. Do not negate the feelings.

2. Help the child to focus on his assets and positive features.

3. Encourage the child to attend support group meetings, such as those designed for transplant patients in his age-group.

4. Encourage the child's siblings and peers to visit.

Rationales

1. Listening provides emotional support and allows the nurse to assess the child's cognitive level regarding his appearance.

2. Focusing on assets and positive features helps to de-emphasize the negative aspects of the child's condition.

3. Support groups help to decrease the child's feelings of isolation by introducing him to other children with similar problems. Such groups also allow the child to see how others are coping with their altered body image.

4. Visits from siblings and peers enable the child to maintain contact with others outside the hospital, thereby fostering a sense of normalcy.

Nursing diagnosis: *Noncompliance with drug regimen related to adverse drug effects*

GOAL: The child and parents will comply with the prescribed drug regimen.

Interventions

1. Instruct the child and parents on the potential adverse effects of immunosuppressive drug therapy, including acne, weight gain, and cushingoid appearance. Explain that these effects should decrease as the dosage is decreased.

2. Instruct the child and parents on how to control weight gain and acne. Teach the importance of proper skin care, monitoring daily fluid intake, and ingesting no more than 2,000 calories/day.

Rationales

1. Knowing this information should decrease the child's and parents' anxiety and encourage them to comply with the medication regimen.

2. Knowing that they can control some of the negative aspects of drug therapy should encourage the child and parents to comply with the medication regimen.

Nursing diagnosis: *Knowledge deficit related to home care*

GOAL: The parents and child will verbalize an understanding of home care instructions.

Interventions

1. Teach the parents and child the signs and symptoms of transplant rejection (see the "Assessment" section at the beginning of this care plan). Tell them to report these signs immediately to the doctor if they should occur.

2. Review with the parents and child their understanding of laboratory values (creatinine, blood urea nitrogen, calcium, and phosphorus levels; white blood cell count; and glomerular filtration rate).

Rationales

1. Early recognition of transplant rejection ensures prompt medical intervention.

2. The parents and child should have a basic understanding of these tests so that they know what the values mean when such tests are performed on an outpatient basis.

Interventions

3. Teach the parents how to take the child's blood pressure and how and when to administer antihypertensive medications. Explain the importance of monitoring for adverse effects and the need to notify the doctor if they should occur.

4. Instruct the parents on the purpose and use of steroids (if applicable), including details on administration, dosages, and potential adverse effects (nausea and vomiting, GI bleeding, increased susceptibility to infection, fluid retention).

5. Instruct the parents on the purpose and use of cyclosporine (if applicable), including details on administration, dosages, and potential adverse effects (hypertension, accelerated hair growth, nephrotoxicity, and diarrhea).

6. Teach the parents and child the signs and symptoms of infection, including fever, increased pain, and increased white blood cell count.

7. Emphasize the child's need to limit his exercise level and to avoid participation in contact sports or long-distance running.

8. Encourage the child and parents to join one or more support groups, such as a hospital transplant support group or the National Association on Hemodialysis and Transplantation.

Rationales

3. Knowing this information helps promote compliance with the medication regimen. Knowing the potential adverse effects (hypotension, bradycardia, faintness, dizziness) should prompt the parents to seek medical advice and attention, when necessary.

4. Knowing this information helps promote compliance with the medication regimen. Knowing the potential adverse effects should prompt the parents to seek medical advice and attention, when necessary.

5. Knowing this information helps promote compliance wth the medication regimen. Knowing the potential adverse effects should prompt parents to seek medical advice and attention, when necessary.

6. Early recognition and reporting of the signs and symptoms of infection ensure prompt treatment to prevent complications.

7. Limiting the child's activities is necessary because heavy exercise may cause dehydration and contact sports or long-distance running may result in trauma to the kidney area.

8. Such groups offer support by enabling the parents and child to meet with others undergoing similar problems.

Documentation checklist

During the hospitalization, be sure to document the following:
___ the child's status and assessment findings upon admission
___ any changes in the child's status
___ pertinent laboratory and diagnostic findings
___ fluid intake and output
___ nutritional intake
___ the child's response to treatment
___ the child's and parents' reaction to the illness and hospitalization
___ patient and family teaching guidelines
___ discharge planning guidelines.

GENITOURINARY SYSTEM

Nephrotic Syndrome

Introduction

A manifestation of a large number of glomerular disorders, nephrotic syndrome is marked by proteinuria, hypoalbuminemia, and edema and sometimes hematuria, hypertension, and a decreased glomerular filtration rate. Often of an unknown etiology, nephrotic syndrome affects more boys than girls, usually between ages 2 and 7.

Usual treatment includes dialysis and the administration of antihypertensives, diuretics, and steroids. Often, children have several relapses throughout treatment. Potential complications include renal disease, renal failure, and congestive heart failure.

Assessment
Genitourinary
• oliguria
• proteinuria
• hematuria

Cardiovascular
• hypertension

Integumentary
• edema of face (in the morning)
• generalized edema of the extremities and abdomen (as the day progresses)
• pallor

Nursing diagnosis: *Potential for impaired skin integrity related to edema and immobility*

GOAL: The child will have no signs of skin breakdown as evidenced by good skin integrity and no muscle wasting.

Interventions

1. Help the child to change position every 2 hours.

2. Provide proper skin care, including daily baths with moisturized soap, massages, position changes, and changing soiled linens and clothing.

3. Assess the child's skin for evidence of irritation and breakdown, such as redness, edema, and abrasions, every 4 to 8 hours.

4. Support or elevate edematous areas, such as the arms, legs, and scrotum, with pillows or bed linens. Use powder to prevent these skin surfaces from rubbing.

5. Perform passive range-of-motion exercises during the acute phase of the disease.

6. Increase the child's activity level as edema subsides.

Rationales

1. Frequent position changes help to prevent skin breakdown by alleviating pressure on body surfaces.

2. Proper skin care helps keep the skin free from irritating substances.

3. Frequent assessments allow for early detection and prompt intervention, when necessary.

4. Elevating or supporting edematous areas helps to decrease edema. Using powder decreases the moisture and friction that often occur when body surfaces rub together.

5. Passive range-of-motion exercises help prevent joint stiffness and muscle wasting.

6. Increased activity helps prevent complications associated with prolonged bed rest, including decreased muscle tone, constipation, muscle wasting, and contractures.

Nursing diagnosis: *Potential for infection related to immunosuppression*

GOAL: The child will remain free of infection as evidenced by lack of temperature elevation, purulent drainage, cough, and sore throat.

Interventions

1. Do not allow visits from anyone with an acute infection.

2. Administer antibiotics, as ordered.

3. Monitor the child on a daily basis for signs of infection, including cough, fever, runny nose, purulent drainage, and sore throat.

Rationales

1. Screening visitors is essential because the child is highly susceptible to infection.

2. Antibiotics, often given prophylactically to immunosuppressed children, help fight or prevent infection.

3. Frequent monitoring ensures early recognition of infection and prompt treatment.

Nursing diagnosis: *Altered tissue perfusion: peripheral related to hypertension*

GOAL: The child will maintain normal tissue perfusion as evidenced by a normal blood pressure, the lack of headaches and seizures, and a brisk capillary refill time.

Interventions

1. Monitor the child's blood pressure every 4 hours.

2. Institute the following seizure precautions:
• Keep a padded tongue depressor, oral airway, and suction equipment near the child's bedside.
• Post a sign above the child's bed and on his door alerting all health care personnel to the child's seizure status.
• Document the child's status on his patient chart.

3. Administer antihypertensive medications, as ordered.

Rationales

1. Frequent monitoring ensures early recognition of hypertension and prompt treatment.

2. Seizure precautions are necessary for children with severe hypertension and hypoxia of the brain.

3. Antihypertensive medications may be ordered to decrease the child's blood pressure and the possiblity of complications, including seizures, stroke, congestive heart failure, and headaches.

Nursing diagnosis: *Altered nutrition: less than body requirements related to disease*

GOAL: The child will have an improved nutritional intake as evidenced by increased intake (eating 80%) of each meal.

Interventions

1. Offer the child small, frequent meals.

2. Serve the child some of his favorite foods provided they are within dietary restrictions.

Rationales

1. Children with this disease often have decreased appetites. Offering small, frequent meals rather than a few large meals does not overfill or tire the child and ensures that the child will eat more at each sitting.

2. The child is more likely to eat more of each meal if he is served some of his favorite foods.

Nursing diagnosis: *Fluid volume excess related to disease process*

GOAL: The child will have no signs of fluid volume excess as evidenced by decreased edema.

Interventions

1. Weigh the child at the same time each day, using the same scale and with the child wearing the same clothes.

2. Carefully monitor the child's fluid intake and output.

3. Place the child on a sodium-restricted diet during the edematous phase of the disease.

4. Administer diuretics, as ordered.

5. Monitor the child for decreased urine specific gravity.

Rationales

1. Daily weights are necessary to determine fluctuations in the child's weight.

2. Careful monitoring is essential to assess the child's current fluid status.

3. Placing the child on a sodium-restricted diet is necessary, as sodium can decrease the elimination of fluid from the cells.

4. Diuretics may be ordered to help eliminate fluid from the child's body. However, they are sometimes ineffective in children with nephrosis.

5. Decreased urine specific gravity indicates diuresis.

Nursing diagnosis: *Knowledge deficit related to home care*

GOAL: The parents will verbalize an understanding of home care instructions.

Interventions

1. Assess the parents' understanding of the disease and prescribed treatment.

2. Instruct the parents on the importance of the child's following a sodium-restricted diet.

3. Advise the parents that the child might demonstrate mood swings and increased irritability. Make sure that they understand that this is normal so that they do not overreact. However, advise them to not allow the child to become overly manipulative.

4. Instruct the parents not to limit the child's activity level unless the child becomes overtired.

Rationales

1. Such assessment serves as a basis on which to begin teaching.

2. Reducing the child's sodium intake is necessary to prevent fluid retention.

3. Mood swings and irritability are common developments related to hospitalization and medication use.

4. Children with nephrotic syndrome usually can tolerate increased activity after the edematous phase has passed.

Documentation checklist

During the hospitalization, be sure to document the following:
___ the child's status and assessment findings upon admission
___ any changes in the child's status
___ pertinent laboratory and diagnostic findings
___ fluid intake and output
___ nutritional intake
___ the child's response to treatment
___ the child's and parents' reaction to the illness and hospitalization
___ patient and family teaching guidelines
___ discharge planning guidelines.

Ureteral Reimplantation

Introduction

Ureteral reimplantation involves the surgical removal of the ureter from the bladder and its subsequent reimplantation (or reimplantation of a synthetic ureter), usually superior to the original site. Used to treat ureterovesical reflux, distal ureteral stricture, and injuries to the lower ureter, ureteral reimplantation enables the proper drainage of urine.

The procedure is more commonly performed on boys than girls. Treatment includes the use of antibiotics and abdominal dressings, and placement of an indwelling (Foley) catheter until the child can void adequately. Potential complications include infection, renal damage, ureteral obstruction, and renal failure. Outcome depends on the degree of ureteral damage before surgery.

Assessment

Genitourinary
- hematuria
- bladder spasms

Neurologic
- restlessness
- irritability

Integumentary
- elevated temperature

Nursing diagnosis: *Potential fluid volume deficit related to surgery or postoperative withholding of oral intake*

GOAL: The child will have an adequate fluid status as evidenced by moist mucous membranes and good skin turgor.

Interventions

1. Monitor the child's fluid intake and output and assess his mucous membranes and skin turgor every 8 hours.

2. Administer I.V. fluids before and after surgery, as ordered.

3. Encourage the child to drink plenty of fluids after nausea subsides, usually within 5 to 12 hours after surgery.

Rationales

1. Frequent monitoring and assessment allow for early detection of changes in the child's fluid status and prompt intervention, when necessary.

2. I.V. fluids help keep the child well hydrated until he can tolerate oral fluids and begins voiding 10 to 30 ml/hour.

3. Increased intake helps prevent dehydration.

Nursing diagnosis: *Altered comfort: pain related to bladder spasms*

GOAL: The child will demonstrate increased comfort as evidenced by decreased guarding behavior, lack of facial tension, and verbalization (if able) of pain relief.

Interventions

1. Assess the severity and location of the child's pain or discomfort.

2. Remove all kinks and dependent loops in the catheter tubing.

3. Be especially careful when handling the child's suprapubic catheter (if one is in place).

Rationales

1. Such assessment is necessary to help determine appropriate nursing measures, including positioning, back rubs, and diversional activities.

2. Removing kinks and loops is necessary to help prevent urine retention and bladder spasms.

3. Manipulating the catheter may cause bladder spasms from irritation of the bladder muscles.

Interventions

4. Monitor the child's urine output.

5. Administer propantheline or B & O Supprettes, as ordered.

6. Use nonpharmacologic measures, such as positioning and distraction, to help control the child's pain.

7. Use pediatric pain assessment tools, such as face interval or number line pain-rating scale, to determine the degree of pain.

Rationales

4. Decreased output may indicate that the catheter is clogged.

5. These medications help relax the smooth muscle of the bladder, thereby decreasing bladder spasms.

6. Using nonpharmacologic measures may help to reduce the amount of medication the child needs to control pain. Changing the child's position alleviates pressure on nerve endings and pressure points. Distraction helps to refocus the child's attention and concentration on thoughts other than his pain.

7. Because some children are too young to verbalize pain, these tools help to identify and assess the intensity of the pain.

Nursing diagnosis: *Potential for infection related to indwelling catheter, incision, and retrograde urinary retention*

GOAL: The child will remain free of infection as evidenced by normal urinalysis results and a temperature between 97.5° and 99° F. (36.5° and 37.2° C.).

Interventions

1. Keep the catheter drainage bag below bladder level and free of kinks or loops in the tubing.

2. Use aseptic technique when emptying the catheter bag.

3. Monitor the child's urine for cloudiness or sedimentation.

4. Encourage the child to drink plenty of fluids, from 2 to 3 oz (60 to 90 ml) per hour.

5. Administer antibiotics, as ordered, and monitor the child's response to therapy.

6. Monitor the child's temperature every 4 hours, and administer antipyretics, as ordered.

7. Provide catheter care every 4 to 8 hours. Be sure to cleanse the urinary meatus with an antimicrobial solution, remove any discharge or crusted material from the catheter, and cleanse the perineal area.

Rationales

1. Keeping the drainage bag in this position helps prevent the backflow of urine into the bladder, which could lead to infection.

2. Using aseptic technique prevents contaminants from entering the urinary system.

3. Cloudiness and sedimentation are indications of possible infection requiring prompt intervention, such as administering antibiotics or changing the catheter.

4. Drinking plenty of fluids helps to dilute the urine, thereby preventing infection.

5. Antibiotics may be given prophylactically to help prevent infection.

6. An elevated temperature may signal infection.

7. Catheter care decreases the risk of bacteria infiltrating the bladder opening.

Nursing diagnosis: *Potential for injury related to catheter dislodgment*

GOAL: The child will suffer no injuries as evidenced by maintaining the catheter's placement until removal by the nurse or doctor.

Interventions

1. Tape the child's catheter (Foley or suprapubic) securely in place. If applicable, tape ureteral stents to the catheter, then secure the catheter to the child's leg.

Rationales

1. A well-secured catheter decreases the risk of accidental dislodgment.

Interventions	Rationales
2. Place restraints on the child's arms.	2. Restraints prevent the child from dislodging the catheter.
3. Attach the catheter drainage bag to side of bed, where it will not interfere with side rails.	3. Attaching the drainage bag in this manner decreases the risk of catheter dislodgment.

Nursing diagnosis: *Potential for infection related to surgical wound*

GOAL: The child will remain free of infection throughout the hospitalization as evidenced by lack of purulent drainage, swelling, and fever.

Interventions	Rationales
1. Use sterile technique when changing the child's incisional dressing.	1. Sterile technique aids in preventing the introduction of contaminants into the wound.
2. Clean the suture line, as ordered.	2. Cleaning the suture line helps to keep the incisional area free of contaminants, thereby decreasing the risk of infection.

Nursing diagnosis: *Knowledge deficit related to home care*

GOAL: The parents will verbalize an understanding of home care instructions.

Interventions	Rationales
1. Instruct the parents on the signs and symptoms of infection, including cloudy urine, elevated temperature, and purulent drainage from the incision site.	1. Knowing this information should prompt the parents to seek medical advice and attention, when necessary.
2. Teach the parents how to perform routine catheter care. Instruct them on cleansing the urinary meatus with an antimicrobial solution, removing any·discharge and crusted material from the catheter, and cleaning the perineal area.	2. Routine catheter care helps reduce the risk of introducing bacteria into the urinary tract.

Documentation checklist

During the hospitalization, be sure to document the following:
___ the child's status and assessment findings upon admission
___ any changes in the child's status
___ pertinent laboratory and diagnostic findings
___ fluid intake and output
___ nutritional intake
___ the child's response to treatment
___ the child's and parents' reaction to the illness and hospitalization
___ patient and family teaching guidelines
___ discharge planning guidelines.

Congenital Hip Dysplasia

Introduction

One of the most common congenital malformations, congenital hip dysplasia refers to displacement of the head of the femur out of the acetabulum, or hip socket. This defect can be categorized into one of three types: acetabular dysplasia, subluxation, or dislocation.

Although the exact etiology is unknown, congenital hip dysplasia may result from fetal malpositioning within the uterus. It is more common in girls and occurs in approximately 1 in every 750 live births.

Usually, the defect can be treated medically, without surgical intervention. Treatment typically includes maintaining abduction of the affected hip using a double diapering technique, Pavlik harness, braces, or a spica cast. The degree of success in correcting this deformity depends on the age at which the deformity is detected (generally, the earlier the deformity is detected, the more successful the treatment will be). Potential complications include shortening of the leg, limping, muscle contractures, and permanent damage to the femur and acetabulum.

Assessment

Musculoskeletal
- immobility of affected hip and leg
- clicking of hip (felt on examination)
- unequal skin folds on buttocks

Nursing diagnosis: *Potential for impaired skin integrity related to immobility, traction, or spica cast*

GOAL: The child will maintain skin integrity as evidenced by warm, pink intact skin and no signs of skin breakdown.

Interventions

1. Frequently inspect the child's skin, especially around bony prominences and cast openings at least once every 4 hours.

2. If the child is in a spica cast, place him in a tilted position on his back or abdomen and turn him every 2 hours. If the child is placed on his abdomen, be sure to position his face so that he can breathe.

3. Bathe the child daily, and massage his skin during baths and every 4 to 6 hours.

4. Pad the cast around the child's perianal area with plastic wrap.

5. Petal the cast after it dries. Use strips of waterproof tape or Op-Site to overlap the cast edges.

Rationales

1. Frequent inspection allows for early detection and prompt treatment of reddened areas to prevent skin breakdown.

2. Turning allows the restoration of circulation to pressure areas.

3. Cleanliness helps prevent skin breakdown. Massage promotes good circulation.

4. Plastic wrap helps keep the cast clean and prevents body fluids from contacting the skin, thereby preventing skin breakdown.

5. Petaling the cast helps keep the cast dry and prevents skin irritation.

Nursing diagnosis: *Altered bowel elimination: constipation related to immobility*

GOAL: The child will have normal bowel elimination as evidenced by regular bowel movements and no sign of constipation.

Interventions

1. Obtain a history of the child's normal bowel habits.

Rationales

1. Knowing the child's normal bowel habits (before hospitalization) helps in assessing the child's current elimination pattern and the need for intervention.

Interventions

2. Maintain a bowel record, including the times of bowel movements, stool consistency and pH, and results of any stool testing.

3. Encourage the child to drink plenty of fluids, especially fruit juices.

4. Administer stool softeners or suppositories, as ordered.

Rationales

2. Recording such information helps to identify the cause of constipation.

3. Increased fluid intake helps prevent constipation. Fruit juices may act as cathartic.

4. These agents stimulate fecal elimination by moisturizing and lubricating the feces to help ease their expulsion.

Nursing diagnosis: *Potential for infection related to break in skin integrity secondary to traction (if pins are used for traction)*

GOAL: The child will remain free of infection as evidenced by pink skin around pin sites, lack of purulent drainage, and no signs of edema.

Interventions

1. Assess the child's skin around pin sites every shift for signs of infection (redness, warmth, edema, and purulent drainage).

2. Cleanse the skin around the pin sites according to hospital policy at least every 8 hours. (Hydrogen peroxide often is used for cleaning.)

3. Use aseptic technique for pin care.

Rationales

1. Frequent assessments allow for early detection of infection and prompt treatment.

2. Routine cleaning around the pin sites helps prevent infection.

3. Aseptic technique is necessary to prevent infection when caring for a break in skin integrity.

Nursing diagnosis: *Potential for injury related to possible mechanical malfunctioning of traction or circulatory compromise*

GOAL: The child will suffer no injuries resulting from mechanical malfunctioning or circulatory compromise as evidenced by a brisk capillary refill time and warm extremities.

Interventions

1. Maintain the traction apparatus by checking the ropes for fraying and making sure the knots are secure. Tighten all bolts, and ensure that weights are hanging freely off the bed.

2. Assess the child's peripheral circulation every 2 hours, noting warmth, movement, capillary refill time, sensation of extremities, and pulse rate.

Rationales

1. The traction apparatus should be set up according to hospital policy and checked routinely to ensure patient safety.

2. Frequent assessments are necessary to allow for early detection of complications (such as tissue necrosis or compartmental syndrome), as the traction device or spica cast may interfere with circulation.

Nursing diagnosis: *Diversional activity deficit related to immobility secondary to traction or spica cast*

GOAL: The child will engage routinely in diversional activities despite his immobility.

Interventions

1. Provide the child with environmental stimulation by placing his bed near a window, occasionally moving the bed outside of the room, placing brightly colored objects on the walls and bed, and placing toys within the child's reach.

2. Provide the child with age-appropriate activities.

3. Provide for increased socialization by encouraging family members to visit or stay with the child, arranging for a volunteer to stay with him (when possible), and encouraging interaction with other children (when appropriate).

Rationales

1. Varying the child's physical environment helps decrease the boredom associated with immobility.

2. Age-appropriate activities provide developmental stimulation and decrease boredom.

3. Increased socialization helps prevent feelings of isolation and loneliness.

Nursing diagnosis: *Knowledge deficit related to home care*

GOAL: The parents will verbalize an understanding of home care instructions.

Interventions

1. Instruct the parents on the following aspects of routine cast care:
• Inspect the skin for redness (especially around bony prominences and cast openings) at least once every 4 hours. If irritation develops, keep the skin clean and dry and apply A & D Ointment to the site.
• Turn the child every 2 hours if he is in a spica cast.

• Bathe the child daily, and massage him during baths and every 4 to 6 hours.

• Pad the cast around the child's perianal area with plastic wrap.

• If the cast edges become soiled, petal the cast by overlapping the edges with strips of waterproof tape or Op-Site.

2. Explain to the parents the importance of maintaining the child on a diet that is high in calories, calcium, and protein. Also explain the benefits of providing fruits, juices, and high-fiber cereals.

3. Instruct the parents to provide environmental and developmental stimulation by:
• placing the child's bed near a window, if possible
• occasionally moving the child's bed outside of his room
• placing brightly colored objects on the walls and bed
• placing toys within the child's reach
• providing the child with age-appropriate activities.

Rationales

1. Routine cast care helps prevent skin breakdown.

• Frequent skin inspection allows for early detection and prompt treatment of irritation that could lead to breakdown.

• Frequent turning promotes the restoration of circulation to pressure areas, thereby preventing skin breakdown.

• Daily bathing cleans the skin thoroughly and helps prevent skin breakdown. Massage promotes good circulation.
• Plastic wrap helps keep the cast clean and prevents body fluids from contacting skin surfaces, thereby preventing skin breakdown.
• Petaling the cast helps keep the cast dry and prevents skin irritation.

2. A diet high in calories, calcium, and protein helps in healing and bone development. Fruits, juices, and high-fiber cereals help prevent constipation, a complication associated with immobility.

3. Varying the child's physical environment helps decrease the boredom associated with prolonged bed rest and immobility. Providing age-appropriate activities helps increase the child's developmental stimulation.

Documentation checklist

During the hospitalization, be sure to document the following:

___ the child's status and assessment findings upon admission
___ any changes in the child's status
___ pertinent laboratory and diagnostic findings
___ nutritional intake
___ growth and development status
___ the child's response to treatment
___ the child's and parents' reaction to the illness and hospitalization
___ patient and family teaching guidelines
___ discharge planning guidelines.

MUSCULOSKELETAL SYSTEM
Craniosynostosis

Introduction
Caused by premature closure of one or more of the skull sutures (commonly the sagittal sutures), craniosynostosis results in abnormal skull development and possible brain damage or mental retardation. Abnormalities usually result from continued brain growth where sutures remained open.

Treatment involves surgical separation of the sutures, usually at age 2 to 3 months. The prognosis is usually favorable the earlier the surgery is performed. Potential complications include increased intracranial pressure, brain damage, and death.

Assessment
Musculoskeletal
• abnormal shape and symmetry of head
• premature closure of skull sutures

Neurologic
• signs and symptoms of increased intracranial pressure (ICP), including papilledema, irritability, possible blindness, and possible mental retardation

Nursing diagnosis: Anxiety (parent) related to lack of knowledge about the infant's condition and need for hospitalization

GOAL: The parents will be less anxious as evidenced by verbalizing an understanding of the infant's condition and need for hospitalization and by participating in child's care.

Interventions

1. Assess the parents' understanding of the infant's condition and need for surgery. Explain the condition and surgical procedure in simple terms.

2. Explain to the parents the preoperative and postoperative events surrounding the surgery, including details on shaving the infant's head, preparation and care of the incisional site, the expected degree of swelling and pain, and the expected length of stay in the intensive care unit (ICU).

3. Allow the parents to visit the ICU before surgery.

4. Allow the parents to ask questions and to express their fears and expectations about the infant's condition and impending surgery.

Rationales

1. Explaining the infant's condition and surgical procedure in simple terms should help to clear up any misconceptions, thereby helping to ease the parents' anxiety.

2. Such explanations help the parents adjust to the infant's need for hospitalization and ease their anxieties by allowing them to anticipate events surrounding the upcoming surgery.

3. Visiting the ICU should help to prepare the parents for the infant's postoperative environment, thereby helping to reduce their anxieties.

4. By allowing the parents to ask questions and express concerns and fears, the nurse can clarify any misconceptions and offer reassurance, thereby helping to reduce the parents' anxieties.

Nursing diagnosis: Altered tissue perfusion: cerebral related to cerebral edema and increased ICP

GOAL: The infant will have no signs or symptoms of cerebral edema or increased ICP as evidenced by stable vital signs and a normal neurologic status.

Interventions

1. Keep the infant's head elevated at all times by elevating the head of the crib 30 degrees.

Rationales

1. Maintaining the infant in this position helps promote venous drainage and decreased swelling.

Interventions

2. Monitor the infant's vital signs hourly, reporting any significant changes (such as hyperthermia, decreased respiratory rate, bradycardia, and hypertension with a widening pulse pressure) immediately to the doctor.

3. Monitor the infant's neurologic status every 2 hours, reporting any significant changes (such as decreased level of consciousness, unilateral or bilateral dilated pupils with decreased response to light, vomiting, irritability, and restlessness) immediately to the doctor.

4. Carefully monitor the infant's fluid intake and output.

5. Turn the infant every 2 hours. If the child is older, encourage him to perform deep-breathing and coughing exercises to maintain respiratory function.

6. When possible, avoid subjecting the infant to the following:
• painful stimuli
• respiratory procedures (especially suctioning)
• procedures involving head rotation or neck flexion and extension
• application of pressure to neck veins.

Rationales

2. Such changes in vital signs indicate increased ICP, which requires prompt intervention.

3. Such changes in neurologic status indicate increased ICP, which requires prompt intervention.

4. Careful monitoring of the infant's fluid intake and output is necessary to prevent fluid overload and cerebral edema, which require fluid restriction.

5. Maintaining respiratory function is essential to prevent hypercapnia or hypoxia.

6. These positions and procedures may result in increased ICP.

Nursing diagnosis: *Potential for infection related to surgical incision*

GOAL: The infant will remain free of infection as evidenced by closed sutures, normal temperature, and no signs of purulent drainage and edema.

Interventions

1. Monitor the infant's temperature every 4 hours, and notify the doctor of any elevation.

2. Observe the infant for signs of cerebrospinal fluid (CSF) leakage (usually from the eye or nose). Check for glucose in the discharge using a Dextrostrip, reporting positive findings immediately to the doctor.

3. Keep the incision site clean and dry, and apply antibiotic ointment (as ordered) to the suture line. Report any signs of redness, swelling, or drainage immediately to the doctor.

Rationales

1. Increased temperature may indicate infection usually requiring the administration of antibiotics and antipyretics.

2. A dural tear during surgery can result in CSF leakage, a potential source of meningeal infection. A positive glucose test indicates CSF.

3. Skin or tissue infection can occur at the operative site and usually requires the administration of antibiotics.

Nursing diagnosis: *Potential for injury related to unstable bone fragments at the surgical site*

GOAL: The infant will suffer no injuries of the operative area.

Interventions

1. Avoid applying pressure anterior to the incision, down to and including the eye orbits and bridge of the nose.

Rationales

1. Pressure on the operative site may disrupt the normal healing process.

Interventions	Rationales
2. Pad the crib side rails.	2. Padding the crib side rails provides a cushion in case the infant accidentally bumps his head.
3. Support the back of the infant's head when lifting him.	3. Supporting the head minimizes pressure at the surgical site, thereby reducing the risk of injury.

Nursing diagnosis: *Altered nutrition: less than body requirements related to postoperative diet*

GOAL: The infant will maintain an adequate nutritional status as evidenced by stable weight and improved nutritional intake (consuming 80% of each feeding).

Interventions	Rationales
1. Weigh the infant daily, using the same scale. Carefully monitor the infant's intake and output on an ongoing basis.	1. Daily weights and careful monitoring of intake and output provide an accurate measure of the infant's current nutritional status.
2. Administer I.V. fluids until the infant can tolerate oral fluids, usually 12 hours after surgery.	2. I.V. fluids help maintain the infant's nutritional status during the immediate postoperative period.

Nursing diagnosis: *Fluid volume excess related to surgery and possible inappropriate antidiuretic hormone secretion*

GOAL: The infant will maintain normal fluid volume as evidenced by the absence of edema, ascites, ICP, headache, and congestive heart failure.

Interventions	Rationales
1. Monitor the infant's fluid intake and output hourly while in the ICU.	1. Frequent monitoring of intake and output allows for early detection and prompt treatment of any problems in the infant's current fluid status.
2. Monitor the infant for decreased serum sodium concentration, high urine osmolality, low urine volume, irritability, and lethargy. Report any of these findings immediately to the doctor.	2. These signs and symptoms may indicate a syndrome of antidiuretic hormone secretion, a common occurrence in neurosurgical procedures involving intracranial manipulation.

Nursing diagnosis: *Altered comfort: pain related to surgical procedure*

GOAL: The infant will maintain a degree of comfort as evidenced by decreased crying and irritability.

Interventions	Rationales
1. Observe the infant for crying, restlessness, loss of appetite, flushing, and increased sweating.	1. Such behavioral changes and physiologic responses indicate pain.
2. Implement appropriate comfort measures (such as positioning, diversional activities, massage, and imagery), and administer pain medication, as needed.	2. Pharmacologic and nonpharmacologic measures should be used to effectively control the infant's pain.

Nursing diagnosis: *Sensory-perceptual alteration: visual related to postoperative orbital edema*

GOAL: The infant will have no signs of visual problems as evidenced by decreased orbital edema.

Interventions

1. Prepare the parents for expected orbital edema (the infant's eyes may be swollen shut for the first few days postoperatively, but should gradually reopen by the 5th day). Offer reassurance during times of peak swelling.

2. Elevate the head of the crib 30 degrees, and apply warm compresses to the orbital area every 4 hours.

3. Help the older child to become oriented to his immediate surroundings. Provide him with a call light and side rails.

Rationales

1. Because of the orbital swelling, the infant may not be able to see for a few days. This can be particularly frightening to the parents, who need continual reassurance.

2. Elevating the head of the crib and applying warm compresses help reduce orbital swelling.

3. The unfamiliar environment and sounds of the ICU can be particularly frightening and potentially unsafe for a child with impaired vision.

Nursing diagnosis: *Knowledge deficit related to home care*

GOAL: The parents will verbalize an understanding of home care instructions.

Interventions

1. Instruct the parents on the importance of the following:
• maintaining routine incisional care by keeping the incision clean (cleansing the site with one-half strength hydrogen peroxide) and dry (with dressings) until sutures are removed and by observing the site for signs and symptoms of infection (purulent drainage, swelling, fever, headache, malaise)
• keeping the head of the crib elevated 30 degrees

• maintaining safety precautions in the home, such as using side rails or bumper pads, placing the infant on a rug or thick blanket when on the floor, and prohibiting roughhousing and running if the child is older.

2. Emphasize the need to keep follow-up appointments, as scheduled.

Rationales

1. The parents need to be informed of the importance of home care.
• Routine incisional care helps decrease the risk of serious complications, such as infection.

• Keeping the head of the bed elevated helps reduce orbital edema.
• Maintaining safety is important to prevent accidental bumping of the infant's head, which could lead to impaired healing.

2. Follow-up is neccessary to monitor any growth or changes in the child's head shape and to evaluate the effectiveness of surgery.

Documentation checklist

During the hospitalization, be sure to document the following:
___ the child's status and assessment findings upon admission
___ any changes in the child's status
___ pertinent laboratory and diagnostic findings
___ fluid intake and output
___ nutritional intake
___ growth and development status
___ the child's response to treatment
___ the child's and parents' reaction to the illness and hospitalization
___ patient and family teaching guidelines
___ discharge planning guidelines.

MUSCULOSKELETAL SYSTEM

Fractures

Introduction

Fractures, usually caused by accidents (such as falls or motor vehicle accidents) during childhood, are classified as follows:
• complete fracture—the bone is broken entirely across, resulting in a break in the continuity of bone (may be further classified as transverse, oblique, spiral, or torsion)
• incomplete fracture—the bone does not break entirely across and does not result in destruction of the continuity of bone
• closed (simple) fracture—the break does not puncture the skin surface
• open (compound) fracture—in which the break causes an external wound on the skin surface.

Common fracture sites include the arm, clavicle, knee, and femur. Treatment includes reduction and immobilization of the fracture and may involve traction, casting, or surgery. The outcome usually depends on the severity of the fracture and the treatment provided. Potential complications include the development of fat emboli, improper bone growth, compartmental syndrome, and infection.

Assessment

Assessment should be based on the history of the injury as well as the physical examination.

Musculoskeletal
• skeletal deformity
• muscle spasm
• pain or tenderness
• bony crepitus

Neurologic
• loss of motor function
• impaired sensation

Integumentary
• swelling
• bruising

Nursing diagnosis: *Altered comfort: pain related to muscle spasm, swelling, or bleeding*

GOAL: The child will have no signs of pain as evidenced by relaxed facial expressions, verbalization of comfort, ability to sleep, and decreased need for analgesics.

Interventions

1. Assess the degree and level of the child's pain using pediatric assessment tools (such as a face interval or line number pain-rating scale).

2. Institute the following comfort measures:
• Keep the child in proper body alignment.

• Provide support above and below the fracture site when moving the child. Move the child carefully, and avoid jarring the bed.

• Monitor for any pressure areas caused by traction, the child's cast, or bedclothes.
• Elevate the area above the level of the heart.

• Apply ice to the fracture site, as ordered.

Rationales

1. Assessing the child's pain allows the nurse to determine the specific area of pain, monitor for changes in the degree of pain before and after interventions, and monitor for complications, such as impaired circulation.

2. Promoting comfort helps to relieve the child's pain.
• Keeping the child in proper body alignment decreases joint strain and prevents contractures.
• Because any movement may potentiate pain, supporting the child above and below the fracture site and avoiding sudden, jerking motions help promote comfort when moving the child.
• Prolonged pressure may cause ischemia, which results in pain.
• Elevating the area above the level of the heart promotes venous return and decreases edema, which exerts pressure on nerve endings, causing pain.
• Applying ice to the fracture site promotes vasoconstriction, which inhibits edema and pain.

Interventions	Rationales
3. Administer analgesics or muscle relaxants (or both), as ordered. Be sure to give medications promptly, especially when the child indicates by verbal complaints, facial expressions, irritability, or body positioning that he is in pain.	3. Analgesics help relieve pain; muscle relaxants help reduce muscle spasms. Giving medications promptly helps ensure that the child's pain will remain controllable.

Nursing diagnosis: *Altered tissue perfusion: peripheral related to bleeding, swelling, cast, or traction*

GOAL: The child will maintain adequate peripheral tissue perfusion as evidenced by decreasing pain; strong pulses distal to the fracture site; pinkish, warm skin, a brisk capillary refill time, and normal sensation in the extremity distal to the fracture site; and pain-free movement of the extremity distal to the fracture site.

Interventions	Rationales
1. Assess the rate and volume of the pulse distal to the fracture site every 2 to 4 hours.	1. Such assessment can indicate whether the fracture has impeded blood flow to the distal extremity, in which case the doctor will replace the cast or readjust the traction device.
2. Assess the color, temperature, and capillary refill time of the affected extremity as compared to that of the unaffected extremity.	2. Assessing the affected extremity as compared to that of the unaffected extremity helps in determining whether the extremity is adequately perfused.
3. Assess the child's sensation distal to the fracture site (using touch, pressure, or the pin prick method) every 15 minutes for the first hour, then hourly for the next 24 hours and every 4 hours thereafter.	3. Such assessment is necessary to determine whether perfusion to the nerves is intact.
4. Assess movement distal to the fracture site every 2 to 4 hours.	4. Such assessment helps in determining whether the fracture has impaired the child's movement, which could result in neurologic damage.
5. Assess the degree and level of the child's pain using pediatric assessment tools (such as a face interval or line number pain-rating scale).	5. Such assessment helps to determine the specific area of pain, monitor any changes in pain before and after intervention, and monitor for complications, such as impaired circulation.
6. Notify the doctor immediately of abnormal signs or symptoms, including decreased sensation, pallor, cool temperature at the fracture site, and decreased peripheral pulses.	6. Early detection ensures prompt treatment to prevent permanent injury resulting from impaired circulation, such as tissue necrosis and nerve damage, leading to permanent damage and possible amputation.

Nursing diagnosis: *Potential for impaired skin integrity related to immobility from cast or traction*

GOAL: The child will maintain skin integrity as evidenced by no signs of irritation or redness and no breaks in the skin.

Interventions	Rationales
1. Assess the child's skin for redness or irritation, especially around pressure points. If redness or irritation is apparent, massage pressure points at least once every 4 hours. Also check to see whether the cast needs trimming or the traction device needs padding.	1. Redness or irritation may signal impending skin breakdown. Relieving pressure points promptly should prevent any further breakdown.

Interventions	Rationales
2. Turn and reposition the child at least once every 2 hours.	2. Turning and repositioning help relieve pressure, thereby preventing skin breakdown.
3. Provide the child with sheepskin padding, an eggcrate mattress, elbow and heel pads, and an overbed trapeze.	3. Padding, such as sheepskin padding and elbow and heel pads, help reduce skin abrasion. An eggcrate mattress helps reduce pressure by distributing body weight evenly on the bed surface. An overbed trapeze allows the child to lift himself without causing abrasions to the skin.
4. Keep the child's skin dry and free of irritants by taking the following measures:	4. Moisture and irritation are potential causes of skin breakdown in children with fractures.
• Use plastic-backed disposable diapers or plastic wrap to tuck around the perianal region to protect the cast from moisture or soiling.	• Protecting the cast from moisture prevents bacterial growth that could lead to infection and skin breakdown.
• Instruct the child to avoid inserting any object under the cast.	• Inserting any object under the cast may break the skin and cause infection.
• Petal the edges of the cast.	• Petaling the cast decreases the likelihood that loose plaster might fall into the cast and irritate the skin.

Nursing diagnosis: *Impaired gas exchange related to complications secondary to the fracture and immobility*

GOAL: The child will develop no signs or symptoms of impaired gas exchange as evidenced by normal vital signs, unlabored respirations, and remaining alert and oriented.

Interventions	Rationales
1. Assess the child's vital signs and neurologic status, noting any wheezing, cyanosis, sluggish pupil response, and lethargy. Report any of these abnormalities immediately to the doctor.	1. Such assessment may indicate complications, such as hypovolemia secondary to hemorrhage or pulmonary embolus, altered level of consciousness secondary to pulmonary embolus or hypovolemia, or respiratory distress secondary to lung secretions or pulmonary embolus.
2. Instruct the child to turn, cough, and deep-breathe every 2 hours.	2. Turning, coughing, and deep breathing help clear secretions and expand the lungs fully.
3. Monitor the child's hematocrit and hemoglobin levels.	3. These levels directly measure the oxygen-carrying capacity of the blood. Low levels may indicate the need for the administration of packed red blood cells.

Nursing diagnosis: *Altered bowel elimination: constipation related to immobility*

GOAL: The child will maintain normal bowel elimination as evidenced by maintaining normal bowel movements and passing softer stools.

Interventions	Rationales
1. Check and record all bowel movements, noting the frequency and consistency of all stools.	1. Monitoring the child's bowel movements helps in determining the need for intervention.
2. Increase the child's fluid and dietary fiber intake, as necessary. Encourage the child to drink plenty of fluids and to eat whole-grain cereals, fruits, and vegetables.	2. Water facilitates the movement of consumed material along the digestive tract. Fiber increases the bulk of feces.
3. Administer stool softeners, as ordered.	3. Stool softeners act as active surface agents that enable water to penetrate fecal material, which allows for easy passage of stool.

Nursing diagnosis: *Potential for activity intolerance related to immobility from cast or traction*

GOAL: The child will participate in self-care and social activities as evidenced by performing activities of daily living (ADLs), exercising, and engaging in age-appropriate activities.

Interventions

1. Encourage the child to perform ADLs (as tolerated) and to participate in decisions concerning his care.

2. Involve the child in a regular exercise program, as ordered. Exercises may include the following:
• active range-of-motion (ROM) exercises on all unaffected joints every 4 hours
• isometric exercises involving the affected area every 2 to 4 hours
• arm-strengthening exercises, if appropriate.

3. Encourage the child to socialize by providing him with a wheelchair or crutches for easy ambulation. If the child cannot ambulate on his own, move him around on a stretcher or move his bed into the playroom.

4. Provide the child with age-appropriate activities, such as toys, games, television, and reading materials.

5. Encourage the parents to bring in the child's school assignments (and a tutor, if necessary) and to arrange for siblings and peers to visit (if age-appropriate).

Rationales

1. Allowing the child to participate in his care promotes independence and feelings of self-control.

2. Regular exercise helps maintain muscle tone and joint mobility and allows the child to prepare for crutch walking, if this is anticipated.

3. Ambulation promotes feelings of independence and increases the likelihood that the child will engage in age-appropriate activities.

4. Such activites are an essential part of the child's normal growth and development.

5. School work and visits from siblings and peers encourage the child to maintain contact with outside interests.

Nursing diagnosis: *Knowledge deficit related to home care*

GOAL: The parents will verbalize an understanding of home care instructions.

Interventions

1. Explain to the parents the normal healing process of a fracture. Also explain the importance of maintaining routine cast care, including:
• protecting the cast from moisture and soil with a plastic-backed diaper or plastic wrap
• petaling the cast to prevent loose plaster from falling into the cast
• notifying the doctor if the cast is loose or broken.

2. Instruct the parents to assess the child's neurovascular status by noting the child's skin color and temperature (should be warm and dry) and capillary refill time (should be 3 to 5 seconds) and by checking for impaired sensation or movement, pain, and swelling.

3. Instruct the parents on providing skin care, especially to the buttocks and back. Tell them to cleanse the skin using a moisturizing lotion and powder and to observe for redness and irritation. Also instruct them to keep the child from inserting objects into the cast.

4. Instruct the parents on the importance of regular exercise, such as active ROM exercises, isometric exercises, and physical therapy (if needed for crutch walking).

Rationales

1. Understanding the normal healing process of a fracture and the importance of cast care should promote compliance with home care.

2. Such assessments are necessary to identify possible complications that require immediate medical attention.

3. Proper skin care is necessary to prevent the risk of infection or trauma to the skin.

4. Regular exercise helps prevent muscle stiffness and contractures.

Interventions

5. Help the parents to assess their home environment to determine the child's special needs. Ask about the location of the child's bed, the bathroom, and stairs and whether the child will require any specialized equipment, such as an overbed trapeze, bedpan, urinal, side rails, shower stool, crutches, or a wheelchair. Also ask about the child's school needs, such as an alternate means of transportation, specialized clothing, and tutoring.

6. Instruct the parents to encourage the child to drink plenty of fluids and to increase his dietary fiber.

7. Offer suggestions for age-appropriate activities.

Rationales

5. Helping to assess the child's home environment enables the parents to anticipate and prepare for the child's special needs.

6. Increased fluid and dietary fiber help prevent constipation, a common complication of immobility.

7. Age-appropriate activities are essential to the child's normal growth and development and help divert the child's attention from his immobility.

Documentation checklist

During the hospitalization, be sure to document the following:
___ the child's status and assessment findings upon admission
___ any changes in the child's status
___ pertinent laboratory and diagnostic findings
___ nutritional intake
___ growth and developmental status
___ the child's response to treatment
___ the child's and parents' reaction to the illness and hospitalization
___ patient and family teaching guidelines
___ discharge planning guidelines.

Osteomyelitis

Introduction

An infection of the bone and marrow, osteomyelitis is caused by septicemia (usually from a *Staphylococcus* infection) resulting from a wound, fracture, surgery, or burn injury. This disease occurs most often in children age 5 to 15, with a higher incidence among boys.

Treatment usually involves administering antibiotics I.V. and immobilizing the infected bone. The prognosis generally depends on the severity of the infection and the response to antibiotic therapy. Potential complications include hematologic, hepatic, or renal damage related to high doses of antibiotics, joint or bone damage, abscesses, and amputation.

Assessment

Musculoskeletal
• localized tenderness (usually over a bone or joint)
• limited range of motion
• guarding of extremity

Neurologic
• generalized malaise
• irritability

Integumentary
• elevated temperature
• increased warmth with edema at affected site

Nursing diagnosis: *Potential for infection related to wound contamination*

GOAL: The child will remain free of further infection as evidenced by decreases in temperature, edema, fever, erythema, warmth at the infection site, white blood cell (WBC) count, and sedimentation rate.

Interventions

1. Use good hand-washing technique before treating the child.

2. Assess the infection site each shift and document any signs of exudate, edema, erythema, or warmth.

3. Monitor the child's vital signs every 4 hours for increases in temperature, heart rate, and respirations.

4. Monitor the child's WBC count, erythrocyte sedimentation rate, and blood cultures. Notify the doctor of any significant changes.

5. Administer antibiotics (cephalosporins and penicillinase-resistant agents are the drugs of choice) and antipyretics, as ordered. Monitor the child for drug compatibility and adverse reactions.

6. Maintain a patent irrigation system, as indicated.

7. Maintain wound and skin precautions when handling infective material.

8. Use sterile technique for all dressing changes.

Rationales

1. Good hand washing decreases the spread of nosocomial infection.

2. Exudate, edema, erythema, and warmth indicate ongoing infection, possibly indicating the need for medication adjustment or change.

3. Such changes in vital signs indicate ongoing infection, possibly indicating the need for medication adjustment or change.

4. Elevations in the WBC count and erythrocyte sedimentation rate indicate ongoing infection. Blood cultures (positive in 60% of children with osteomyelitis) indicate an ongoing systemic infection.

5. Antibiotics help fight bacterial infections. Antipyretics help decrease fever.

6. Proper drainage prevents the risk of tissue damage from accumulation of purulent exudate or clots.

7. Such precautions are necessary to help prevent the risk of contamination.

8. Sterile technique helps prevent the introduction of bacteria into the wound.

Nursing diagnosis: *Impaired skin integrity related to infection*

GOAL: The child will have no signs of skin breakdown as evidenced by decreased edema and new skin growth at the surgical site.

Interventions

1. Elevate the affected extremity 30 degrees.

2. Assess the peripheral pulses, skin color, and sensation of the affected extremity every 4 hours. Also check the capillary refill time of the extremity distal to the splint or cast every 4 hours.

3. Monitor the amount of drainage, especially bloody drainage, around the cast or splint every 4 hours. Notify the doctor if the drainage soaks through the cast.

4. Use sterile technique when changing dressings.

5. Provide the following cast or splint care, as needed:

• Petal the child's cast.

• Keep the cast or splint dry.

• Instruct the child to avoid putting objects into the cast or splint.

Rationales

1. Elevation ensures venous return, thereby decreasing edema and the risk of skin breakdown.

2. In edematous or splinted extremities, frequent assessment of pulses, skin color, and sensation is necessary to ensure adequate circulation and prevent nerve impairment. Capillary refill time should be 3 seconds.

3. Monitoring is essential to determine the amount of wound drainage. Excessive bloody drainage may indicate hemorrhage or infection.

4. Sterile technique decreases the risk of contamination and possible skin breakdown. Frequent dressing changes keep the wound clean and dry and allow the nurse to evaluate the wound.

5. Proper care of casts or splints is essential to prevent breaks in the child's skin integrity.

• Petaling the cast helps to prevent loose plaster from falling into the cast, which could cause irritation and possible breakdown.

• Keeping the cast dry is essential because moisture can lead to skin breakdown.

• Putting objects, such as food or toys into the cast or splint can cause injury or irritation to the skin.

Nursing diagnosis: *Altered comfort: pain related to inflammation and infection*

GOAL: The child will have decreased pain as evidenced by decreased irritability, verbalizations of decreased pain, and relaxed behavior when interacting with others.

Interventions

1. Assess and document characteristics of the child's pain, including location, type, duration, and pattern. To determine the severity of pain, have the child use a face interval or number line pain-rating scale.

2. Administer analgesics, as ordered or needed. Document the child's response.

3. Elevate the affected extremity 30 degrees.

4. Move the affected extremity smoothly and gently.

5. Use distraction techniques, such as television, music, or games, to help comfort the child.

6. Promote periods of quiet and rest.

7. Document the most effective strategy for pain relief in the child's record.

Rationales

1. Frequent assessment and documentation help to determine the need for intervention or to evaluate the effectiveness of previous interventions.

2. Analgesics help relieve pain.

3. Elevating the affected extremity decreases edema and pain by promoting venous return.

4. Any sudden or abrupt movements may increase the child's pain.

5. Distraction helps to divert the child's attention from his pain and enables him to focus on other activities.

6. Quiet and rest are important because fatigue can lessen the child's tolerance for pain.

7. Documentation helps ensure consistent pain control by all team members caring for the child.

Nursing diagnosis: *Impaired physical mobility related to infection*

GOAL: The child will demonstrate optimal mobility (as allowed or tolerated) as evidenced by performing passive range-of-motion (ROM) exercises and moving his extremities.

Interventions

1. Maintain immobility of the affected extremity using a splint or cast, as ordered.

2. Assess the skin color, sensation, and movement of the affected extremity every 4 hours.

3. Consult a physical therapist or occupational therapist, as necessary, to develop an effective exercise program that includes ROM and isometric exercises.

Rationales

1. Immobilization with a splint or cast helps maintain proper bone alignment, thereby ensuring proper healing and optimal mobility of the recovered extremity.

2. Such assessment is necessary to prevent circulatory or nerve impairment and to evaluate the effectiveness of keeping the extremity immobile.

3. An effective exercise program is necessary to maintain muscle strength, ensure optimal recovery, and prevent potential complications associated with immobility, such as contractures, limb shortening, and limping.

Nursing diagnosis: *Altered nutrition: less than body requirements related to increased metabolic needs for wound healing*

GOAL: The child will have an improved nutritional intake as evidenced by maintaining a stable weight and consuming at least 80% of each meal.

Interventions

1. Assess the child's nutritional and emotional status, noting any sign of apathy, irritability, pallor, edema, or cachexia.

2. Monitor the child's intake and output, reporting urine output of less than 1 ml/kg/hour.

3. Document and evaluate the child's food intake every shift.

4. Serve the child small, frequent high-calorie meals and drinks. Consult the hospital dietitian, as necessary, to ensure that the child receives a well-balanced diet and the proper number of calories.

5. Serve some of the child's favorite foods, if they are within dietary restrictions.

Rationales

1. Assessing for such findings may indicate bowel obstruction or constipation, possibly contributing to the child's unstable weight.

2. Oliguria, a sign of dehydration, often occurs in osteomyelitis.

3. Knowing the child's food intake helps in determining whether the child is receiving adequate nutrition for wound healing.

4. Small, frequent meals do not overfill the stomach, enabling the child to eat more of each meal. A high-calorie diet helps in the normal healing process.

5. Serving the child some of his favorite foods helps ensure compliance with the dietary regimen.

Nursing diagnosis: *Ineffective family coping: compromised related to prolonged hospitalization*

GOAL: The child and parents will demonstrate appropriate coping and support mechanisms as evidenced by maintaining communcation among family members and significant others.

Interventions

1. Encourage the parents and other family members to assist in planning the child's daily activities. Designate at least two activities each day for the family to do with the child.

Rationales

1. Family involvement in the child's activities helps foster a sense of family unity, thereby enabling them to cope with the child's hospitalization.

Interventions

2. Arrange for a foster grandparent or volunteer to stay with the child when the parents are away from the child's hospital room.

3. Use a treatment room when performing any invasive procedure on the child.

4. Encourage the parents to help the child to continue his schoolwork by bringing in the child's assignments and arranging for a tutor, if necessary.

5. Update the parents each day on the child's current status.

Rationales

2. The parents may need time away from the child to rest and to take care of other family matters. Time away from the hospital also allows them to use diversionary methods of coping with the child's hospitalization.

3. Performing invasive procedures in a treatment room rather than the child's hospital room allows the child to maintain a sense of security while in his own room, thereby helping him to cope with the hospitalization.

4. Continuing with schoolwork allows the child to cope with the hospitalization by maintaining his school standing and contact with outside interests.

5. Daily updates help the parents to cope by decreasing anxiety and fostering trust in the health care team.

Nursing diagnosis: *Knowledge deficit related to home care*

GOAL: The parents will verbalize an understanding of home care instructions.

Interventions

1. Explain to the parents the basic etiology and pathophysiology of osteomyelitis.

2. Review with the parents the signs and symptoms of recurring infection (see the "Assessment" section at the beginning of this care plan).

3. Instruct the parents on the purpose and use of antibiotics, including details on administration, dosage, and potential adverse effects.

4. Instruct the parents on the importance of providing a well-balanced diet.

5. Instruct the parents on the importance of maintaining cast or splint care, including details on:
• petaling the cast edges
• keeping the cast or splint dry
• instructing the child to avoid placing objects in the cast or splint.

6. Instruct the parents on the importance of keeping all follow-up appointments.

7. Refer the parents to the school nurse or a home health nurse, as necessary.

Rationales

1. Such explanations should help to prevent recurrence of the infection.

2. Knowing the signs and symptoms helps in early detection and prompt treatment of infection, which decreases the risk of complications.

3. Knowing this information helps promote compliance with the medication regimen and should alert the parents to the need for medical advice and assistance, when necessary.

4. A well-balanced diet provides essential vitamins, calories, protein, and calcium to promote healing.

5. Maintaining proper cast or splint care helps in preventing complications of the skin or affected extremities.

6. Follow-up appointments are necessary to evaluate the clinical progress of the disease and to help prevent reinfection.

7. A school nurse or home care nurse can monitor the child's progress and compliance with the overall treatment regimen.

Documentation checklist

During the hospitalization, be sure to document the following:
___ the child's status and assessment findings upon admission
___ any changes in the child's status
___ pertinent laboratory and diagnostic findings
___ nutritional intake
___ growth and development status
___ the child's response to treatment
___ the child's and parents' reaction to the illness and hospitalization
___ patient and family teaching guidelines
___ discharge planning guidelines.

Rheumatoid Arthritis

Introduction

Juvenile rheumatoid arthritis—characterized by inflammation of the joints resulting in decreased mobility, pain, and swelling—may be classified according to one of three forms: polyarticular, pauciarticular, or systemic.

Polyarticular arthritis, which involves many joints (particularly the small joints of the hands), occurs more frequently in girls. *Pauciarticular* arthritis, which primarily affects only a few joints (such as the knees, ankles, and elbows), occurs more frequently in girls. *Systemic* arthritis, which characteristically involves a high fever, rheumatoid rash, and polyarthritis, equally affects boys and girls.

Although the exact cause of rheumatoid arthritis is unknown, it is believed to be linked to certain immunodeficiencies. Peak onset is associated with two different age-groups: children age 2 to 5 and children age 9 to 12.

Treatment may include the administration of corticosteroids, nonsteroidal anti-inflammatory agents, gold salts, and penicillamine as well as physical therapy and joint replacement surgery. Potential complications include joint deformity and adverse reactions resulting from medication use, including bleeding, GI distress, ulcers, blindness, and death. Although the prognosis usually depends on the severity of the disease, many children have some form of joint disability.

Assessment

Musculoskeletal
- joint pain
- joint swelling
- decreased mobility
- joint inflammation

Hematologic
- elevated erythrocyte sedimentation rate

Nursing diagnosis: Altered comfort: pain related to inflamed joints, joint immobility, and gastric irritation secondary to aspirin use

GOAL: The child will have decreased pain as evidenced by the ability to do range-of-motion (ROM) exercises, verbalization of decreased pain, and absence of gastric irritation.

Interventions

1. Assess the intensity and location of the child's pain as well as the relationship of the pain to the time of day and activities performed. Use pediatric pain assessment tools, such as a face-interval or line number pain-rating scale, in your evaluation.

2. Provide a warm bath or shower (approximately 100° F. [37.8° C.]) each morning for 10 to 12 minutes.

3. Administer analgesics and anti-inflammatory medications, as ordered (most commonly, aspirin four times daily). To prevent stomach irritation or pain, administer aspirin with food, milk, or an antacid about half an hour before the child rises in the morning.

4. Monitor the child for signs and symptoms of aspirin toxicity, including ringing in the ears, decreased hearing, drowsiness, nausea, vomiting, irritability, unusual behavior, and rapid, deep breathing.

5. Help the child perform active and passive ROM exercises after first consulting with the physical therapist. Encourage ambulation during play activities.

Rationales

1. Knowing this information helps in determining the type and amount of pain medication needed.

2. Heat helps relieve pain and joint stiffness. Because joint stiffness usually is worse in the morning, a warm shower is often helpful at that time.

3. Aspirin provides pain relief and decreases the joint inflammation associated with arthritis. Administering aspirin with food or milk decreases the risk of gastric irritation; giving it in the early morning is most effective, as joint stiffness usually worsens upon rising.

4. Monitoring for such signs and symptoms is important, as the child may require a dosage reduction or discontinuation of aspirin therapy.

5. Moving the joints helps relieve joint stiffness; however, excessive exercise may worsen the pain. Consulting the physical therapist is necessary to plan an individualized program for the child.

Interventions	Rationales
6. Maintain the child's proper body alignment by propping him with pillows when in bed.	6. Maintaining proper body alignment helps ease pain and prevents contractures.
7. Consult the physical therapist about the use of splints. Set up a schedule for when splints should be put on and when they should be taken off.	7. Splints may be necessary to help prevent contractures. They should be taken off at regular intervals to ease pain and prevent skin breakdown.

Nursing diagnosis: *Self-care deficit related to pain, immobility, and joint contractures*

GOAL: The child will have no self-care deficits as evidenced by his ability to perform activities of daily living (ADLs).

Interventions	Rationales
1. Assess the child's current level of self-care.	1. Such assessment is necessary to establish a baseline of the child's current abilities for further comparison and evaluation of his progress.
2. Help the child to establish a self-care program based on mutual goals and expectations. Be sure to consult the occupational therapist and physical therapist before completing the plan.	2. Allowing the child to help design a self-care plan fosters a sense of control over the situation and encourages participation and compliance. An occupational therapist can provide advice and therapy regarding the child's ADLs and need for adaptation devices, such as bathroom and bedside support bars, tongs (to lift and reach objects), and fasteners (to help buckle and button clothing). A physical therapist can help to individualize an exercise program designed to maintain ROM of the affected joints.
3. Encourage independence in performing ADLs; however, be sure to provide assistance, when necessary.	3. The child's degree of independence in performing ADLs may vary depending on the severity of his pain.

Nursing diagnosis: *Disturbance in self-concept: body image related to the effects of the chronic illness and the disabling nature of the disease*

GOAL: The child will have no disturbance in self-concept as evidenced by verbalizing an acceptance of his altered body image.

Interventions	Rationales
1. Establish a therapeutic relationship with the child and encourage him to express his feelings about his body image.	1. Establishing a therapeutic relationship helps the child to develop a feeling of trust, thereby opening the lines of communication. Having the child express his feelings allows the nurse to determine the child's current cognitive and emotional level.
2. Correct any misconceptions the child may have concerning his condition and help to build on his positive feelings and coping skills.	2. The child may feel overwhelmed and need help in sorting out the facts from his preconceived perceptions. He also may need help in coping and dealing with his negative feelings.
3. Encourage the child to interact with his peers, family, and the hospital staff.	3. Interaction with and acceptance by others helps build a positive self-concept.
4. Consult social services, a child-life worker, or a psychologist, as needed.	4. Such professionals can help to identify the child's needs to help improve his self-concept by using play therapy and teaching appropriate coping skills.
5. Provide time for the child and parents to express their feelings related to the crippling effects of the disease.	5. The child and parents undoubtedly have certain feelings about the disabling nature of the disease that they need to express to help them cope more effectively.

Nursing diagnosis: *Ineffective family coping: compromised related to the effects of the child's chronic illness*

GOAL: The family will exhibit effective coping skills as evidenced by expressing their feelings about the child's chronic illness and by stating what resources are available to them.

Interventions

1. Assess the family's dynamics and interactions, including role expectations and boundaries.

2. Assess the family's knowledge and current use of support systems.

3. Encourage the family to express their feelings, and help them to deal with such threatening feelings as guilt, anger, hopelessness, grief, and anxiety.

4. Help the family to recognize ineffective coping patterns and to find alternate means of dealing with their problems.

5. Refer the family to available resources within the hospital and the community, such as social services and the Juvenile Arthritis Foundation.

Rationales

1. Such assessment may reveal ineffective family communication patterns and unrealistic expectations.

2. Support systems, such as extended family, friends, and church and community resources, help the family remain healthy and intact. Knowing how the family uses these resources is essential before the nurse can suggest alternate coping and support systems.

3. Families with chronically ill children often harbor negative feelings, which they need to express to receive emotional support.

4. Identifying ineffective behavior is the first step toward change. Assisting the family with problem-solving skills encourages them to discover alternate solutions.

5. Families need to be aware of what resources are available to them for support in their current situation.

Nursing diagnosis: *Knowledge deficit related to home care*

GOAL: The parents will verbalize an understanding of home care instructions.

Interventions

1. Explain to the parents the purpose and use of pain medications, including details on administration, dosages, and potential adverse effects.

2. Explain to the parents the importance of regular exercise, including active and passive ROM exercises.

3. Stress to the parents the importance of promoting self-care.

4. Instruct the parents and child on the use of adaptive devices, such as fasteners and tongs.

5. Refer the parents to appropriate community resources, such as the Juvenile Arthritis Foundation.

Rationales

1. Understanding the purpose and use of pain medications helps the parents to comply with the medication regimen. Knowing the potential adverse efffects should prompt them to seek medical advice and attention, when necessary.

2. Regular exercise is necessary to help relieve joint stiffness and prevent contractures.

3. Depending on the degree of pain, the child should be encouraged to perform self-care activities to promote self-esteem.

4. Knowing how to use such devices promotes independence and improved self-esteem.

5. Community resources provide information and support to families of chronically ill children.

Documentation checklist

During the hospitalization, be sure to document the following:

___ the child's status and assessment findings upon admission
___ any changes in the child's status
___ pertinent laboratory and diagnostic findings
___ nutritional intake
___ growth and development status
___ the child's response to treatment
___ the child's and parents' reaction to the illness and hospitalization
___ patient and family teaching guidelines
___ discharge planning guidelines.

Cleft Lip and Cleft Palate

Introduction

Congenital defects of the lip and palate, cleft lip and cleft palate may occur separately or together. Caused by the failure or incomplete union of embryonic facial structures, these defects tend to be hereditary but may result from nongenetic factors. Often, they are associated with other anomalies as well. The incidence of these defects is 1 in 750 live births.

Cleft lip, which is more common in girls, may range from a slight indentation to an open cleft. Treatment involves surgical repair to correct the child's cosmetic appearance, usually between ages 1 and 3 months. Cleft palate, which is more common in boys, may involve only the soft palate or may extend to the hard palate and nose. Treatment for this defect involves surgical repair, usually between ages 1 and 2, before the child's speech is well developed.

Potential complications include infection, otitis media, hearing loss, and lack of parental attachment. The expected outcome for these defects is generally favorable; however, children with cleft palate often have speech and dental problems.

Assessment

EENT
• abnormal separation of the upper lip or palate (or both)
• separation of the upper gum
• impaired dentition

Respiratory
• respiratory distress with aspiration
• possible dyspnea

Gastrointestinal
• difficulty feeding

Psychosocial
• impaired parent-infant bonding

Nursing diagnosis: *Altered nutrition: less than body requirements related to impaired feeding (preoperative)*

GOAL: The infant will maintain adequate nutritional status as evidenced by gaining the appropriate weight (1 to 2 lb/month).

Interventions

1. Use an appropriate nipple and bottle (soft, cross-cut nipples or those especially designed for premature infants; Breck feeder) to feed the infant.

2. Place the nipple in the infant's mouth on the side opposite the cleft, toward the back of the tongue.

3. Feed the infant in a relaxed upright or semisitting position.

4. Burp the infant after every ½ to 1 oz (15 to 30 ml); however, avoid removing the nipple frequently during the feeding process.

5. Schedule the feedings so that the infant consumes the appropriate amount of calories within a 30- to 45-minute period.

Rationales

1. Because of his inability to create a vacuum, an infant with cleft palate may have an ineffective sucking reflex. Use of an appropriate nipple and bottle helps facilitate feeding. The specific type of nipple depends on the severity of the cleft.

2. Placing the nipple in this manner facilitates the infant's "stripping" action (pressing the nipple against the tongue and the roof of the mouth to expel milk) by which he obtains formula from the bottle.

3. Feeding in this position prevents nasal regurgitation and choking.

4. Burping is essential because the infant may swallow more air than usual, causing discomfort. Removing the nipple frequently may cause him to tire and become frustrated, resulting in incomplete feedings.

5. Limiting the feedings to 30 to 45 minutes' duration is important because feeding for a longer period often tires the infant and results in poor weight gain.

Nursing diagnosis: *Potential for infection related to the defect (preoperative)*

GOAL: The infant will have no signs of infection as evidenced by a normal temperature and no signs of ear drainage or redness.

Interventions

1. Offer the infant ⅛ to ⅜ oz (5 to 10 ml) of water after each feeding.

2. Remove crusted formula or milk with a moist cotton-tipped applicator or a 1:2 solution of hydrogen peroxide and water.

3. After each feeding, place the infant in an infant seat or position him in his crib on his right side with the head of the bed elevated 30 degrees.

4. Inspect the infant's eardrums for signs of infection, including ear drainage, odor, and redness. Begin administering antibiotics, as ordered.

Rationales

1. Water helps to clean the nasal passages and palate and prevents the collection of milk in the eustachian tubes, thereby preventing the growth of bacteria that could lead to infection.

2. Loosening and removing crusted material helps to keep the cleft clean and free of bacterial growth, thereby decreasing the risk of infection.

3. Positioning the infant in this manner helps prevent aspiration of formula that could lead to pneumonia.

4. Recurring otitis media, resulting from abnormal eustachian tube functioning, is associated with cleft lip and cleft palate.

Nursing diagnosis: *Potential for altered parenting related to the stress of hospitalization (preoperative)*

GOAL: The parents will incorporate the infant's care into their normal life-style and verbalize their feelings about the infant's appearance.

Interventions

1. Provide opportunities for the parents to hold and cuddle the infant and to practice caregiving tasks before discharge.

2. Encourage the parents to prepare the family, including siblings and other relatives, for the infant's arrival home. Advise them to explain to the family the infant's appearance in simple terms, to show them pictures, and to have them visit the infant in the hospital.

3. Encourage the parents to treat the infant as a normal family member and to incorporate his care into their daily routine.

4. Encourage the parents to seek the participation of other family members or friends in the infant's feeding and routine care.

5. Refer the parents to an appropriate support group, if available.

Rationales

1. Providing such opportunities allows for increased parent-infant bonding and preparation for home care.

2. Preparing the family in this manner allows them to adjust to the shock of the infant's appearance and enables the parents to focus on the infant's immediate needs.

3. The parents need to think of their infant as a normal child with a cleft lip or cleft palate, not as a sick child, to provide adequate home care and to preserve family unity.

4. Having others help in the infant's feeding and routine care allows the parents to rest and focus on their own needs, when necessary.

5. Support groups offer opportunities for the parents to share their feelings and experiences with other parents in similar situations, which helps decrease anxiety and enhance their coping and problem-solving skills.

Nursing diagnosis: *Anxiety (parent) related to impending surgery (preoperative)*

GOAL: The parents will be less anxious as evidenced by verbalizing an understanding of the need for surgery and by participating in the infant's or child's preoperative and postoperative care.

Interventions

1. Assess the parents' understanding of the defect and the need for surgery.

2. Explain to the parents the preoperative and postoperative procedures surrounding the surgery, including the surgical procedure, length of surgery, and the infant's or child's expected postoperative appearance.

3. Demonstrate to the parents the proper feeding technique to use after surgery (placing a tube toward the back of the infant's mouth and squirting small amounts of formula through a syringe); allow them to practice the technique. Also demonstrate the proper use of arm restraints, which prevent the child from touching and disturbing the incision.

Rationales

1. Such assessment serves as a basis on which to begin teaching.

2. Such explanations prepare the parents for the perioperative events and the infant's or child's expected outcome, thereby helping to relieve anxiety.

3. Demonstrating the proper feeding technique and use of arm restraints allows the parents to become familiar with postoperative care, thereby helping to decrease their anxiety.

Nursing diagnosis: *Ineffective airway clearance related to the effects of anesthesia, postoperative edema, and excessive mucus production*

GOAL: The infant or child will remain free of respiratory complications as evidenced by maintaining clear, regular respirations.

Interventions

1. Assess the infant's or child's respiratory status every 4 hours for abnormal breath sounds, cyanosis, retractions, grunting, or nasal flaring.

2. Reposition the infant or child every 2 hours.

3. Place the infant or child in a mist tent, as ordered.

Rationales

1. These signs of respiratory distress may indicate pneumonia, which requires antibiotic therapy.

2. Frequent repositioning facilitates the drainage of secretions from the lungs.

3. Cool, humidified air helps to liquefy secretions, thereby helping the child to breathe easier.

Nursing diagnosis: *Altered nutrition: less than body requirements related to new feeding technique and postoperative dietary changes*

GOAL: The infant or child will continue to maintain adequate nutrition as evidenced by adapting to the new diet and feeding methods and continuing to gain weight.

Interventions

1. If the infant or child has undergone cleft lip repair, feed him through a syringe and soft rubber tubing placed inside the cheek and away from the suture line by squirting small amounts of formula into his mouth. If he has undergone cleft palate repair, use a syringe and tubing or a regular drinking cup (if he is developmentally ready to use one). In either case, avoid placing a nipple in the child's mouth.

2. Encourage small, frequent feedings at first, then progress to the appropriate age-designated fluid intake.

Rationales

1. Sucking on a nipple causes too much pressure on the suture line.

2. The infant or child may require smaller feedings while adapting to the new feeding method.

Interventions	Rationales
3. If the child has undergone cleft palate repair, instruct the parents to feed him a full liquid diet (such as high-calorie drinks) for the first 3 weeks postoperatively.	3. A liquid diet is necessary during this time to prevent damage to the incision site.

Nursing diagnosis: *Impaired skin integrity related to surgical incision*

GOAL: The infant or child will suffer no break in skin integrity as evidenced by an intact incision and no signs of infection.

Interventions	Rationales
1. Provide the following suture line care after feedings and as needed: • Clean the suture line with 1:2 solution of hydrogen peroxide and water with a cotton-tipped applicator. • Apply an antibiotic ointment, as ordered, to moisturize the mouth and prevent separation of the sutures. • Offer small amounts of water after feedings to rinse the mouth of any milk residue that could lead to bacterial growth.	1. Proper suture line care ensures cleanliness, decreases the risk of infection, and reduces the amount of crusted material around the suture line that might result in an enlarged scar.
2. Apply arm restraints, as ordered.	2. Arm restraints are necessary to prevent the infant or child from rubbing the suture line or placing objects in his mouth until the incision is healed.
3. After surgery, position the infant or child on his side or back, never on his stomach, keeping the head of the bed elevated.	3. This position prevents the infant or child from rubbing his lip on the bed linens, reducing the risk of rupture.
4. Anticipate the child's needs to decrease his crying. Maintain placement of a Logan bow across the child's lip if one was applied after surgery.	4. Crying causes tension on the suture line, which could lead to rupture. A Logan bow prevents separation of the sutures by relieving stress on the suture line.

Nursing diagnosis: *Altered comfort: pain related to surgery*

GOAL: The infant or child will maintain a degree of comfort as evidenced by decreased crying and irritability.

Interventions	Rationales
1. Assess the infant or child for irritability, loss of appetite, and disturbances in his sleep pattern every 2 hours after surgery.	1. Because the infant or child may be too young to verbalize discomfort, the nurse needs to rely on behavioral cues for indications of pain.
2. Administer analgesics, as ordered.	2. Analgesics help to decrease pain.
3. Provide diversional activities, such as games, cards, videotapes, and reading materials, for the older child.	3. Diversional activities refocus the child's attention, thereby reducing his perception of pain.

Nursing diagnosis: *Knowledge deficit related to home care*

GOAL 1: The parents will verbalize an understanding of preoperative home care instructions.

Interventions	Rationales
1. Explain to the parents the pathophysiology of the defect and the need for follow-up care.	1. Such explanations help decrease anxiety and increase compliance with the prescribed treatment and impending surgery.

Interventions

2. Instruct the parents on the following feeding techniques:
• Feed the infant with an appropriate nipple and bottle (soft, cross-cut nipples or those specially designed for premature infants; regular or squeeze bottles; Breck feeders).
• Position the nipple in the child's mouth opposite the cleft and toward the back of the tongue.

• Keep the infant in an upright or semisitting position.

• Burp the infant after every ½ to 1 oz (15 to 30 ml).

• Clean the cleft immediately after feeding.

3. Explain to the parents the purpose and use of an apnea monitor if one is prescribed for home care.

Rationales

2. Because of the defect, the parents need to pay particular attention to the infant's feeding.

• Because of the infant's defect, he may have an ineffective swallow reflex. Using an appropriate feeding device helps ensure that the infant retains each feeding.
• Placing the nipple in this manner facilitates the "stripping" action the infant uses to obtain the formula from the bottle.
• Positioning the infant upright or semisitting prevents nasal regurgitation and choking.
• Frequent burping reduces the amount of air swallowed during feeding, thereby reducing the infant's discomfort.
• Cleaning the cleft immediately after feedings helps decrease the risk of infection.

3. An apnea monitor may be prescribed to help the parents detect apneic episodes related to respiratory difficulty from aspiration of feedings.

GOAL 2: The parents will verbalize an understanding of postoperative home care instructions.

Interventions

1. Instruct the parents on the following feeding techniques:
• Use a spoon, not a fork, to feed the child solid foods and a rubber-tipped syringe or a cup (if appropriate) to feed the infant or child fluids.
• Do not allow the child to use a straw.

2. Instruct the parents on the following suture line care:
• Use a 1:2 solution of hydrogen peroxide and water and a cotton-tipped applicator to clean the suture line.
• Apply antibiotic ointment, as ordered, to cover the incision.
• Offer small amounts of water after feedings to rinse away any milk residue that could lead to bacterial growth and infection.

3. Instruct the parents on the importance of keeping the infant's or child's arms restrained.

4. Instruct the parents to position the infant or child on his side or back—never on his stomach—with head of bed elevated.

5. Advise the parents to learn to anticipate the infant's or child's needs to decrease his crying. Instruct them to maintain placement of the Logan bow if one was applied after surgery.

6. Explain to the parents the importance of follow-up care, including the need for ear inspections and hearing evaluations every 2 to 4 months and routine checkups and immunizations.

7. Discuss the possibility of further follow-up care, including speech therapy, orthodontal care, and surgery.

Rationales

1. Using a spoon for solid foods and a rubber-tipped syringe for fluids reduces the risk of trauma to the suture line. Using a straw can traumatize the suture line.

2. Proper suture line care ensures cleanliness, reduces the risk of infection, and reduces crust formation that may result in an enlarged scar.

3. Arm restraints prevent the infant or child from rubbing the suture line or placing objects in his mouth.

4. Positioning the infant or child in this manner prevents him from rubbing his lip on the bed linens.

5. Prolonged crying causes tension on the suture line. Using a Logan bow helps to prevent stress on the sutures that could lead to separation of the sutures.

6. Frequent ear inspections and hearing evaluations are necessary because abnormal eustachian tube function predisposes the infant or child to frequent attacks of otitis media, which may lead to hearing loss. Routine checkups and immunizations are necessary to maintain optimal health.

7. Children with cleft palate often have speech impediments and dental problems that require surgery. Depending on the severity of the defect, the child may need extensive care.

Documentation checklist

During the hospitalization, be sure to document the following:

__ the infant's or child's status and assessment findings upon admission

__ any changes in the infant's or child's status

__ pertinent laboratory and diagnostic findings

__ nutritional intake

__ growth and development status

__ the infant's or child's response to treatment

__ the child's and parents' reaction to the illness and hospitalization

__ patient and family teaching guidelines

__ discharge planning guidelines.

Myringotomy

Introduction

Myringotomy is the surgical incision of the inferior portion of the tympanic membrane to drain fluid from the middle ear. The insertion of myringotomy (tympanostomy) tubes facilitates the continuous drainage of fluid and encourages the equalization of pressure in the middle ear.

Surgery, which is usually indicated for children with recurring ear infections (common in children under age 3), can be performed on an outpatient basis. The expected outcome depends on the effectiveness of the myringotomy tubes in preventing recurrent infections. Potential complications include hearing loss and infection.

Assessment
EENT
• chronic ear infections (usually at least four per year)
• ear pain
• yellowish green drainage from the ear
• pain upon swallowing

Nursing diagnosis: *Anxiety (child and parent) related to the surgical procedure and perioperative events*

GOAL: The child and parents will be less anxious as evidenced by verbalizing an understanding of the surgical procedure and the preoperative and postoperative events surrounding surgery.

Interventions

1. Explain the surgical procedure to the child and parents in simple terms. Be sure to mention that, if the child undergoes local anesthesia, he will be awake during the procedure so that the surgeon can test his hearing. Answer any questions simply and honestly.

2. Explain that, depending on the time of surgery, the child may not be given anything to eat or drink after midnight on the day of surgery to prevent vomiting and aspiration during surgery.

3. Explain to the parents that surgery may not be performed if the child has signs and symptoms of an acute infection, including elevated temperature, runny nose, and ear pain, on the day of surgery.

4. Inform the parents about the expected length of surgery and where they may wait during the actual procedure and recovery period. Make sure they know who will contact them when the procedure is over.

5. Explain to the child and parents the expected postoperative events, including expectant ear drainage, hearing loss, and pain.

Rationales

1. Such information helps to decrease fear and anxiety by preparing the child and parents for the anticipated surgical events.

2. The child may become frightened if he is denied food or drink throughout the night or on the morning of surgery. Explaining this to him beforehand should help to lessen his anxiety and fear.

3. Surgery is avoided under these circumstances to prevent the risk of septicemia or rampant infection.

4. Parents sometimes become unduly anxious during the operative period, especially if they do not know how long the surgery might take. Knowing the anticipated length of surgery and with whom they will confer after the procedure should help to reduce their fear and apprehension.

5. The parents and child should be aware of the child's expected postoperative condition so that they do not become overly concerned and anxious.

Nursing diagnosis: *Potential for injury (hemorrhage) related to surgery*

GOAL: The child will have no signs of hemorrhage resulting from surgery as evidenced by lack of bleeding, normal hemoglobin and hematocrit levels, and pink mucous membranes.

Interventions	**Rationales**
1. Monitor the amount of ear drainage during the post-operative period.	1. A small amount of reddish drainage is normal during the first few days after surgery. However, any bleeding that is heavier or that occurs after the 3 days is abnormal and should be reported to the surgeon immediately.
2. Administer antihistamines and decongestants, as ordered.	2. These agents act to constrict vessels to reduce the amount of bleeding.

Nursing diagnosis: *Knowledge deficit related to home care*

GOAL: The parents will verbalize an understanding of home care instructions.

Interventions	**Rationales**
1. Instruct the parents to report any evidence of fever, increased bloody drainage, or increased pain immediately to the doctor.	1. These signs and symptoms may indicate infection or hemorrhage and should be brought to the doctor's attention immediately.
2. Instruct the parents to avoid getting water in the child's ears. Advise them to place cotton balls or earplugs in the child's ears during baths and shampoos until the tubes fall out or the doctor states otherwise. Also advise them against allowing the child to swim during this time.	2. Because of the tube placement, water can easily enter the middle ear, resulting in infection.
3. Instruct the parents to cover the child's ears when exposed to cold, windy weather.	3. Exposure to cold may result in ear pain.
4. Advise the parents that they may need to speak clearer and slightly louder and to face the child when talking to him.	4. The child may have some hearing loss during the first few weeks after surgery.
5. Instruct the parents on the purpose and use of antibiotics and analgesics, including administration, dosages, and adverse effects. Warn them not to give the child aspirin.	5. Antibiotics may be prescribed to reduce the risk of postoperative infection. Analgesics help to control pain. Aspirin should be avoided, as it may cause bleeding.
6. Describe the tubes' appearance and explain that they may protrude from the child's ear. Emphasize that this is normal and painless, but that expulsion of the tubes should be reported to the doctor.	6. Parents need to report the expulsion of tubes, as this may cause the ear to drain ineffectively, possibly resulting in infection.

Documentation checklist

During the hospitalization, be sure to document the following:
___ the child's status and assessment findings upon admission
___ any changes in the child's status
___ pertinent laboratory and diagnostic findings
___ nutritional intake
___ the child's response to treatment
___ the child's and parents' reaction to the illness and hospitalization
___ patient and family teaching guidelines
___ discharge planning guidelines.

EYE, EAR, NOSE, AND THROAT

Tonsillectomy and Adenoidectomy

Introduction

Tonsillectomy and adenoidectomy—usually performed simultaneously—involve the removal of the tonsils and adenoids because of repeated infections and the increased risk of airway obstruction. Repeated infections often occur because of the development of increased resistance to antibiotic therapy with each episode of tonsillitis.

Surgery, which is rarely performed on children under age 3 except when airway obstruction is a serious threat, significantly decreases the incidence of throat infections and apneic spells. However, it is associated with certain minor complications, including possible respiratory distress and hemorrhage.

Assessment

EENT
• recent sore throat

Respiratory
• recent rhinorrhea
• history of obstructive apnea

Cardiovascular
• history of cardiovascular complications, including murmurs and valvular disease

Hematologic
• history of prolonged bleeding or excessive bruising

Integumentary
• recent fever

Nursing diagnosis: Anxiety (child and parent) related to surgical procedure and perioperative events

GOAL: The child and parents will be less anxious as evidenced by verbalizing an understanding of the surgical procedure and the perioperative events.

Interventions

1. Explain the surgical procedure to the child and parents and answer all questions simply and honestly.

2. Describe to the child the usual sights and sounds associated with the operating room, including the hospital masks and gowns, equipment, and anesthetic apparatus.

3. Inform the parents about the anticipated length of surgery and where they should wait during the actual procedure and recovery period. Make sure they know who will contact them when the procedure is over.

4. Explain to the child and parents the postoperative events, including details on the child's diet and anticipated pain and bleeding. Explain that the child may be allowed clear (not red-colored) liquids immediately after surgery followed by a soft diet of pudding, ice cream, Jell-O, and mashed potatoes when he can tolerate liquids well. Also explain that the child may be given analgesics and an ice collar to control pain. Tell the parents to report any frequent swallowing or vomiting of bright red blood (indications of hemorrhage) to the doctor.

Rationales

1. Understanding the surgical procedure and answering all questions should promote a feeling of security, thereby helping to lessen anxiety.

2. Because the operating room can be particularly frightening to a young child, preparing him for the usual sights and sounds should help to lessen his anxiety.

3. Some parents become unduly anxious during the surgical procedure, especially when they do not know how long the surgery might take. Knowing the anticipated time frame and with whom they can confer after the procedure should help to lessen their fear and apprehension.

4. The parents and child should be aware of the usual postoperative events so that they do not become unduly anxious and unable to provide proper home care. The parents need to know the signs of potential complications so that they can seek medical advice and attention, when necessary.

Nursing diagnosis: *Potential for injury (hemorrhage) related to surgery*

GOAL: The child will have no signs of bleeding as evidenced by stable vital signs and lack of excessive swallowing and restlessness.

Interventions	Rationales
1. Assess the child's vital signs hourly.	1. Increased pulse and respiratory rates and decreased blood pressure may indicate hemorrhage, which requires prompt medical attention.
2. Assess the child's ability to swallow at least every 2 hours.	2. Frequent swallowing is one of the first indications of hemorrhage, which requires prompt medical attention.
3. Assess the child's throat and vomitus for evidence of bleeding.	3. Bright red blood indicates fresh bleeding from the site and requires prompt medical attention.
4. Apply an ice collar to the child's neck.	4. Ice helps to decrease swelling and bleeding.

Nursing diagnosis: *Altered comfort: pain related to surgical procedure*

GOAL: The child will exhibit adequate pain control as evidenced by decreased irritability and restlessness.

Interventions	Rationales
1. Administer analgesics and antipyretics, as ordered, 30 minutes before meals.	1. Analgesics help control pain; antipyretics help reduce fever. Administering these medications before meals helps ensure compliance with the dietary regimen.
2. Apply an ice collar to the child's neck for 10 to 15 minutes at a time.	2. Ear pain—referred throat pain—is common during the first postoperative week. Ice helps to relieve this pain.

Nursing diagnosis: *Potential for infection related to surgical incision*

GOAL: The child will have no signs of infection as evidenced by lack of fever and decreased throat pain.

Interventions	Rationales
1. Administer antibiotics, as ordered.	1. Antibiotics help to fight postoperative infection.
2. Monitor the child for elevated temperature, increasing swallowing difficulty, and increased pain.	2. These signs and symptoms indicate infection, which requires the initiation of antibiotic therapy or dosage adjustment if such therapy has been started.

Nursing diagnosis: *Knowledge deficit related to home care*

GOAL: The parents will verbalize an understanding of home care instructions.

Interventions	Rationales
1. Instruct the parents to monitor the child for increased swallowing, vomiting bright red blood, increased pain, persistent earache after the first 2 or 3 postoperative days, and continuous elevated temperature.	1. These signs and symptoms are indicative of complications, such as hemorrhage, edema, and infection, and should be reported immediately to the doctor.
2. Instruct the parents to discourage the child from coughing.	2. Coughing can dislodge the clot covering the surgical site and put stress on the sutures.

Interventions

3. Instruct the parents to encourage the child to consume cool, clear fluids (such as Popsicles, Gatorade, apple juice, Jell-O, or soda—not milk or milk products) the same day after surgery. Advise them to avoid giving the child fluids that contain red food coloring and to avoid giving the child a straw.

4. If the child tolerates liquids well, instruct the parents to give the child a soft diet (pudding, yogurt, macaroni, mashed potatoes) on the day after surgery.

5. Instruct the parents to avoid giving the child hard, scratchy foods (crackers, popcorn, potato chips, raw vegetables), spicy or salty foods, and citrus fruits for 3 weeks after surgery.

6. Instruct the parents to limit the child's activity as follows:
• During the 1st postoperative week, the child should be confined to bed.
• During the 2nd week (if the doctor approves), the child may return to school with limited activity.
• After the 3rd week, the child may resume recess and gym classes.

7. Instruct the parents to give the child mild analgesics (not aspirin) and to apply an ice collar to help control throat pain.

Rationales

3. Cool fluids are soothing to the throat. However, milk and milk products make throat secretions difficult to clear and can cause nausea. Red food coloring may be confused with bleeding. Using a straw can traumatize the operative site.

4. Soft foods are less irritating to a child's sore throat, yet provide adequate nutrition.

5. Hard foods are uncomfortable to swallow and may dislodge formed clots, which could lead to recurrent bleeding. Spicy or salty foods and citrus fruits may irritate the throat.

6. Tonsillectomy is a major assault on the body system. Returning to a strenuous activity level too quickly may lead to hemorrhage and the need for a longer recuperative period, possibly resulting in complications related to immobility, including muscle weakness and skin breakdown.

7. Analgesics and an ice collar help to reduce throat pain. Aspirin should not be given because it may increase the risk of bleeding.

Documentation checklist

During the hospitalization, be sure to document the following:
___ the child's status and assessment findings upon admission
___ any changes in the child's status
___ pertinent laboratory and diagnostic findings
___ fluid intake and output
___ nutritional intake
___ the child's response to treatment
___ the child's and parents' reaction to the illness and hospitalization
___ patient and family teaching guidelines
___ discharge planning guidelines.

EYE, EAR, NOSE, AND THROAT

Tympanoplasty

Introduction

Tympanoplasty, the surgical reconstruction of the hearing mechanism of the middle ear, often is used to repair ruptured eardrums resulting from frequent ear infections. The expected outcome is generally favorable; however, some children experience permanent hearing loss.

Assessment

EENT
• chronic ear infections (usually more than four per year)
• hearing loss
• ear pain
• drainage from ears

Nursing diagnosis: *Anxiety (child and parent) related to surgical procedure and perioperative events*

GOAL: The child and parents will be less anxious as evidenced by verbalizing an understanding of the surgical procedure and preoperative and postoperative events surrounding the surgery.

Interventions

1. Explain the surgical procedure to the child and parents and answer any questions honestly and simply. Also explain that, if the child is to undergo local anesthesia, he will be awake during surgery so that the surgeon can test his hearing.

2. Explain that, depending on the time of surgery, the child may not be permitted to eat or drink anything after midnight on the day of surgery to prevent the risk of vomiting and aspiration.

3. Explain to the parents that surgery may not be performed if the child has signs and symptoms of an acute infection, including elevated temperature, runny nose, and ear pain.

4. Inform the parents about the expected length of surgery and where they should wait during the actual procedure and recovery period. Make sure they know who will contact them when the procedure is over.

5. Explain to the child and parents the usual postoperative events, including details on expected pain, bleeding, and hearing loss. Explain that the child can expect some pain, which is usually controlled with analgesics, and that he may have a minimal amount of bleeding, probably in the form of bloody drainage. Also explain that the child's hearing may decrease initially but that it will improve in time.

Rationales

1. Explaining the surgical procedure and answering questions should promote a sense of security, thereby helping to lessen anxiety and fear.

2. The child may become frightened if he is denied food or drink during the night or on the morning of surgery. Explaining this to him beforehand should help lessen his fear and anxiety.

3. The parents may become alarmed if the surgery is suddenly postponed.

4. Some parents become unduly anxious during the surgical procedure, especially if they do not know how long the procedure should take. Knowing the anticipated time frame and with whom they will confer after the procedure should help to ease their anxiety and apprehension.

5. Offering such explanations helps to prepare the child and parents for the child's expected postoperative condition, thereby helping to relieve their anxiety and fear.

Nursing diagnosis: *Potential for injury (hemorrhage) related to surgery*

GOAL: The child will have no signs of bleeding as evidenced by a lack of drainage and normal hemoglobin and hematocrit levels.

Interventions	Rationales
1. Check the child's dressing every 1 to 2 hours for signs of excessive bleeding.	1. A minimal amount of bleeding sometimes occurs after surgery. However, excessive bleeding may indicate hemorrhage and should be reported immediately to the doctor.
2. Elevate the head of the bed 30 degrees.	2. Raising the head of the bed reduces intracranial pressure, thereby decreasing the risk of bleeding.
3. Apply a pressure dressing for the first 24 hours after surgery.	3. Pressure dressings help to decrease postoperative bleeding and swelling.
4. Instruct the child to cough and sneeze with an open mouth, avoid blowing his nose, and avoid exposure to loud noises or music.	4. Coughing or sneezing, nose blowing, and exposure to loud sounds produce increased pressure on the ears and may precipitate bleeding.

Nursing diagnosis: *Knowledge deficit related to home care*

GOAL: The parents will verbalize an understanding of home care instructions.

Interventions	Rationales
1. Instruct the parents to monitor the child for fever, increased bloody drainage, and increased pain.	1. These may be signs of infection or hemorrhage and require immediate medical attention.
2. Instruct the parents to avoid getting water in the child's ears. Tell them to avoid washing the child's hair for 1 week after surgery, to place cotton balls or earplugs in the child's ears during baths or showers, and to prohibit the child from swimming until the doctor approves.	2. Water in the ear may cause the absorbable packing to be absorbed prematurely or to break down. It also can be painful and lead to an infection.
3. Instruct the parents to give the child mild analgesics (not aspirin) for pain.	3. Analgesics help to control pain; aspirin increases the risk of bleeding.
4. Advise the parents that they may need to speak slower and louder to the child and turn up the volume on the radio or television.	4. The child may have impaired hearing in the operative ear for 3 to 6 weeks after surgery.
5. Advise the parents to instruct the child to avoid elevator trips of more than eight floors, or, if elevators are unavoidable, to go eight floors, then get out and wait until equilibrium is restored.	5. High altitudes increase pressure in the eustachian tube and inner ear, possibly resulting in dislodgment of the tympanic membrane graft.

Documentation checklist

During the hospitalization, be sure to document the following:
___ the child's status and assessment findings upon admission
___ any changes in the child's status
___ pertinent laboratory and diagnostic findings
___ nutritional intake
___ the child's response to treatment
___ the child's and parents' reaction to the illness and hospitalization
___ patient and family teaching guidelines
___ discharge planning guidelines.

Acquired Immunodeficiency Syndrome

Introduction

Acquired immunodeficiency syndrome (AIDS), caused by human immunodeficiency virus (HIV), results in weakened immunity to numerous opportunistic infections, including *Pneumocystis carinii,* cytomegalovirus, herpesvirus, toxoplasmosis, and Kaposi's sarcoma. The virus may be transmitted through sexual contact with an infected person, contact with an infected person's body fluids, sharing I.V. needles and syringes with an infected person, or the transfusion of contaminated blood products. AIDS also may be contracted congenitally from an HIV-positive mother, through placental transfer or breast milk.

Because of the incidence of the disease among hospital care workers, the Centers for Disease Control recommends that all health care personnel who care for an AIDS patient take special precautions when handling the patient's blood or body fluids (see *Caring for an AIDS Patient: CDC Guidelines*).

AIDS has a high mortality rate and, as of this time, no cure. Treatment usually includes measures to control symptoms, such as the administration of antibiotics, antifungal agents, and pain medications. Zidovudine (formerly AZT) therapy, which slows the progression of the disease in some children, has met with some success.

Assessment

Immunologic
• lymphadenopathy
• decreased number of T cells

Respiratory
• respiratory distress
• *Pneumocystis carinii* pneumonia

Gastrointestinal
• hepatomegaly
• hepatitis (fungal)

Musculoskeletal
• malaise

Hematologic
• anemia

Integumentary
• elevated temperature

CARING FOR AN AIDS PATIENT: CDC GUIDELINES

When caring for a patient with acquired immunodeficiency syndrome (AIDS), the Centers for Disease Control (CDC) suggests the following:
• Provide the patient with a private room if he has profuse diarrhea or fecal incontinence or if he exhibits altered behavior secondary to central nervous system infections.
• Avoid accidentally wounding yourself with sharp instruments contaminated with potentially infected materials.
• Avoid contacting open skin lesions with potentially infected materials.
• Wear disposable gloves and a gown when handling blood specimens, blood-soaked articles, body fluids, and secretions as well as any areas exposed to them.
• If your hands become contaminated, wash them immediately and thoroughly. Also wash your hands after removing gowns and gloves and before leaving the patient's room.
• Label all blood and other specimen containers with a warning, such as "AIDS precaution." Be sure to clean the outside of the specimen container with a disinfectant and to examine it for cracks or leaks. Clean blood or other spills with a disinfectant as well. Transport blood or specimens in an impervious container.
• Put soiled articles in an impervious bag that is clearly labeled, or use a colored plastic bag designed for infectious waste disposal.
• Sterilize all lensed instruments after use.
• Use disposable needles—preferably needle-locking syringes or one-piece units—to aspirate fluid so that collected fluid can be safely discharged through the needle. If reusable syringes are used, decontaminate them before reprocessing.
• Avoid puncturing yourself with needles by discarding them in a puncture-resistant container. Do not bend the needles or reinsert them into their original sheaths.

Nursing diagnosis: *Potential for infection related to immunosuppressed state*

GOAL: The child will have no sign of infection as evidenced by normal temperature and lack of pain or purulent drainage.

Interventions

1. Assess the child for fever, rash, cough, and purulent drainage.

Rationales

1. These signs indicate infection, which requires the administration of antibiotics.

Interventions	Rationales
2. Institute reverse isolation precautions, as necessary, to prevent the child's exposure to further infection.	2. Isolation precautions may be necessary because, in the child's immunosuppressed state, he is highly susceptible to nosocomial infections.

Nursing diagnosis: *Disturbance in self-esteem related to disease and isolation*

GOAL: The child will have improved self-esteem as evidenced by expressing positive feelings about himself to his parents and significant others.

Interventions	Rationales
1. Explain to the child, in appropriate terms, the nature of the disease and the need for reverse isolation precautions (if applicable).	1. The child may not understand the seriousness of his disease and the need to protect him from further infection. Such explanations should help to increase his awareness of the condition and promote increased self-esteem.
2. If the child is not in reverse isolation and poses no risk to other children on the unit, allow him to leave his room.	2. Isolation usually is age-dependent and necessary only when the child is at risk for infection and when he poses a risk to others because of contaminated body fluids. Allowing the child to interact with others is necessary for normal growth and development and helps to improve self-esteem.
3. Allow the child to help with his own care, if appropriate.	3. Performing self-care helps increase the child's self-esteem by fostering a sense of control over the disease and hospitalization.
4. Explain all procedures to the child.	4. Explaining the reason for and steps involved in procedures helps alleviate fear and fosters a sense of control over the situation.
5. Encourage the child to express his feelings.	5. Such encouragement helps the child to ventilate his anxieties, frustrations, and fears—emotions that may be hampering his self-esteem.

Nursing diagnosis: *Fear (child and parent) related to life-threatening implications of the child's disease*

GOAL: The child and parents will exhibit less fear as evidenced by demonstrating decreased anxiety and by asking appropriate questions about the child's condition.

Interventions	Rationales
1. Explain to the parents and child, in appropriate terms, the nature of the child's illness and the need for hospitalization. Answer all questions simply and honestly.	1. The parents and child need to understand the reason for hospitalization and the seriousness of the child's condition. However, they also need reassurance that the child is receiving the best medical and nursing care and that researchers are constantly searching for new treatments and a cure.
2. Encourage the parents and child to express their feelings.	2. Allowing the parents and child to ventilate their fears, anxieties, and frustrations helps them to face the seriousness of the child's illness and to develop new ways of coping. The parents may feel an overwhelming sense of guilt, especially if the child contracted the disease congenitally, and may need special counseling.

Interventions	Rationales
3. Explain all procedures to the parents and child.	3. Explaining the reason for and steps involved in procedures helps to lessen fear and apprehension about the child's care.
4. Encourage the parents and child to join a local AIDS support group. Offer referrals, as needed.	4. Support groups allow the parents and child to interact with other families facing similar circumstances. Knowing that they are not alone and can turn to others for emotional support should help to lessen their fear.

Nursing diagnosis: *Knowledge deficit related to home care*

GOAL: The parents will verbalize an understanding of home care instructions.

Interventions	Rationales
1. Explain to the parents the importance of keeping the child from interacting with other children and family members with infections.	1. Avoiding contact with infected children and family members is essential because the child's immunosuppressed state makes him highly susceptible to further infection.
2. Instruct the parents to provide a diet high in calories and protein.	2. A diet high in calories and protein is necessary to replenish the child's diminished reserves and to help him fight infection.
3. Advise the parents to encourage the child to interact socially with other noninfectious children and to return to school (if applicable).	3. Social interaction and education are important aspects of normal development. As long as the child poses no risk to other children, he should be encouraged to keep up developmentally with his peers.

Documentation checklist

During the hospitalization, be sure to document the following:
___ the child's status and assessment findings upon admission
___ any changes in the child's status
___ pertinent laboratory and diagnostic findings
___ fluid intake and output
___ nutritional intake
___ the child's response to treatment
___ the child's and parents' reaction to the illness and hospitalization
___ patient and family teaching guidelines
___ discharge planning guidelines.

HEMATOLOGIC AND IMMUNOLOGIC SYSTEMS

Hemophilia A

Introduction

A congenital bleeding disorder usually transmitted as an X-linked recessive trait (some cases result from spontaneous gene mutation), hemophilia A (classic hemophilia) is caused by a deficiency of Factor VIII. This type of hemophilia accounts for 80% of all affected children and may be classified as mild, moderate, or severe.

Mild hemophilia is generally marked by prolonged bleeding, easy bruising, and a tendency toward epistaxis (nosebleeds) and bleeding gums. Moderate hemophilia is marked by more frequent and prolonged bleeding episodes and possible hemarthrosis (bleeding into the joints). The severe form is marked by excessive bleeding (sometimes spontaneous), subcutaneous and intramuscular hemorrhage, and bleeding into the joint cavities.

Treatment includes the administration of cryoprecipitate and steroids as well as physical therapy. Potential complications include joint deformity, hemorrhage, and death. The prognosis depends on the severity of the disease.

Assessment

Hematologic
• hemorrhage and prolonged bleeding
• superficial bruises

Genitourinary
• spontaneous hematuria

Musculoskeletal
• signs and symptoms of deep muscle bleeding (pain, guarding of the affected area, limited range of motion, increased temperature and edema at the bleeding site)
• signs and symptoms of hemarthrosis (pain, limited range of motion, increased temperature and edema at the bleeding site)

EENT
• epistaxis
• bleeding gums

Nursing diagnosis: *Altered tissue perfusion related to prolonged bleeding*

GOAL: The child's bleeding will stop as evidenced by no observable bleeding, no increase in the circumference of the bleeding site, no increase in pain, stable vital signs, rising Factor VIII level, and a decreasing partial thromboplastin time (PTT).

Interventions

1. Apply direct pressure to the bleeding site (such as an abrasion or a laceration) for at least 15 minutes.

2. Immobilize the bleeding site.

3. Elevate the bleeding site above the level of the heart for 12 to 24 hours.

4. Apply ice to the affected area.

5. Administer cryoprecipitate or Factor VIII concentrate (antihemophilic factor), as ordered. Allow the parents or child to administer the agent if they wish to and are already familiar with the administration method. If they require instruction, teach them how to insert an I.V. line, prepare the skin site, secure the I.V. setup, prepare the mixture, and start the infusion.

6. Monitor the child's vital signs, noting any signs of bradycardia, tachycardia, decreased blood pressure, increased respiratory rate, or elevated temperature. Report any of these signs immediately to the doctor.

Rationales

1. Pressure applied directly to the bleeding site facilitates clot formation.

2. Immobilization decreases blood flow to the bleeding site and prevents clot dislodgment.

3. Elevating the bleeding site decreases blood flow to the area and promotes clot formation.

4. Coldness promotes vasoconstriction.

5. Administering cryoprecipitate or Factor VIII concentrate allows for completion of the clot formation. Having the parents or child administer the agent allows them to practice the technique for home use.

6. These signs indicate potential complications, including hypovolemia secondary to bleeding and circulatory overload or transfusion reaction secondary to administration of cryoprecipitate or Factor VIII concentrate.

Interventions

7. Measure the circumference of the bleeding site, marking the skin to ensure consistent measurements. Remeasure the site every 8 hours.

8. Monitor the child's Factor VIII and PTT levels at least once daily. Report any abnormalities to the doctor.

9. Administer aminocaproic acid, as ordered, if the child is scheduled for surgery.

10. Follow the Centers for Disease Control guidelines for handling blood or body fluids of children at high risk for acquired immunodeficiency syndrome (see *Caring for an AIDS patient: CDC Guidelines*, page 162).

Rationales

7. Any increase in the circumference indicates continued bleeding, which requires immobilization of the site and the application of ice packs.

8. Monitoring these laboratory values helps determine the child's current clotting status and the need for further intervention, if necessary.

9. This agent (not used on a routine basis) inhibits clot destruction.

10. Hemophiliacs are at high risk for AIDS because of their use of I.V. drugs and blood products.

Nursing diagnosis: *Altered comfort: pain related to bleeding and swelling*

GOAL: The child will be have no signs of pain as evidenced by a relaxed facial expression, verbalization of comfort, ability to sleep, and no need for analgesics.

Interventions

1. Assess the child's degree and level of pain using pediatric pain assessment tools.

2. Administer analgesics (not salicylates or aspirin-containing products), as ordered

Rationales

1. Such assessment provides essential data for determining changes in pain before and after intervention and monitoring the child's bleeding status, as consistent or increasing pain can indicate continued bleeding.

2. Analgesics relieve pain, the mode of action depending on the specific agent ordered. Salicylates and aspirin prolong the prothrombin time and inhibit platelet aggregation.

Nursing diagnosis: *Impaired physical mobility related to decreased range of motion secondary to bleeding and swelling*

GOAL: The child will achieve maximum range of motion (ROM) in the affected joint as evidenced by the ability to perform prescribed exercises.

Interventions

1. Encourage the child to perform isometric exercises, as ordered.

2. Consult the physical therapist on the need for supportive devices, such as braces, and on developing a passive and active ROM exercise program.

3. Assess the child's need for pain medication before beginning each exercise session.

Rationales

1. Isometric exercises help maintain muscle strength through muscle tension without joint movement.

2. Supportive devices help maintain functional position of muscles and joints and prevent or decrease the degree of physical deformity. Passive and active ROM exercises increase muscle tone and strength around the joint and help prevent muscle atrophy and disability.

3. Administering pain medication before exercise promotes comfort and cooperation.

Nursing diagnosis: *Potential for injury related to hospitalization or procedures (or both)*

GOAL: The child will suffer no injuries resulting from the hospitalization or procedures as evidenced by the absence of hematomas, bruising, and hemorrhaging.

Interventions	Rationales
1. Pad the bed's side rails, if age-appropriate.	1. Padding the side rails decreases the risk of injury, such as bruises, that may result from accidental bumps.
2. Make sure the child uses any protective equipment (such as a plastic helmet and elbow and knee pads) that he brought with him from home. Also ensure that he uses a soft-bristled toothbrush for cleaning his teeth.	2. Using protective equipment helps decrease the risk of injury from falls caused by accidents or routine play. A soft-bristled toothbrush decreases the risk of bleeding gums.
3. When collecting blood specimens, use a fingerstick rather than a venipuncture, when possible. When giving injections, use the subcutaneous (not intramuscular) route, when possible. Afterward, apply pressure to the site for at least 5 minutes.	3. Using a fingerstick rather than a venipuncture decreases the risk of excessive blood loss because capillaries are smaller than veins and contain less blood. Using the subcutaneous route allows for use of a smaller-gauge needle, thereby reducing the risk of blood loss from a larger puncture site. Also, subcutaneous tissue is less vascular than muscle.
4. After any bleeding episode, immobilize the bleeding site, then elevate the site above the level of the heart for 12 to 24 hours. Then, apply ice to the area.	4. Immobilization and elevation above the heart level decrease blood flow to the bleeding site and prevent clot dislodgment. Applying ice promotes vasoconstriction and decreases pain.
5. Inspect the child's toys for sharp edges.	5. Sharp-edged toys could lacerate or puncture the child's skin.

Nursing diagnosis: *Disturbance in self-esteem related to chronic illness and hospitalization*

GOAL: The child will maintain a positive self-image as evidenced by his ability to verbalize capabilities as well as his limitations, participation in self-care, and continued involvement in age-appropriate activities (such as play, schoolwork, and contact with peers).

Interventions	Rationales
1. Encourage the child to participate in his care, as appropriate. Allow him to perform activities of daily living, administer cryoprecipitate or Factor VIII concentrate, and participate in decisions affecting his care, when possible.	1. Encouraging the child to participate in his care promotes independence and fosters a sense of control over the situation.
2. Encourage the child to express his feelings about the hospitalization and his disease.	2. Such encouragement allows the child to ventilate such feelings as frustration and anxiety that may be hampering his self-esteem.
3. Provide the child with age-appropriate play activities for use in the playroom or when confined to bed.	3. Play, an essential part of normal growth and development, can help divert the child's attention from his condition, thereby helping to improve his self-esteem.
4. Encourage the parents to bring in school assignments and to arrange for the child's siblings and peers to visit, if age-appropriate.	4. Contact with others promotes normal interactions and decreases feelings of isolation, thereby helping to improve the child's self-esteem.

Nursing diagnosis: *Ineffective family coping: compromised related to repeated hospitalizations and the child's chronic illness*

GOAL: The parents and other family members will demonstrate effective coping skills as evidenced by interacting with the child and staff and helping with some of the child's required care.

Interventions

1. Explore with the parents and other family members their feelings about the child's chronic condition and its implications on their life-style.

2. Refer the family to a social worker and other appropriate support groups (such as the National Hemophilia Foundation), as needed.

Rationales

1. Such discussions allow the nurse to assess the family's needs and their usual coping methods.

2. Parents of children with chronic diseases often need extensive emotional and financial support. If still of child-bearing age, the parents may also need genetic counseling to help them understand the hereditary aspects of the disease.

Nursing diagnosis: *Knowledge deficit related to home care*

GOAL: The parents verbalize an understanding of home care instructions.

Interventions

1. Explain to the parents the importance of providing a safe home environment for the child. Stress the need for the following safety precautions:
• padding side rails and sharp corners on furniture
• inspecting all toys for sharp edges
• making the child wear a plastic helmet and elbow and knee pads during play
• carpeting all floors.

2. Instruct the parents on the importance of taking the following precautionary health measures:

• making the child wear a Medic Alert identification bracelet or necklace identifying him as a hemophiliac

• ensuring that the child undergoes routine dental checkups

• consulting a dietitian on the child's iron needs

• restricting the use of salicylates and aspirin-containing compounds

• conferring with the child's teachers, school nurse, and coaches on the child's condition and need for certain restrictions

• promoting the child's participation in appropriate physical activities, such as swimming rather than football.

3. Instruct the parents to take the following measures to control the child's bleeding:
• Apply direct pressure to the bleeding site for at least 15 minutes.
• Immobilize the bleeding site and elevate the area above the level of the heart.

Rationales

1. Implementing these safety measures helps decrease the risk of injury and bleeding from bumps, falls, and accidental lacerations and punctures.

2. Certain precautionary measures are needed to ensure that the child avoids situations leading to potential bleeding episodes.
• Wearing a Medic Alert bracelet or necklace identifies the child as a hemophiliac and alerts rescuers to the child's need for emergency care.
• Routine dental checkups and care are necessary to help prevent tooth and gum disease that can lead to bleeding.
• Children with hemophilia are prone to iron deficiency and often require a diet high in iron.
• Salicylates and aspirin-containing products can increase the bleeding time and inhibit platelet aggregation.
• The child's teachers, school nurse, and coaches need to be aware of the seriousness of the child's condition so that they can enforce health and safety precautions, yet allow the child to develop to his highest potential.
• Encouraging the child to participate in less hazardous sports and activities ensures his developmental growth, yet protects him from the risk of bleeding episodes.

3. Taking appropriate measures during bleeding episodes helps prevent life-threatening hemorrhage.
• Applying direct pressure stops blood flow to the bleeding site and allows for clot formation.
• Immobilizing the site and elevating the area above the heart reduces the flow of blood to the bleeding site and prevents clot dislodgment.

Interventions

• Apply ice to the bleeding site.

• Administer Factor VIII concentrate.

4. Instruct the parents on the purpose and use of Factor VIII concentrate, including details on administration, dosage, and potential adverse effects. Also explain how to store and mix the agent, set up an I.V. line, perform a venipuncture, adjust the infusion rate, and document any transfusion reactions.

Rationales

• Applying ice to the bleeding site promotes vasoconstriction.

• Administering Factor VIII concentrate ensures completion of the clotting process.

4. Knowing this information helps ensure correct use and administration for emergency home care.

Documentation checklist

During the hospitalization, be sure to document the following:

___ the child's status and assessment findings upon admission

___ any changes in the child's status

___ pertinent laboratory and diagnostic findings

___ nutritional intake

___ growth and development status

___ the child's response to treatment

___ the child's and parents' reaction to the illness and hospitalization

___ patient and family teaching guidelines

___ discharge planning guidelines.

Hyperbilirubinemia

Introduction

Hyperbilirubinemia is caused by excess concentrations of bilirubin in the blood, often resulting in jaundice. In the neonate, hyperbilirubinemia may be caused by physiologic immaturity of the liver or by blood group incompatibility.

Physiologic jaundice, which occurs during the first 48 to 72 hours of life, is marked by a slightly elevated bilirubin level of 8 to 12 mg/dl. Treatment usually is not indicated; however, daily follow-up evaluation is recommended for the first 3 days, even if the infant has been discharged. If necessary, the infant may require home phototherapy.

Physiologic jaundice of the premature infant usually follows the same course as that of a term infant; however, diagnosis is based on serum bilirubin levels adjusted to the infant's gestational age and weight.

Exaggerated jaundice, marked by a serum bilirubin level >12 mg/dl during the first 72 hours of life, usually requires treatment with phototherapy and monitoring of serial bilirubin levels. Breast-feeding may be contraindicated until the levels begin to decline. Further evaluation differentiates this type of jaundice from pathologic jaundice.

Pathologic jaundice is marked by a rapid rise in serum bilirubin levels during the first 24 hours of life, usually resulting from an underlying disease, such as hemolytic disease, an infection, excessive breakdown of blood products, a metabolic disorder, an anatomic abnormality, or inadequate caloric intake.

Treatment for this type of jaundice includes phototherapy or exchange transfusions (or both). Additional blood studies and X-rays help diagnose the specific underlying disease.

Assessment

Hematologic
• elevated bilirubin levels
• enlarged liver

Gastrointestinal
• yellowish orange feces

Genitourinary
• dark orange urine

Musculoskeletal
• lethargy

Integumentary
• jaundice
• dry skin

Nursing diagnosis: *Potential for injury related to phototherapy*

GOAL: The infant will suffer no injury from phototherapy as evidenced by normal bilirubin levels within 24 to 48 hours after treatment is discontinued and a body temperature of between 97.6° and 99° F. (36.4° and 37.2° C.).

Interventions

1. Monitor the infant's serum bilirubin levels daily.

2. Place eye shields over the infant's eyes whenever the infant is under the phototherapy lamp. Remove the shields every 4 to 8 hours to assess his eyes.

3. Remove all of the infant's clothing during phototherapy treatment. (*Note:* Some hospitals recommend placing a covering over the scrotal area to protect the testes.) Monitor the infant's body temperature every 2 to 4 hours, or use skin probes to monitor the temperature continuously. Keep all of the Isolette portholes closed.

Rationales

1. Frequent monitoring helps determine the need for phototherapy treatment to help prevent bilirubin toxicity and kernicterus.

2. Because phototherapy uses bright fluorescent light to break down bilirubin in the bloodstream, eye shields are necessary to prevent retinal damage and infection.

3. During phototherapy treatment, the entire body surface area is exposed fluorescent light. Because this places the infant at risk for hypothermia (through loss of body heat) or hyperthermia (through dehydration), careful temperature monitoring is essential. Keeping the Isolette portholes closed during treatment helps decrease the amount of body heat lost through convection.

Nursing diagnosis: *Potential for fluid volume deficit related to phototherapy treatment*

GOAL: The infant will maintain adequate fluid volume as evidenced by no signs of dehydration.

Interventions

1. Increase the infant's fluid intake by 20% to 25%.

2. Assess the infant's urine output, skin turgor, and fontanels every 2 to 4 hours.

3. If the mother wishes to breast-feed her infant, obtain a doctor's order before beginning feeding.

Rationales

1. Adequate hydration helps in the excretion of bilirubin through urine and feces and decreases the amount of fluids lost through dehydration.

2. Such assessment is necessary to determine the infant's current hydration status. Dehydration, which is characterized by poor skin turgor, sunken fontanels, and decreased urine output, requires prompt treatment, including the administration of I.V. fluids for rehydration.

3. Breast-feeding may be contraindicated until the infant's bilirubin level begins to decline, as breast milk contains an enzyme that prohibits the breakdown of bilirubin.

Nursing diagnosis: *Potential for injury (kernicterus) related to high bilirubin levels*

GOAL: The infant will have no signs of kernicterus as evidenced by lack of feeding difficulties, lethargy, irritability, seizures, and brain damage.

Interventions

1. Monitor the infant's bilirubin level two or three times daily if levels are >10 mg/dl.

2. Assess the infant every 8 hours for signs of lethargy, feeding difficulties, and irritability possibly leading to seizures.

3. Take the following measures for exchange transfusions:
• Monitor the infant's vital signs to determine baseline levels.
• Prepare the infant for umbilical access.
• Make sure that blood for transfusion is warmed to prevent venous spasms and hypothermia.
• Record the amount of blood being exchanged.
• Assess the infant's general condition throughout the transfusion process.

4. Monitor the infant for signs and symptoms of transfusion reactions, including hemolytic reactions (hematuria, fever, shock), circulatory overload (congestive heart failure, wheezing, crackles, rhonchi), hypothermia (decreased temperature, increased respiratory rate), and febrile reactions (increased temperature).

Rationales

1. Because bilirubin levels >20 mg/dl place the infant at risk for kernicterus, frequent monitoring is essential for early detection and prompt treatment.

2. These are signs indicative of kernicterus.

3. Exchange transfusions may be necessary to lower the infant's total bilirubin level and prevent kernicterus.

4. Such monitoring allows for the early recognition and prompt treatment of potentially serious complications.

Nursing diagnosis: *Knowledge deficit related to home care*

GOAL: The parents will verbalize an understanding of home care instructions.

Interventions

1. Explain to the parents the causes and usual course of neonatal jaundice and hyperbilirubinemia. Also explain the usual treatments recommended for home therapy.

Rationales

1. Knowing this information should help to lessen the parents' anxiety about the child's condition and ensure compliance with home therapy.

Interventions

2. Explain to the parents that the infant's yellowish orange skin color is normal for his condition and that it should disappear within days after treatment.

3. Explain to the parents the importance of increasing the infant's fluid intake.

4. If phototherapy is ordered for home use, instruct the parents on the following:
• setting up the equipment
• using eye shields
• keeping the infant's skin uncovered
• monitoring the infant's temperature
• avoiding the use of lotions
• monitoring for complications.

Rationales

2. Some parents may become unduly alarmed by the infant's appearance and may mistake it for hepatitis.

3. Increased fluids help in the excretion of bilirubin.

4. Phototherapy is not always used at home because of the potential risks, including blindness, burns, and dehydration. Parents may have to sign a waiver to cover the risk of complications.

Documentation checklist

During the hospitalization, be sure to document the following:
___ the infant's status and assessment findings upon admission
___ any changes in the infant's status
___ pertinent laboratory and diagnostic findings
___ fluid intake and output
___ nutritional intake
___ the infant's response to treatment
___ the parents' reaction to the illness and hospitalization
___ family teaching guidelines
___ discharge planning guidelines.

Sickle Cell Anemia

Introduction

An incurable autosomal recessive disease that predominantly affects blacks, sickle cell anemia is characterized by the abnormal formation of red blood cells (RBCs) that, under certain circumstances, appear sickle-shaped. Because of the cells' fragility and inflexibility, the disease results in occlusion of the small blood vessels and increased RBC destruction.

Treatment for this potentially life-threatening disease usually is supportive unless the child is in sickle cell crisis (usually caused by decreased oxygen levels, stress, infection, or extreme exercise), in which case medical intervention is necessary. Supportive measures include pain control, physical therapy, blood replacement, and rehydration therapy. The prognosis for this disease depends on the extent of the crises and bleeding episodes. Potential complications include splenic infarction, infection, and death.

Assessment

Hematologic
• anemia
• enlarged spleen
• enlarged liver

Neurologic
• numbness in the fingers and toes
• anxiety

Gastrointestinal
• abdominal pain
• thirst
• vomiting

Genitourinary
• frequent urination

Musculoskeletal
• muscle weakness
• edematous joints
• joint and back pain

Psychosocial
• delayed growth and development

Integumentary
• jaundice
• elevated temperature

Nursing diagnosis: *Altered tissue perfusion related to blood vessel obstruction secondary to sickling of RBCs*

GOAL: The child will have adequate tissue perfusion as evidenced by decreased cyanosis, warm extremities, and a stable blood pressure.

Interventions

1. Encourage complete bed rest during the acute phase of the illness.

2. Perform passive range-of-motion exercises every 4 to 6 hours, or provide other age-appropriate activities that the child can perform in bed, such as isometric exercises.

3. Avoid or limit the number of activities and situations that may cause emotional stress.

4. Coordinate caregiving activities to minimize interrupting the child's sleep and rest periods.

Rationales

1. Bed rest is necessary because exercise increases cellular metabolism, resulting in tissue hypoxia and increased sickling.

2. Passive ROM exercises and isometric exercises promote mobility without stressing the joints and causing pain.

3. Increased cellular metabolism results in tissue hypoxia and increased sickling. Adrenaline released during stress further constricts vessels.

4. Adequate rest and sleep are necessary during the acute phase of the illness.

Nursing diagnosis: *Fluid volume deficit related to decreased fluid intake and the kidneys' inability to concentrate urine*

GOAL: The child will maintain adequate hydration as evidenced by adequate urine output, moist mucous membranes, decreased thirst, stable weight, and flat fontanels (in infants).

Interventions	Rationales
1. Encourage the child to drink fluids every 2 hours.	1. Adequate hydration is necessary to prevent increased sickling of cells.
2. Carefully monitor the child's fluid intake and output, including the administration of any I.V. fluids.	2. Accurate measurements are necessary to assess the child's current fluid balance, which is critical for evaluating kidney function, hemodilution, and circulatory overload.
3. Weigh the child daily.	3. Daily weight is the most accurate measure of the child's hydration status.
4. Observe the child every 2 to 4 hours for signs of dehydration, including dry skin, poor skin turgor, and decreased urine output. Administer increased fluids if dehydration occurs.	4. Dehydration, a common cause of further sickling, requires increased fluid intake necessary for rehydration.
5. Monitor laboratory results for pH, hematocrit, hemoglobin, PCO_2, and PO_2 levels.	5. Acid-base imbalances may indicate that the child is dehydrated.
6. Make sure that the child is not dressed too warmly.	6. Dressing the child too warmly may cause overheating, resulting in fluid loss.

Nursing diagnosis: *Altered comfort: pain related to vascular occlusion and tissue hypoxia*

GOAL: The child will have no signs of pain as evidenced by decreased verbalization of pain, restful sleep periods, and relaxed facial expressions.

Interventions	Rationales
1. Assess the child's need for pain medication every 3 to 4 hours. Check for restlessness, tense facial expressions, decreased appetite, crying when touched, and grunting.	1. Frequent assessment is necessary to help determine the child's degree and type of pain and need for medication.
2. Administer analgesics and narcotics, as ordered. Evaluate the child's response to pain control measures.	2. Pain management can be difficult to achieve. The child may require experimentation with various types of analgesics and narcotics to achieve the desired response.
3. Apply warmth to the affected site every 3 to 4 hours.	3. Heat causes vasodilation, moving sickled cells through occluded areas and thereby promoting comfort.
4. Maintain the child in a comfortable position with his joints supported in alignment with the rest of the body. Be careful to handle his extremities gently and to avoid bumping or jarring the bed.	4. Proper positioning promotes comfort in painful joints.

Nursing diagnosis: *Potential for infection related to sickling of cells and splenic infarction*

GOAL: The child will have no signs of infection as evidenced by absence of fever and cough and a normal white blood cell count.

Interventions

1. Isolate the child from all known sources of infection.

2. Monitor the child's temperature every 4 hours.

3. Check the child's immunization record and administer vaccines, as ordered.

4. Administer antibiotics, as ordered.

5. Provide a high-calorie, high-protein diet served in small, frequent meals.

Rationales

1. The child is especially susceptible to infection because of the spleen's inability to filter bacteria as a result of infarction.

2. An elevated temperature is an indication of infection.

3. Children with sickle cell anemia have a markedly increased susceptibility to *Pneumococcus* and *Hemophilus influenzae* infections and should receive scheduled immunizations. (*Note:* Pneumococcal vaccines are recommended at age 2; Hemophilus b polysaccharide vaccine, at age 18 months.)

4. Antibiotics help in fighting and preventing infections.

5. This type of diet helps the child to fight infection and enables proper growth and development, as sickled cells interfere with the use of nutrients. Serving small, frequent meals helps prevent the child from tiring and ensures that he will eat more of each meal.

Nursing diagnosis: *Knowledge deficit related to home care*

GOAL: The parents will verbalize an understanding of home care instructions.

Interventions

1. Instruct the parents on the anatomy and physiology of normal RBCs and on the pathophysiology of sickle cell disease.

2. Instruct the parents on the signs and symptoms of developing crisis, including anorexia, joint pain, epigastric pain, fever, and vomiting.

3. Instruct the parents on the importance of taking the following measures during a sickle cell crisis:
• Maintain adequate hydration.
• Prevent infection by isolating the child from known causes.
• Administer antibiotics, as ordered.
• Avoid exposing the child to low-oxygen environments (such as flying in unpressurized airplanes).

Rationales

1. Understanding the normal functioning of RBCs and the nature and course of the disease should encourage compliance with the overall treatment plan.

2. Knowing this information should prompt the parents to seek medical advice and attention, when necessary.

3. Taking such measures helps prevent further complications associated with sickle cell crisis.

Documentation checklist

During the hospitalization, be sure to document the following:
___ the child's status and assessment findings upon admission
___ any changes in the child's status
___ pertinent laboratory and diagnostic findings
___ fluid intake and output
___ nutritional intake
___ the child's response to treatment
___ the child's and parents' reaction to the illness and hospitalization
___ patient and family teaching guidelines
___ discharge planning guidelines.

ENDOCRINE SYSTEM

Cushing's Syndrome

Introduction

Cushing's syndrome, a clinical manifestation of the prolonged overproduction of glucocorticoid (in particular, cortisol), is characterized by truncal obesity, short stature, and hypertension. Although rare in children (more common in girls), this disorder usually results from prolonged or excessive administration of adrenocorticotropic hormone (ACTH) but also may result from long-term steroid use, oversecretion of the adrenal glands, or an adrenal neoplasm. Depending on the specific cause, excessive mineralocorticoids and androgens also may be excreted.

Usual treatment includes the gradual decrease of steroid use and surgery (when necessary). Potential complications include osteoporosis, hypertension, arteriosclerosis, amenorrhea, and psychoses.

Assessment

Endocrine
- obesity
- hyperglycemia
- amenorrhea

Cardiovascular
- hypertension

Musculoskeletal
- fatigue
- loss of muscle mass

Integumentary
- characteristic fat distribution (moon face, buffalo hump)
- fragile skin
- edema
- hirsutism
- bruising
- poor wound healing

Nursing diagnosis: *Potential for injury (hyperglycemia) related to the anti-insulin properties of glucocorticoids*

GOAL: The child will suffer no injury from hyperglycemia as evidenced by maintaining stable glucose levels.

Interventions

1. Monitor the child's serum glucose levels at least twice daily for hyperglycemia.

2. Begin the child on a diabetic diet, and instruct the parents to continue the diet after the child is discharged from the hospital.

Rationales

1. The child may develop hyperglycemia as a result of the anti-insulin properties of glucocorticoids.

2. A diabetic diet, which includes a balance of complex carbohydrates, protein, and fat to meet the child's daily metabolic needs, may be necessary until the syndrome resolves to help control hyperglycemia.

Nursing diagnosis: *Potential for infection related to the immunosuppressive action of glucocorticoids*

GOAL: The child will remain free of infection as evidenced by maintaining a normal temperature and stable vital signs.

Interventions

1. Take necessary measures to protect the child from potential sources of infection. Screen all visitors with respiratory or other infections.

Rationales

1. Because glucocorticoids suppress the child's normal body response to infection, the child should be protected from all possible contaminants.

Interventions	Rationales
2. Assess the child on a daily basis for signs of infection, including slight temperature elevation, rhinitis, cough, and ear or wound drainage.	2. Because normal signs of infection, such as elevated temperature and swelling, may be absent in a child with excessive glucocorticoid levels, careful observation is necessary to detect any subtle signs.

Nursing diagnosis: *Fluid volume excess related to excess corticosteroids*

GOAL: The child will maintain fluid homeostasis as evidenced by good skin turgor and a brisk capillary refill time.

Interventions	Rationales
1. Measure and record the child's blood pressure every shift.	1. Excessive mineralocorticoid activity may result in sodium retention and depletion of serum potassium levels. Hypertension may result from an exaggerated response to catecholamines, the constriction of peripheral vessels, and sodium retention.
2. Weigh the child daily and assess for pitting edema in dependent areas.	2. Monitoring the child's daily weight and assessing for edema help to determine whether the child is retaining any fluid.
3. Monitor the child's daily fluid intake and output.	3. Decreased output may be caused by excessive mineralocorticoid activity resulting in the retention of sodium and fluid.
4. Monitor the child's electrolyte levels.	4. Excessive mineralocorticoid activity causes sodium retention and potassium depletion.
5. Restrict the child's sodium intake, as ordered.	5. The child may require sodium restriction to help prevent fluid retention.

Nursing diagnosis: *Potential for injury related to excessive corticosteroid production*

GOAL: The child will suffer no injuries as evidenced by no signs of soft tissue damage or trauma.

Interventions	Rationales
1. Protect the child from injury by padding the sharp corners of all furniture in the child's room. Also, inspect all toys for sharp edges or other potentially dangerous features.	1. Such precautions are necessary, as the child's skin is extremely fragile because of protein catabolism associated with excessive corticosteroid levels. The child is especially at risk for hemorrhaging because of the fragility of blood vessel walls.
2. After giving an injection, hold the venipuncture site for 3 to 5 minutes.	2. This prevents hemorrhaging and hematoma formation.

Nursing diagnosis: *Disturbance in self-concept: body image related to excessive corticosteroid levels*

GOAL: The child will exhibit an improved self-concept as evidenced by verbalizing an acceptance of his current body image.

Interventions	Rationales
1. Explain to the child, in age-appropriate terms, the reason for the changes in his physical appearance, stressing that such changes are usually only temporary.	1. The child may not understand that the changes in his body's appearance are temporary and caused by controllable factors. Knowing this information should help to improve his self-esteem.

Interventions	Rationales
2. Encourage the child to express his feelings about his altered appearance.	2. By expressing his feelings and discussing his condition, the child may be better able to accept his altered body image.

Nursing diagnosis: *Knowledge deficit related to home care*

GOAL: The parents will verbalize an understanding of home care instructions.

Interventions	Rationales
1. Instruct the parents on the importance of the child's following a diabetic diet and limiting the number of snacks.	1. A strict dietary regimen helps to control glucose levels, thereby preventing the risk of hyperglycemia.
2. Instruct the parents on the importance of preventing infection, including having the child avoid crowds and infected individuals, carefully managing wounds, and observing for signs and symptoms of infection (ear or wound drainage, fever, rhinorrhea, swelling, and pain).	2. The child is at increased risk for infection because of his immunosuppressed state.

Documentation checklist

During the hospitalization, be sure to document the following:

___ the child's status and assessment findings upon admission
___ any changes in the child's status
___ pertinent laboratory and diagnostic findings
___ fluid intake and output
___ growth and development status
___ the child's response to treatment
___ the child's and parents' reaction to the illness
___ patient and family teaching guidelines
___ discharge planning guidelines.

ENDOCRINE SYSTEM

Diabetes Mellitus

Introduction

Diabetes encompasses a group of disorders characterized by glucose intolerance resulting from insulin deficiency. Type I (insulin-dependent) diabetes mellitus can occur at any age but usually manifests during adolescence, between ages 11 and 12, and affects about 10% to 20% of the entire diabetic population. Type II (non-insulin-dependent) diabetes mellitus usually manifests after age 40.

Although the exact cause of Type I diabetes has not been confirmed, it may be associated with an autoimmune disorder activated by a virus. Treatment for this type includes a diabetic diet, use of insulin, glucose monitoring, and exercise. Potential complications include blindness, renal disease, and peripheral vascular disease. Life expectancy may be shortened by 10 to 20 years.

Assessment

Endocrine
- lack of endogenous insulin
- unstable blood glucose levels

Neurologic
- irritability

Gastrointestinal
- increased appetite
- increased thirst
- weight loss
- abdominal pain

Genitourinary
- frequent urination
- urinary tract infections
- sugar and acetones in urine
- enuresis

Musculoskeletal
- malaise
- lethargy

Neurologic
- irritability

Integumentary
- dry skin
- poor wound healing
- dehydration

Nursing diagnosis: *Potential for injury related to disease*

GOAL: The child will suffer minimal injury from the disease as evidenced by the absence of severe hypoglycemia and ketoacidotic responses.

Interventions

1. Monitor the child's blood glucose levels three or four times daily.

2. Assess the child for signs and symptoms of hypoglycemia (weakness, ataxia, anxiety, irritability, short attention span, rapid heart rate, tremors, and pale, moist skin) or hyperglycemia (fruity breath, glycosuria, lethargy, decreased level of consciousness, polydipsia, dehydration, and polyuria). Take the following measures, as necessary:
- If the child is hypoglycemic, give him one or two Lifesavers, one sugar cube, or one spoonful of honey to place in his mouth. Repeat every 10 to 15 minutes.
- If the child is hyperglycemic, check his glucose level and give the ordered amount of insulin.

3. If hyperglycemia progresses to diabetic ketoacidosis (marked by increased thirst, increased urine output, dehydration, electrolyte imbalance, and a sweet or fruity breath odor), administer a continuous infusion of insulin and provide fluid and electrolyte replacement.

Rationales

1. Frequent monitoring helps determine the effectiveness of insulin and dietary therapy.

2. Hypoglycemia (which may result from too-high insulin levels, lack of food, extreme exercise, headache, or illness) requires prompt action to raise the child's glucose level quickly. Hyperglycemia (which may result from improper eating, a missed insulin dose, or illness) requires the prompt administration of insulin to raise the child's insulin level.

3. Ketoacidosis, which occurs as a result of lowered insulin levels, may be life-threatening if not treated promptly.

Interventions	Rationales
4. Instruct the child to wear a Medic Alert bracelet or necklace identifying himself as a diabetic.	4. Wearing a Medic Alert necklace or bracelet enables emergency medical personnel to provide appropriate treatment.

Nursing diagnosis: *Potential for injury related to noncompliance with the dietary regimen*

GOAL: The child will suffer no diet-related injury as evidenced by following dietary restrictions as closely as possible.

Interventions	Rationales
1. Instruct the child and parents on the importance of following a strict dietary regimen. Explain that the diet must be consistent and that food must be eaten at regular intervals.	1. The child and parents need to understand the importance of following a strict diet to ensure compliance with the dietary regimen. They also need to understand that dietary consistency and regularly-timed meals help keep blood glucose and insulin levels within acceptable ranges.
2. Consult the hospital dietitian about the child's food preferences and current eating patterns.	2. Consulting the hospital dietitian allows the nurse to incorporate some of the child's favorite foods into each meal, thereby helping to ensure compliance with the dietary regimen.
3. Provide the child and parents with a list of appropriate food exchanges and a sample menu that includes acceptable food choices. Stress the importance of reading labels on all purchased food items.	3. The child and parents need to know which foods are included in the dietary plan to enable them to make appropriate choices. They also need to understand the importance of reading food labels to identify potentially dangerous substances that might alter the glucose-insulin balance.

Nursing diagnosis: *Potential for injury related to exercise*

GOAL: The child will suffer no exercise-related injuries as evidenced by the absence of hypoglycemia.

Interventions	Rationales
1. Encourage the child to participate in a regular exercise program.	1. Regular exercise is important for normal growth and development and usually is not limited unless the child has other problems, such as injuries, infections, or renal disease.
2. Instruct the child to eat a snack (something high in protein and carbohydrates, such as cheese or peanut butter and crackers) before exercising.	2. Snacks are important because exercise decreases blood glucose levels.

Nursing diagnosis: *Ineffective family coping: compromised related to new diagnosis of chronic illness*

GOAL: The child and family will demonstrate effective coping skills as evidenced by complying with the treatment regimen.

Interventions	Rationales
1. Encourage the child and parents to express their feelings about the child's illness and its effect on their life-style.	1. The child and parents may have fears and anxieties that are hindering their ability to cope with their new situation. Younger children may be fearful of blood tests and insulin injections. Parents may be fearful of not

Interventions	Rationales
	only the immediate threats of the disease but also the long-term effects on the child's health.
2. Instruct the child and parents on the controllable factors of the disease, including diet, insulin, and regular exercise. Explain that adhering to a strict regimen may help to prevent the onset or severity of complications.	2. The child and parents may identify diabetes with the onset of complications or even death. Emphasizing the importance of the controllable factors of the disease should help them to cope with the illness.
3. Refer the parents to a local support group or chapter of the American Diabetes Association or Juvenile Diabetes Foundation. If possible, arrange for the parents and child to meet with another family with a diabetic child of the same age.	3. Such groups provide support and information, which should help the family to cope with the child's illness. Meeting another family that is coping well with the disease should encourage the child and parents that the disease can be managed.

Nursing diagnosis: *Knowledge deficit related to home care*

GOAL: The child and parents will verbalize an understanding of home care instructions.

Interventions	Rationales
1. Assess the child's and parents' knowledge of the disease and their readiness to learn.	1. Families displaying high levels of fear, denial, and stress may need to discuss their feelings before beginning teaching sessions.
2. Arrange to hold specific teaching sessions with the child and parents. Encourage all family members to participate in learning about diabetes.	2. Unlike many diseases, diabetes requires the development of specific home management skills. Encouraging all family members to attend the teaching sessions helps stress the importance of learning these skills and ensures compliance with the home care regimen.
3. Provide information on the cause of the child's disease and on ways to manage it, including: • dietary regimen (eating a well-balanced diet, using the proper number of exchanges from each food group) • insulin use (administered by subcutaneous injection into the arm, thigh, or abdomen or by a metered pump) • glucose testing (checking the glucose level in blood, usually by a fingerstick method) • preventive care (snacking before exercise, managing sores or wounds, preventing infection).	3. Providing such information is essential to ensure compliance with the treatment regimen.
4. Explain to the child and parents the importance and action of insulin within the body. Explain to the younger child that insulin acts as a key that opens cell doors to allow glucose to enter the cells to supply them with energy.	4. Age-appropriate analogies can help the child and parents understand the need for insulin and the importance of complying with the medication regimen.
5. Instruct the child and parents on recognizing the signs and symptoms of hypoglycemia (weakness, ataxia, anxiety, irritability, short attention span, rapid heart rate, tremors, and pale, moist skin) and hyperglycemia (fruity breath, glycosuria, lethargy, decreased level of consciousness, polydipsia, dehydration, and polyuria). Explain what measures to take if the child suddenly exhibits signs of either of these conditions.	5. The child and parents need to know the signs and symptoms of hypoglycemia and hyperglycemia to ensure prompt treatment.
6. Instruct the child and parents on the proper way to mix insulin and give injections. For a younger child, demonstrate the injection procedure on a cloth doll and ask the child to repeat your actions. Have the parents practice giving injections by administering saline solution injections to each other. If a continuous infusion pump is to be used, demonstrate the proper administration technique.	6. Administering injections is an important part of home care. Encouraging the child and parents to practice giving injections reinforces what they learned during the teaching session, thereby helping to ensure their compliance with the medication regimen.

Interventions

7. Instruct the child and parents on proper injection sites and on the need for rotating sites. Explain that they should use the same anatomic area (common sites include the thigh, arm, or abdomen) for injections and that they should rotate the site so that each subsequent injection is 1 inch away from the previous site. Instruct the child to keep a chart of the sites used.

8. Instruct the child and parents on the purpose and procedure for home glucose monitoring. Have the parents demonstrate the procedure to the child by testing their own blood.

9. Instruct the child and parents on sick-day management and urine ketone testing.

10. Help the parents to plan for the child's return to school by creating a daily schedule for glucose testing, insulin administration, and meals and snacks. Encourage them to set up an appointment with the child's teacher or school nurse to explain the child's condition.

11. Explain to the child and parents the importance of maintaining proper hygiene. Advise the child to avoid walking in bare feet and to keep his toenails cut straight across, being careful not to nick the skin. Also advise him to keep his perineal area clean and dry.

12. Emphasize to the parents the importance of having the child's eyes checked at least yearly.

13. Advise the child to wear a Medic Alert necklace or bracelet that identifies him as a diabetic.

Rationales

7. Rotating the sites helps to prevent hypertrophy of the muscles.

8. Home glucose monitoring enables the child and parents to check the child's blood glucose levels on a regular basis, thereby ensuring that levels are within the acceptable range (usually between 80 and 120 mg/dl). Having the parents rather than the nurse demonstrate the procedure is less frightening to the child and helps ensure compliance with the technique.

9. During times of illness, insulin dosages may need to be adjusted to compensate for the child's decreased appetite and unstable blood glucose levels. Urine ketone testing, together with blood glucose monitoring, is effective in determining the child's insulin needs during this time.

10. A schedule helps to prioritize the child's daily needs and helps ensure compliance with the home care regimen. Meeting with the child's teacher or school nurse alerts the proper authorities to the child's condition in case emergency intervention is necessary.

11. Proper hygiene is important, as diabetics are poor healers and more susceptible than the general population to infection.

12. Yearly eye examinations are important, as diabetics are at risk for certain vision problems, such as diabetic retinopathy.

13. Such identification is necessary in case the child requires emergency treatment.

Documentation checklist

During the hospitalization, be sure to document the following:
___ the child's status and assessment findings upon admission
___ any changes in the child's status
___ fluid intake and output
___ nutritional intake
___ blood and urine glucose levels
___ insulin dosages and injection sites
___ the child's response to treatment
___ the child's and parents' reaction to the illness
___ patient and family teaching guidelines
___ discharge planning guidelines.

ENDOCRINE SYSTEM
Graves' Disease

Introduction
An autoimmune disease of unknown etiology, Graves' disease is characterized by thyrotoxicosis with diffuse goiter, exophthalmos, or pretibial myxedema (or any combination of the three) resulting from the overproduction of thyroid hormones. The disease affects more girls than boys. Peak incidence is during adolescence (ages 12 to 14).

Assessment
Endocrine
• goiter with bruit
• elevated levels of triiodothyronine (T_3) or thyroxine (T_4) (or both)
• low levels of thyroid-stimulating hormone (TSH)

Cardiovascular
• tachycardia
• wide pulse pressure
• systolic hypertension
• murmurs

Neurologic
• nervousness
• irritability
• recent poor school performance
• hyperactivity

Gastrointestinal
• increased appetite
• diarrhea
• weight loss

Musculoskeletal
• tall stature (if undiagnosed for a long period)
• fine hand tremors
• muscle weakness

EENT
• exophthalmos
• eyelid retraction (stare)
• visual disturbances

Integumentary
• excessive sweating
• warm, moist skin
• fine hair texture
• heat intolerance

Nursing diagnosis: *Altered nutrition: less than body requirements related to increased metabolic state*

GOAL: The child will maintain an adequate nutritional status as evidenced by improved nutritional intake and weight gain.

Interventions

1. Serve the child small, frequent meals that are high in carbohydrates and protein.

2. Try to incorporate some of the child's favorite foods into each meal, and encourage the parents to bring in some of these foods when visiting.

3. Arrange for the hospital dietitian to meet with the parents before the child is discharged from the hospital.

Rationales

1. Eating small, frequent meals is less tiring to the child and helps ensure that he will eat more of each meal. A high-carbohydrate, high-protein diet provides essential nutrients and calories to help with normal growth and development.

2. Serving the child's favorite foods helps ensure that he will eat more of each meal.

3. The parents will require special counseling on the child's caloric intake once the hyperthyroidism is controlled, as continued excessive intake can lead to obesity.

Nursing diagnosis: *Sleep-pattern disturbance related to hypermetabolic state*

GOAL: The child will receive adequate rest as evidenced by sleeping 8 to 10 hours each night and taking one nap during the day.

Interventions

1. Encourage the child to go to bed at a regular time and to comply with the unit's lights-out schedule. Instruct him to stay in bed, but allow him to play quietly if he is not sleepy.

2. Schedule one or two nap periods during the day based on the child's individual activity cycle. Make sure the room is dark and quiet at this time.

3. Maintain the child's room at a cool temperature.

Rationales

1. Children with Graves' disease often have insomnia and need to maintain a regular schedule for sleep.

2. Scheduling nap time will depend on the child's normal activity cycle. Providing a dark, quiet environment helps induce sleep.

3. Heat intolerance, a frequent symptom of Graves' disease, may contribute to sleeplessness.

Nursing diagnosis: *Disturbance in self-concept: personal identity related to hypermetabolic state*

GOAL: The child will have an improved self-image as evidenced by identifying his unique and desirable qualities and verbalizing an acceptance of his altered body image.

Interventions

1. Help the child to identify his unique talents or skills rather than concentrate on his physical appearance.

2. Encourage the parents to bring in the child's schoolwork on a regular basis.

3. Provide various age-appropriate activities to direct the child's energies. Avoid activities that are strenuous or intense or that require a long attention span.

4. Explain to the child that changes in his activity level, attention span, and emotional lability are disease-related and that, as hyperthyroidism is controlled, his previous behavioral patterns will reemerge.

Rationales

1. Graves' disease, when undetected for a long period, can result in such physical changes as eyelid retraction, exophthalmos, goiter, fine hand tremors, excessive sweating, and excessive growth. These changes can be especially disturbing to an adolescent. Getting the child to identify his unique talents and skills helps to divert his attention from his appearance and allows him to build self-esteem.

2. The child may have fallen behind in his studies because of his poor attention span, which is characteristic of hyperthyroidism. Allowing the child to work on school assignments for short intervals enables him to keep up with his peers and promotes a feeling of accomplishment and improved self-esteem.

3. Such activities help to combat boredom and promote normal growth and development. Providing nonstrenuous activities that require little intensity and a short attention span promote self-assurance and are less tiring to the child.

4. The child may not understand that his behavioral changes are transient and disease-related and may be confused or overly anxious about his current state. Reassuring him that such changes are temporary and caused by his illness can help improve his self-esteem.

Nursing diagnosis: *Anxiety (child and parent) related to surgery*

GOAL: The child and parents will be less fearful as evidenced by verbalizing an understanding of the need for surgery and an awareness of the perioperative events.

Interventions

1. Explain to the child and parents the reason for surgery. (Thyroidectomy usually is required because of poor physiologic response to medication or noncompliance with the medical regimen.)

2. Verify that the child and parents are aware of the potential adverse effects of the procedure, including parathyroid damage, hoarseness, and hypothyroidism. Explain that, although a small portion of the thyroid gland may be left postoperatively, the child may be hypothyroid and require replacement thyroid medication. He also may be hypocalcemic from trauma or manipulation of the parathyroid gland and require replacement calcium medication.

3. Explain to the child and parents that, before thyroidectomy can be scheduled, the child must be euthyroid. Hospitalization sometimes is required for 10 days to 2 weeks before the procedure to monitor and suppress thyroid function.

Rationales

1. Understanding the reason for surgery should help the child and parents feel less anxious about the procedure.

2. Being aware of the potential for such postoperative problems helps to decrease anxiety should these problems actually occur.

3. Explaining this to the child and parents helps them to anticipate the need for further medications and special monitoring before surgery (such as monitoring for hyperglycemia and hypertension), thereby helping to lessen their anxiety.

Nursing diagnosis: *Potential for infection related to surgery*

GOAL: The child will have no signs of postoperative wound infection as evidenced by a lack of foul odor and purulent drainage and by stable vital signs.

Interventions

1. Change the child's surgical dressing every 24 hours. Observe wound for redness, swelling, bleeding, and drainage. Record the time of each dressing change.

2. Monitor the child's temperature, as ordered. Notify the doctor if the child's temperature is elevated.

Rationales

1. Redness, swelling, or drainage may indicate infection and the need for antibiotic therapy.

2. An elevated temperature may indicate infection.

Nursing diagnosis: *Potential for injury related to surgery*

GOAL: The child will have no signs of further injury as evidenced by lack of excessive bleeding or swelling at surgical site and no signs of hoarseness or respiratory difficulty.

Interventions

1. Place a small rolled towel under the child's neck to keep the neck slightly flexed.

2. Assess the child for hoarseness or respiratory difficulty every 1 to 2 hours for 48 hours.

Rationales

1. Maintaining the child in this position helps prevent strain on the sutures.

2. Hoarseness or respiratory difficulty may indicate nerve damage or increased swelling from bleeding or edema at the surgical site, possibly indicating the need for intubation.

Nursing diagnosis: *Knowledge deficit related to home care*

GOAL: The parents will verbalize an understanding of home care instructions.

Interventions

1. Review with the parents the medications ordered for the child and help them to devise a schedule for regular administration. Advise them to contact the school nurse to help with administration during school hours.

2. Instruct the parents on recognizing and reporting the adverse effects of antithyroid medications (skin rash, urticaria, arthritis-like symptoms, and fever) and the signs and symptoms of hypothyroidism (dry skin, puffiness around the eyes, constipation, and decreased energy level).

3. Instruct the parents on the purpose and use of propranolol, including details on administration, dosage, and potential adverse effects (bradycardia and hypoglycemia). Explain that propranolol may be given for 5 to 7 days, then tapered as the child's symptoms of hypermetabolism are controlled. Caution them against stopping the medication suddenly, and advise the child to avoid strenuous physical activity.

4. Instruct the parents to notify the doctor immediately if the child has a recurrence of signs and symptoms of hyperthyroidism, including nervousness, irritability, heat intolerance, excessive sweating, tachycardia, fine hand tremors, diarrhea, and warm, moist skin.

5. Explain to the parents the importance of keeping all follow-up medical and laboratory appointments.

Rationales

1. It is important that antithyroid medications, such as propylthiouracil and methimazole, are given as scheduled. A missed or delayed dose may compromise the suppressive action of the medication on the thyroid gland.

2. Children who take antithyroid medications are at high risk for adverse effects, such as agranulocytosis.

3. Understanding the purpose and use of the medication should help the parents and child to comply with the medication regimen. Knowing the potential adverse effects should prompt them to seek medical advice and attention, when necessary.

4. Symptoms may recur despite the child's adherence to the medication regimen. Thyroid storm, although rare in children, is an extreme metabolic imbalance caused by excessive thyroid hormone levels and stress. It may follow untreated hyperthyroidism.

5. Regular follow-up care is essential to evaluate the child's thyroid function. Laboratory studies (such as a complete blood count and T_3, T_4, and thyroid-stimulating hormone studies) help to evaluate the effectiveness of medication therapy.

Documentation checklist

During the hospitalization, be sure to document the following:
___ the child's status and assessment findings upon admission
___ any changes in the child's status
___ pertinent laboratory and diagnostic findings
___ fluid intake and output
___ nutritional intake
___ growth and development status
___ cardiovascular status
___ the child's response to treatment
___ the child's and parents' reaction to the illness and hospitalization
___ patient and family teaching guidelines
___ discharge planning guidelines.

Anorexia Nervosa

Introduction

Anorexia nervosa is a complex emotional disorder characterized by severe weight loss and body image disturbances, preoccupation with food, and a morbid fear of obesity. Although the exact etiology is unknown, the disorder, which usually affects adolescent girls, can be linked to some underlying psychological or behavioral problem.

Treatment may include the use of I.V. replacement therapy, total parenteral nutrition, and long-term psychotherapy. Potential complications include cardiovascular damage, hypothermia, dehydration, and death. The expected outcome is variable, as anorexics are difficult to treat and often have relapses.

Assessment
Psychosocial
- intense fear of becoming obese
- refusal to maintain weight
- distorted body image (overestimation of weight)
- moodiness
- social isolation
- feelings of insecurity and helplessness

Cardiovascular
- bradycardia
- hypotension

Musculoskeletal
- weight loss of over 25% of body weight

Endocrine
- amenorrhea

Integumentary
- lanugo
- dry skin
- hypothermia

Nursing diagnosis: *Altered nutrition: less than body requirements related to fear of obesity*

GOAL: The child will have an improved nutritional intake as evidenced by gaining 2 lb/week.

Interventions

1. Provide a well-balanced, high-calorie diet (increasing the caloric intake by 200 to 300 calories/day, to a total of 3,000 calories/day).

2. Weigh the child daily without revealing the actual weight gain to the child.

3. Stay with the child during and after meals.

4. Enforce bed rest until the life-threatening period (marked by fluid and electrolyte imbalance, bradycardia, and extreme weakness) is over.

5. Establish a written contract that clearly defines the child's responsibilities as well as those of the hospital staff regarding diet and activities. Avoid any discussion of food.

6. Use a nasogastric tube to feed the child if she continues to lose rather than gain weight.

Rationales

1. A high-calorie diet is necessary to help reverse the anorexic effects of the disorder and to ensure that the child gains weight. However, giving more than 3,000 calories/day can lead to cardiac arrest.

2. Monitoring the daily weight is an important assessment tool for gauging the child's current nutritional status. Keeping the actual weight gain from the child helps to prevent any manipulative behavior (such as eating meals, then vomiting or taking laxatives) that could lead to a dietary setback.

3. Being present during and after meals ensures that the child does not dispose of food or resort to self-induced vomiting.

4. Bed rest reduces the amount of energy required to maintain vital organs and promotes steady weight gain.

5. A written contract provides limits and structure. Avoiding discussions of food is important, as such discussions may increase the child's anxiety or lead to power struggles with nursing and other staff members.

6. Tube feeding may be necessary to ensure that the child receives adequate calories and nutrients to sustain life.

Nursing diagnosis: *Disturbance in self-concept: body image related to the psychological effects of the disorder*

GOAL: The child will demonstrate a positive self-image as evidenced by remarking positively about her image and performing activities of daily living.

Interventions

1. Encourage the child to engage in activities that will help her become aware of body sensations, such as discussions on appetite before and after meals.

2. Use analogies and storytelling that demonstrate appropriate communication and interfamily relationships to help the child change her self-perception.

3. Encourage the child to recognize her strengths, talents, and skills in a warm, caring manner.

4. Ensure that the child receives consistent care by the same health care members throughout the hospitalization.

Rationales

1. Anorexics are often unaware of such body sensations as hunger and satiety and need to be reminded that they exist.

2. Because of the child's distorted self-image, she may not respond to direct discussions about her appearance and the disorder.

3. Such encouragement helps the child to build self-confidence and self-acceptance and to overcome the intense feelings of rejection often associated with this disorder. It also enables her to focus on her inner strengths rather than on her physical appearance.

4. Anorexics require consistent care and a highly structured environment to promote behavioral changes.

Nursing diagnosis: *Social isolation related to role conflict*

GOAL: The child will exhibit decreased social isolation as evidenced by the ability to make friends and to perform age-appropriate role behaviors.

Interventions

1. Discuss with the child her perceived family and societal roles, and assess the appropriateness of her role behaviors.

2. Use role playing to help the child learn appropriate family and societal role behaviors. Provide positive reinforcement.

3. Help the child to select role behaviors that meet her personal needs rather than the perceived needs of others.

4. Teach the child to use problem-solving skills to help her accomplish age-appropriate developmental tasks.

Rationales

1. Such discussions and assessments enable the nurse to determine the child's cognitive state and to evaluate her feelings of isolation in relation to role conflicts.

2. Role playing can effectively teach the child to learn new age-appropriate behaviors, thereby helping to decrease feelings of isolation.

3. By selecting behaviors that concentrate on fulfilling personal needs, the child should feel less threatened and isolated.

4. Mastering such skills promotes a feeling of competence in dealing with life's demands and problems.

Nursing diagnosis: *Impaired social interaction related to low self-esteem*

GOAL: The child will demonstrate improved social interaction as evidenced by exhibiting feelings of love and support and by communicating effectively with parents and significant others.

Interventions

1. Encourage the child to express her feelings and needs.

2. Help the child learn to distinguish between dependent and independent behaviors and to strive for a balance between the two.

Rationales

1. Getting the child to talk about herself opens the lines of communication and forces her to acknowledge her true feelings and needs.

2. The balance between dependency and aggressive drives positively influences the ability to love and be loved (that is, an overabundance of dependency or aggressive behavior affects the child's ability to develop satisfactory relationships).

Interventions

3. Teach the child effective communication and socialization skills.

4. Provide consistent verbal and nonverbal feedback when interacting with the child.

5. Coordinate the support of the child's family and friends.

Rationales

3. Learning these skills helps the child to develop a mastery over herself and her environment and enables her to interact in a socially acceptable manner.

4. Consistent feedback helps the child to build a trusting therapeutic relationship.

5. A strong support system provides nurturing, which is essential to the child's developing a sense of self-identity and self-esteem.

Documentation checklist

During the hospitalization, be sure to document the following:

___ the child's status and assessment findings upon admission
___ any changes in the child's status
___ pertinent laboratory and diagnostic findings
___ fluid intake and output
___ nutritional intake
___ behavioral contract
___ weight gain
___ family involvement and therapy
___ discharge planning guidelines.

PSYCHOSOCIAL AND OTHER PROBLEMS

Autism

Introduction

Autism is a developmental disability usually manifested before age 2½ and characterized by disturbances in speech and language, mobility, perception, and interpersonal relationships. The disorder occurs in 5 out of every 10,000 children, affecting boys more than girls.

Treatment includes behavioral modification therapy and a structured environment usually provided in a specialized care unit. Potential complications include abuse, neglect, and the breakdown of family relationships.

Assessment

Psychosocial
• withdrawal and unresponsiveness to parents
• extreme resistance to change
• inappropriate attachment to objects
• self-stimulating behavior
• irregular sleep patterns
• stereotypic play
• destructive behavior toward self and others
• frequent tantrums
• attention to soft sounds rather than speech
• decreased verbalization
• refusal to eat lumpy foods

Neurologic
• inappropriate responses to stimuli
• poor sucking reflex
• failure to cry when hungry

Nursing diagnosis: *Impaired communication: verbal related to stimulus confusion*

GOAL: The child will communicate his needs as evidenced by his ability to use simple, concrete words.

Interventions

1. When communicating with the child, speak in one- to three-word sentences and repeat commands, as necessary. Tell the child to look at you when you speak, and closely observe his body language.

2. Use rhythms, music, and body movements to foster communication until the child can understand language.

3. Help the child to recognize the relationship between cause and effect by naming specific feelings and identifying the cause of or stimulus behind them.

4. When communicating with the child, be sure to differentiate reality from fantasy in clear, simple terms.

Rationales

1. Communicating through the use of simple, repetitive sentences is necessary because the child may not progress beyond the stage of concrete operational thought. Direct eye contact forces the child to focus his attention on the speaker and helps him to correlate speech with language and communication. Because of the child's inarticulateness, body language may be his only means of communicating his acknowledgment or comprehension of speech.

2. Physical movements and sound help the child to recognize body integrity and boundaries, thereby reinforcing his separate identity from objects and other people.

3. Understanding the concept of cause and effect helps the child to establish a sense of separateness apart from objects and other people and allows him to verbalize his needs and feelings.

4. Often, autistic children do not differentiate between reality and fantasy and fail to acknowledge pain or other sensations and life events in a meaningful way. By emphasizing the difference between reality and fantasy, the nurse can help the child to express his real needs and feelings.

Nursing diagnosis: *Potential for violence: self-directed or directed at others related to hospitalization*

GOAL: The child will exhibit decreased tendencies toward violent or self-destructive behavior as evidenced by decreased tantrums and episodes of aggression or destruction and increased ability to cope with frustration.

Interventions

1. Provide a structured environment and as much routine as possible throughout the hospitalization.

2. When performing nursing interventions, provide care in short, frequent sessions. Be sure to approach the child in a gentle, friendly manner, and explain what you are about to do in clear, simple terms. If necessary, demonstrate the procedure first on the parents.

3. Use physical restraint during procedures, when necessary, to ensure the child's safety and to redirect his anger and frustration. For example, to prevent the child from banging his head repeatedly against a wall, restrain his upper body but allow him to slap a pillow.

4. Use appropriate behavior modification techniques to reward positive behavior and punish negative behavior. For example, reward positive behavior by giving the child a favorite food or toy; punish negative behavior by ignoring the child or sending him to stand in a corner of the room. ·

5. When the child is behaving in destructive ways, ask him if he is trying to tell you something, such as that he would like something to eat or drink or that he needs to go to the bathroom.

Rationales

1. Autistic children thrive on structure and routine and often cannot cope with changes in their lives. Maintaining order is necessary to help prevent feelings of frustration that could lead to violent episodes.

2. Short, frequent sessions allow the child to become familiar with the nurse and the hospital environment. Maintaining a calm, friendly manner and demonstrating procedures on parents can help direct the child to accepting interventions as nonthreatening measures, thereby preventing destructive behavior.

3. Physical restraint may be necessary to prevent the child from engaging in self-destructive behavior. Allowing the child to engage in less harmful behavior, such as pillow slapping, enables him to redirect his anger yet still express his frustration.

4. Reward and punishment may an effective means of altering the child's behavior to prevent violent episodes.

5. Any increase in aggressive behavior may indicate that the child is feeling increased stress, possibly from the need to communicate something.

Nursing diagnosis: *Potential for altered parenting related to the disorder*

GOAL: The parents will demonstrate normal parenting skills as evidenced by verbalizing their concerns about the child's condition and seeking advice and help.

Interventions

1. Encourage the parents to express their feeling and concerns.

2. Refer the parents to a local autistic support group and to a specialized school, as necessary.

Rationales

1. Allowing the parents to express their feelings and concerns about the child's chronic condition may help them to better cope with the frustrations involved in raising an autistic child.

2. Support groups allow the parents to meet with parents of other autistic children to share information and provide emotional support. Specialized schools provide a structured environment in which to implement behavioral modification therapy.

Documentation checklist

During the hospitalization, be sure to document the following:

___ the child's status and assessment findings upon admission

___ any change in the child's status

___ fluid intake and output

___ nutritional intake

___ environmental structure

___ behavioral modification therapy

___ family involvement and therapy

___ discharge planning guidelines.

Bulimia

Introduction

Bulimia refers to a syndrome characterized by self-induced vomiting or laxative use and powerful urges to overeat. The child, typically an older adolescent girl, usually has an obsessive fear of obesity and may even resort to intermittent periods of starvation to avoid becoming fat.

Treatment usually involves I.V. fluid replacement, total parenteral nutrition, psychotherapy, and behavioral modification. Potential complications include fluid and electrolyte imbalances, cardiovascular disorders, muscle weakness, and anemia. The outcome is variable, as bulimics are often difficult to treat.

Assessment

Psychosocial
• recurrent binging during which high-calorie foods are consumed
• self-induced vomiting
• laxative and diuretic abuse
• hiding of food

Neurologic
• morbid fear of the inability to control food intake
• depression after binges

Gastrointestinal
• gastric dilation
• esophagitis

Musculoskeletal
• weight fluctuations

EENT
• erosion of enamel on inner surface of teeth

Endocrine
• painless swelling of salivary glands
• menstrual irregularities

Nursing diagnosis: *Altered nutrition: less than body requirements related to bulimic behavior*

GOAL: The child will maintain an adequate nutritional intake as evidenced by eating the prescribed diet, maintaining weight within standard limits, and having no episodes of self-induced vomiting.

Interventions

1. Establish a written contract with the child regarding her diet and activity.

2. Stay with the child during and after meals.

3. Encourage the child to discuss her feelings.

Rationales

1. Written contracts provide structure and limitations necessary for the bulimic child while decreasing the level of dietary manipulation (such as eating, then vomiting or taking laxatives).

2. Staying with the child is important to provide needed support and to ensure that she does not resort to self-induced vomiting.

3. Getting the child to ventilate her feelings is an important part of the overall therapy, as bulimic children often use eating as a means of coping with problems.

Nursing diagnosis: *Disturbance in self-concept: personal identity related to weight loss*

GOAL: The child will demonstrate an improved self-concept as evidenced by verbalizing an acceptance of her body image and appropriate weight.

Interventions	Rationales
1. Encourage the child to discuss her feelings about her family, friends, and self-image.	1. Such discussions help the nurse to assess the child's cognitive and emotional state and to begin building a therapeutic relationship with the child.
2. Assess the child for signs and symptoms of sexual abuse (such as overt sexual behavior and language, increased masturbation, isolation, and withdrawal from adults).	2. Bulimic children sometimes exhibit signs and symptoms of sexual abuse that may account for their negative self-concept and low self-esteem.
3. Assess the child's usual coping mechanisms.	3. Such assessment helps the nurse to determine which coping mechanisms are maladaptive, possibly contributing to the child's condition and underlying negative self-concept.
4. Help the child to establish and achieve realistic short- and long-term goals.	4. Achieving clearly defined, realistic, and measurable goals is important for normal growth and development, especially for a child suffering from chronic low self-esteem.
5. Reinforce the child's strengths and skills.	5. Reinforcing strengths and skills helps the child to focus on the positive aspects of her personality rather than on the negative aspects that might be contributing to her bulimia.
6. Teach the child necessary role behaviors that will enhance her sense of competency.	6. Role adequacy supports a sense of self-esteem.
7. Coordinate the support of family and friends to provide realistic, positive feedback.	7. A strong support system helps provide the nurturing needed to reinforce the child's sense of self-esteem.

Documentation checklist

During the hospitalization, be sure to document the following:

__ the child's status and assessment findings upon admission
__ any change in the child's status
__ fluid intake and output
__ nutritional intake
__ behavioral contract
__ weight gain
__ family involvement and therapy
__ discharge planning guidelines.

Burn Injuries

Introduction

Thermal injuries caused by intense heat, electrical shock, chemical burns, or radiation are the third leading cause of accidental death in children. About 80% of all burn injuries occur within the home, most of which result from exposure to flames or scalding with extremely hot water.

Major burns affect not only the integumentary system but also the respiratory, cardiovascular, musculoskeletal, and other body systems and present a special challenge to the nursing and medical team.

Treatment usualy involves fluid replacement, burn treatment (using sterile dressings, debridement, and topical ointments), and physical therapy. Potential complications include contractures, kidney damage, respiratory disease, and death. The expected outcome depends on the severity of the burn.

Assessment

Integumentary
• reddened, blistered, or blackened skin
• edema
• exudate

Cardiovascular
• decreased cardiac output (initially)
• shock

Respiratory
• respiratory distress
• hoarseness

Genitourinary
• decreased urine output initially, followed by increased urine output
• hematuria

EENT
• singed nasal hairs
• soot-coated tongue

Hematologic
• anemia

Nursing diagnosis: *Impaired gas exchange related to edema of the upper airway*

GOAL: The child's respiratory status will remain stable as evidenced by normal rate, depth, and ease of breathing.

Interventions

1. Assess child for singed nasal hair, soot-coated tongue, wheezing, soot-laden sputum, or hoarseness. Then determine where and how the injury occurred. Note whether the child has a history of previous respiratory problems.

2. Monitor the child's respiratory status hourly, noting the rate and depth of respirations, hoarseness, nasal flaring, retractions, and changes in arterial blood gas (ABG) levels (such as increased PO_2 and decreased PCO_2 levels).

3. Gently suction the child, as needed.

4. Assist with endotracheal intubation, as necessary.

Rationales

1. These signs indicate injury resulting from smoke inhalation, direct thermal injury to the respiratory tract, or shock. Knowing the exact cause of the injury is essential to providing immediate and appropriate treatment.

2. Increased respiratory rate and effort and developing hoarseness are indications of increasing airway obstruction. ABG studies indicate the child's current oxygen, carbon dioxide, and pH levels.

3. Suctioning is necessary because respiratory injury is accompanied by increased secretions and decreased ciliary action.

4. Prophylactic intubation may be performed in children with known smoke inhalation or facial burns.

Nursing diagnosis: *Fluid volume deficit related to fluid lost through thermal burns*

GOAL: The child will maintain adequate fluid balance as evidenced by good skin turgor, a brisk capillary refill time, no mental confusion, moist mucous membranes, and a urine output of 1 ml/kg/hour.

Interventions

1. Maintain I.V. patency and administer I.V. fluids, including plasma and electrolyte solutions, as ordered.

2. Monitor the child's urine output and urine specific gravity hourly, observing for trends.

3. Monitor the child's mental state, vital signs, peripheral perfusion, and urine volume.

4. Monitor the child's daily weight.

Rationales

1. I.V. patency is crucial to allow for administration of replacement fluids during the first 24 to 48 hours after burn injury. During this time, profuse amounts of plasma begin leaking from the vasculature to the interstitial spaces, resulting in decreased circulatory volume.

2. Changes in urine output (output usually is 0.5 to 1 ml/kg/hour) may indicate renal failure, fluid shifts, or diuresis related to various stages of burn injury. Specific gravity (should be 1.005 to 1.030) increases with significant protein breakdown. Trends lasting over 2 hours are more significant than a single reading.

3. Such monitoring helps to determine the child's current fluid status and the need for adjustments in therapy.

4. Daily weight monitoring is a major indication of the child's current fluid status.

Nursing diagnosis: *Impaired skin integrity related to the burn wound (pregrafting)*

GOAL: The child will have no indication of impaired skin integrity as evidenced by new skin growth and reduction in the size of the burn and no signs of infection.

Interventions

1. Bathe the child with an antiseptic solution, such as povidone-iodine solution or bleach, one or two times daily.

2. Remove the eschar using a soft sponge, forceps, and scissors.

3. Observe the wound for changes in the amount, color, or odor of drainage and for other signs of bacterial infection (such as fever).

4. Apply a topical antimicrobial ointment or solution, such as silver sulfadiazine or silver nitrate, as ordered.

5. After debridement, inspect the homograft, xenograft, or synthetic wound dressing for purulence or further necrosis.

Rationales

1. Bathing promotes gentle separation of the eschar and dilutes and removes surface bacteria.

2. Removing eschar decreases the risk of bacterial infection.

3. Changes in the wound appearance may indicate developing sepsis and may signal problems with the potential graft site.

4. Topical antimicrobials may be ordered to decrease the risk of bacterial infection.

5. Purulent areas of the dressing should be removed to prevent bacterial invasion and burn wound sepsis.

Nursing diagnosis: *Ineffective thermoregulation related to skin damage and heat loss*

GOAL: The child will maintain normal thermoregulation as evidenced by maintaining a temperature between 99° and 100° F. (37.2° and 37.8° C.).

Interventions

1. Monitor the child's temperature hourly until stable.

Rationales

1. Frequent monitoring ensures the early detection and prompt treatment of hypothermia to prevent the risk of potential life-threatening adverse effects, such as sepsis and renal failure.

Interventions

2. Maintain a warm environment. Make sure that the water temperature for hydrotherapy remains at 98° F. (36.7° C.) and that the room temperature remains at 88° F. (31.1° C.).

3. Use an overhead radiant heat lamp, and cover the child with blankets, making sure the blankets are tented around the child's body and not lying directly on the skin surface.

Rationales

2. A warm environment and constant water temperature minimizes the reduction of core body temperature by reducing radiant heat loss.

3. Use of an overhead heat lamp and blankets further reduces the amount of radiant heat lost and increases body temperature.

Nursing diagnosis: *Potential for infection related to changes in skin integrity*

GOAL: The child will have no signs of systemic infection as evidenced by stable vital signs and normal wound cultures.

Interventions

1. Monitor the child's vital signs every 1 to 2 hours, noting any changes in the heart and respiratory rate or body temperature.

2. Monitor the child for nausea, vomiting, and abdominal distention.

3. Test the child's stools for occult bleeding using a guaiac preparation (such as Hemoccult).

4. Assess the child for changes in neurologic status or behavior.

5. Assess the burn wound for changes in color, drainage, and odor.

6. Assist with obtaining skin biopsies for culturing, as ordered.

7. Administer antibiotics and fluid, electrolyte, and plasma replacements, as ordered.

8. Screen all visitors for signs and symptoms of infection before they enter the child's room, and institute isolation precautions, as necessary.

Rationales

1. Increased heart and respiratory rates and increased or decreased body temperature may be early signs of sepsis.

2. Impaired intestinal motility is a common early complication of burn injury. Ileus occurring later in the hospitalization may indicate sepsis.

3. Evidence of occult bleeding may indicate that the child has a stress ulcer, which is commonly associated with septicemia.

4. A change from an alert state to one of lethargy, confusion, or delerium may indicate sepsis.

5. Changes such as foul odor and purulent drainage may indicate bacterial infection.

6. Surgery may be required to remove the source of infection if biopsy reports indicate 7 to 10 microorganisms per 1 gram of vital tissue.

7. Such supportive measures usually are instituted as soon as sepsis is suspected. Antibiotics help to fight infection. Fluid, plasma, and electrolytes help to stabilize the circulatory system to fight infection by supplying the tissues with nutrients.

8. Such precautions are necessary to reduce the risk of infection.

Nursing diagnosis: *Impaired skin integrity related to the burn wound (postgrafting)*

GOAL: The child will have no signs of impaired skin integrity as evidenced by an intact autograft and a pink skin color.

Interventions

1. Determine what type of graft (autograft, homograft, xenograft, isograft) was applied to the burn wound.

2. Roll sheet grafts every 1 to 2 hours with a cotton-tipped applicator.

Rationales

1. The type of graft determines the nursing care required.

2. Rolling sheet grafts removes excess plasma and promotes adherence of the graft to the wound.

Interventions	**Rationales**
3. Assess the color, amount, and type of drainage from the graft, and note whether the graft appears to be adhering to the wound.	3. Within 48 to 72 hours after graft placement, the graft should become vascularized. Purulent or bloody drainage and swelling indicate that the wound is not fully vascularized.
4. Blot any excess blood or plasma from graft.	4. Removing excess blood minimizes crust formation and promotes adherence.
5. Use a bed cradle or reposition the child so that the graft does not come in contact with sheets or bed linens.	5. New grafts must be protected from rubbing to ensure adherence to the wound.

Nursing diagnosis: *Altered comfort: pain related to skin damage and destruction*

GOAL: The child will have minimal pain as evidenced by stable vital signs, decreased verbalization of pain, and decreased restlessness and irritability.

Interventions	**Rationales**
1. Assess the child for tachycardia, tachypnea, crying, withdrawal, decreased appetite, and inability to sleep.	1. Because children are sometimes too embarrassed to complain about pain, they may try to hide their discomfort. Changes in vital signs, emotional level, appetite, and ability to sleep may signal increased discomfort.
2. Administer pain medication, such as meperidine hydrochloride or morphine, as ordered.	2. Pain medication effectively controls the degree of pain.
3. Prepare the child for all treatments by explaining the procedures beforehand.	3. Knowing what to expect gives the child a greater sense of control over the situation and increases his tolerance of pain.
4. Allow the child to practice self-care, such as allowing him to bathe himself and to remove dressings, whenever possible.	4. The child's participation in routine care helps promote a sense of control over the situation and increases his tolerance of pain.
5. Institute additional pain-relief measures, such as relaxation and hypnosis, as needed.	5. Nonpharmacologic pain-control measures have proven effective in relieving pain from burn injuries.
6. Administer pain medication, such as meperidine hydrochloride or morphine, before such procedures as bathing and debridement.	6. Bathing and debridement are painful procedures and require premedication to help ease the pain.
7. Provide age-appropriate diversional activities.	7. Diversional activities help distract the child from his pain.
8. Use a bed cradle to keep bed linens away from the wound site.	8. Keeping the wound site free from contact with other surfaces helps prevent pain.

Nursing diagnosis: *Altered nutrition: less than body requirements related to increased caloric requirements*

GOAL: The child will maintain adequate nutritional status as evidenced by maintaining or increasing his weight and by eating most (at least 80%) of all meals.

Interventions	**Rationales**
1. Obtain a dietary history, including the child's usual food intake, food allergies, food preferences, and chewing and swallowing difficulties.	1. Such information, usually obtained from the parents (or the child, if age-appropriate) should be incorporated into the nutritional plan.

Interventions

2. Administer oral fluids or nasogastric feedings, as necessary.

3. Administer enteral fluids, such as Ensure, via a Silastic feeding tube.

4. Check gastric residual volumes before each feeding or every 4 hours if the child is being fed continuously by a nasogastric tube. Also assess bowel sounds.

5. Administer total parenteral nutrition, as necessary.

6. Offer the child a diet high in calories, protein, and carbohydrates.

7. Weigh the child daily.

8. Monitor the child's fluid intake and output hourly.

Rationales

2. Caloric requirements can be met by administering fluids (such as Ensure or an acceptable substitute).

3. Using a Silastic feeding tube is less irritating to the child's esophagus and helps to ensure that he receives adequate nutrition.

4. Checking for residual volume helps prevent unnecessary gastric dilation and vomiting. Children should not be fed if the residual volume is over one-half the amount of the proposed feeding or if bowel sounds are absent. Presence of bowel sounds indicates that the bowels are functioning.

5. High-protein, high-calorie parenteral feedings may be necessary if the child cannot tolerate enteral feedings.

6. Extra calories and protein help to replenish nutrients to allow for optimal tissue growth. Extra carbohydrates help to combat malnutrition.

7. Daily weight monitoring is a direct measure of the child's nutritional status.

8. Such monitoring is necessary to determine whether the child requires fluid replacement.

Nursing diagnosis: *Impaired physical mobility related to scar formation*

GOAL 1: The child will maintain physical mobility before grafting as evidenced by having full range of motion (ROM) and minimal contractures.

Interventions

1. Position the child as follows to minimize contracture formation:
• neck—slightly extended with no pillow
• ankles—placed at a 90-degree angle on a foot board
• elbows and knees—placed in a three-point splint to keep the joint extended
• hands—placed in a thermoplastic splint to maintain a functional position
• burned extremity—elevated 20 to 30 degrees.
Also, encourage ambulation several times per day (if not contraindicated by the extent or severity of burns).

2. Depending on the degree of pain or edema, perform ROM exercises every 4 hours for 15 minutes, then reapply splints.

Rationales

1. Preventing contractures requires the application of forces to overcome the intrinsic pull of myofibroblasts.

2. ROM exercises are necessary to prevent joints from becoming stiff.

GOAL 2: The child will maintain physical mobility after healing as evidenced by having full ROM and minimal contractures.

Interventions

1. Apply splints and pressure bandages to all areas of deep second- and third-degree burns.

2. Perform ROM exercises, as ordered.

Rationales

1. Applying constant pressure helps minimize the formation of scars.

2. ROM exercises are necessary to help increase muscle tone and prevent contractures.

Nursing diagnosis: *Knowledge deficit related to home care*

GOAL: The parents will verbalize an understanding of home care instructions.

Interventions

1. Instruct the parents on proper wound care, including details on medication administration, cleansing techniques, debridement, dressing changes, and sterile technique. Have them demonstrate such care before the child is discharged from the hospital.

2. Instruct the parents to perform ROM exercises, such as moving all joints (knees, elbows, wrists, shoulders, and ankles) through their normal range of motion, every 4 hours for 15 minutes.

3. Explain to the parents the need for a diet high in calories, protein, and carbohydrates.

4. Encourage the parents to provide emotional support by allowing the child to perform self-care (when appropriate), encouraging him to express his feelings, and providing nonpharmacologic pain-control measures (such as hypnosis and guided imagery).

Rationales

1. Knowing this information and demonstrating techniques before discharge enables the parents to provide adequate home care.

2. ROM exercises, which increase the return of mobility to injured muscles and limbs, are an important part of the child's home care.

3. A high-calorie, high-protein diet provides essential nutrients to repair damaged tissue. A high-carbohydrate diet supplies necessary calories to combat malnutrition.

4. Burn injuries can be physiologically and psychologically devastating to the child, who requires much patience and support to work through his feelings of fear, anger, frustration, and body-image difficulties.

Documentation checklist

During the hospitalization, be sure to document the following:
___ the child's status and assessment findings upon admission
___ any changes in the child's status
___ pertinent laboratory and diagnostic findings
___ fluid intake and output
___ nutritional intake
___ the child's response to treatment
___ graft response
___ patient and family teaching guidelines
___ discharge planning guidelines.

Child Abuse and Neglect

Introduction

Child abuse and neglect involves chronic physical, mental, or emotional maltreatment of an infant or a child, usually resulting in physical trauma, sexual molestation, or nutritional or medical neglect. In recent years, the number of reported child abuse cases has risen sharply—as many as 25% of all children are considered abused or neglected in some way. Such abusive behavior may be triggered by stress, socioeconomic pressures, or other psychosocial problems. In many cases, the abusive parent or caregiver was abused as a child.

Treatment involves immediate medical attention to correct the child's physical problems (such as fractures, burns, or head or spinal cord injuries) and psychotherapy or family therapy. Part of the nurse's duty involves reporting all cases of known or suspected abuse to the proper authorities. Potential complications include brain damage, muscle and bone damage, coma, and death.

This care plan focuses on the psychosocial aspects of child abuse and neglect. For more information on the physical aspects, see the individual care plans on fractures, head injury, spinal cord injury, and burn injuries in this book.

Assessment

Psychosocial
- evidence of neglect (dirty clothes and hair, diaper rash, foul smell)
- failure to thrive
- delayed development (cognitive, psychomotor, psychosocial)

Integumentary
- circular lesions (usually caused by cigarette burns)
- scalded skin or burns
- bruises or abrasions
- unexplained human bite marks
- unexplained injuries
- soft-tissue swelling

Diagnostic tests

The following tests may be ordered, depending on the extent of injuries noted in the assessment:
- X-rays—to detect broken bones or dislocated joints
- vaginal and anal smears—to detect sexual abuse
- blood tests—to detect sexually transmitted disease.

Nursing diagnosis: *Ineffective family coping: compromised related to factors (specify) that contribute to child abuse*

GOAL: The parents and family will demonstrate improved coping mechanisms within 6 months after diagnosis.

Interventions

1. Identify factors leading to the breakdown of the family's coping mechanisms, such as the parents' age, the number of children in the family, the parents' socioeconomic status, the developmental level of all family members, the use or lack of support systems, and any other triggering events.

2. Consult appropriate health care personnel and social services regarding the family's problems. Offer referrals for individual or family therapy, as needed.

3. Encourage the child and family to express their feelings about what might be causing the abusive behavior.

4. Instruct the parents on the normal development and management of children at various age levels.

Rationales

1. Identifying such factors enables the nurse to determine the need for interventions and referral to appropriate health care and social services organizations.

2. Families affected by child abuse or neglect often require therapeutic care by a multidisciplinary team. Support groups, such as Parents Anonymous and Alcoholics Anonymous, can help with specific problems related to the dysfunctional mechanism involved.

3. Such encouragement allows the family to discuss their problems and to explore ways of modifying their behavior.

4. The parents may have unrealistic expectations regarding the normal growth and development of children, possibly affecting their ability to cope with the stresses of parenting.

Nursing diagnosis: *Altered growth and development related to inadequate caregiving*

GOAL: The child will demonstrate developmental advancement pertinent to age in cognitive, psychomotor, and psychosocial areas within 6 months after diagnosis.

Interventions

1. Administer age-appropriate developmental testing to determine the child's current developmental level.

2. Discuss test findings with the parents and child.

3. Initiate activities (such as reading, bicycling, and discussions on feelings) with the parents and child to enhance the development of deficient psychomotor skills, cognitive abilities, and psychosocial functioning.

4. Reassess the child's developmental levels at appropriate intervals, such as 1 month, 2 months, 6 months, and 1 year.

Rationales

1. Test results can be used as a baseline from which to gauge the child's progress over the projected course of teaching and therapy.

2. The parents and child should be aware of test findings so that they can plan for the achievement of short- and long-term goals.

3. Often, abused children experience developmental delays because of impaired family functioning. Initiating such activities helps to correct any problems resulting from dysfunctional relationships.

4. Assessing the developmental level at periodic intervals helps to determine whether the child is progressing as expected.

Nursing diagnosis: *Potential for violence (parent or abusive family member): directed at others related to maladaptive behavior and development*

GOAL: The parent or abusive family member will demonstrate a decreased level of violence within 2 to 4 weeks after diagnosis.

Interventions

1. Identify the abuser's violent behavior patterns, such as demonstrating abusive behavior while using alcohol or drugs or while unemployed.

2. Explore with the abuser the triggering factors that may have precipitated his violent episodes, such as alcohol or drug use.

3. Provide counseling on a multidisciplinary level, including referral to a psychologist and appropriate community organizations (such as Alcoholics Anonymous and Parents Anonymous).

4. Initiate family therapy (involving role playing and effective communication skills) by referring the family to an appropriate therapist.

5. Report all incidents of actual or suspected abuse to the proper authorities.

Rationales

1. Identifying such abusive behavior patterns provides a baseline from which to determine appropriate interventions and to gauge improvement.

2. Identifying such factors enhances the abuser's awareness of which situations might precipitate violent behavior, thereby helping him to prevent further recurrences.

3. Counseling is necessary to help the abuser develop effective coping skills to deal with and eliminate from his life-style the precipitating factors leading to abusive behavior.

4. Family therapy stresses the involvement and support of the entire family in helping to prevent recurrences of violent behavior patterns.

5. Nurses have a legal responsibility to report all such cases and to keep accurate records of physical evidence for further investigation.

Nursing diagnosis: *Altered parenting related to the abusive parent's inability to attach or bond with the child*

GOAL: The abusive parent will demonstrate appropriate and effective parenting patterns as evidenced by appropriate touching and the ability to communicate without yelling or screaming.

Interventions

1. Discuss normal attachment and bonding with the abusive parent.

2. Provide role models for the parent to emulate.

3. Encourage the parent to enroll in specific classes that teach appropriate parenting skills.

4. Refer the parent to appropriate support services (such as Parents Anonymous, Alcoholics Anonymous, or Al-Anon) for routine intervention and counseling, as needed.

Rationales

1. Making the parent aware of the normal attachment and bonding process may help him to become interested in developing appropriate parenting skills.

2. Role models allow the parent to imitate appropriate parenting behavior.

3. Such classes provide examples and practice forums for developing effective parenting skills.

4. The parent may need to rely on support services during times of crisis to help him cope with stressful events and situations that might trigger another abusive episode.

Documentation checklist

During the hospitalization, be sure to document the following:
___ the child's status and assessment findings upon admission
___ discharge planning guidelines.
___ parental involvement in the child's care
___ the child's response to the family
___ social services involvement
___ reports of abuse to the appropriate authorities.

Depression

Introduction

Depression is a mood disturbance disorder characterized by feelings of sadness, despair, and discouragement usually resulting from some loss or disappointment. The disorder is more common among adolescents than younger children and tends to run in families.

Acute depression that last from days to weeks may be normal and usually requires no medical or therapeutic intervention. Chronic depression, however, requires therapeutic measures, including psychotherapy and use of antidepressants. Potential complications include anorexia, bulimia, and suicide.

Assessment

Psychosocial
• impulsiveness
• self-destructive or self-demeaning behaviors
• attention-getting behaviors
• feelings of hopelessness, helplessness, and worthlessness
• withdrawal
• loss of interest in usual activities

Neurologic
• excessive sleep or insomnia

Gastrointestinal
• weight gain or loss

Nursing diagnosis: *Disturbance in self-concept related to low self-esteem*

GOAL: The child will demonstrate an improved self-concept as evidenced by demonstrating increased interest in interpersonal interactions, school, and social activities and by verbalizing an increased ability to cope with the future.

Interventions

1. Establish a trusting therapeutic relationship with the child.

2. Encourage the child to recognize and express his feelings, especially those of shame and loss, and to forgive himself and others.

3. Teach the child acceptable social skills (such as communication skills, proper hygiene, and appropriate dress) and role behaviors (family and societal) and provide positive feedback.

4. Carefully examine the child's belief systems and expectations about the future.

5. Identify the child's maladaptive coping mechanisms and encourage him to use alternative methods in times of crisis.

6. Coordinate peer and family support.

Rationales

1. Establishing a trusting relationship with the child is essential before treatment can begin. The child must feel comfortable enough to discuss his problems and usually will not share them with a total stranger.

2. A depressed child tends to internalize feelings. Getting him to express feelings of shame, loss, and forgiveness allows for progression through the normal stages of the grieving process, which is prerequisite to becoming well.

3. Learning to interact successfully with others and receiving positive feedback should increase the child's self-esteem and encourage him to feel hopeful about the future.

4. Such examination may reveal that the child has unrealistic expectations, possibly a source of much anxiety and stress and a contributing factor in his depression.

5. Learning to use appropriate coping mechanisms should help to improve the child's self-esteem through use of self-control.

6. A strong support system provides security, love, and a sense of belonging, which are necessary to building self-esteem.

Nursing diagnosis: *Potential for violence: self-directed or directed at others related to the inability to cope with negative feelings*

GOAL: The child will demonstrate decreased aggressiveness and violence as evidenced by not harming himself or others.

Interventions

1. Assess the child's potential for destructive behavior, and take necessary precautions to ensure his safety and the safety of others (including observing the child on an hourly basis and removing potentially harmful objects from his room).

2. Encourage the child to use alternative methods for coping with his negative feelings.

3. Help the child to recognize the cause and effect relationship of his violent behavior.

4. Teach the child appropriate problem-solving skills.

Rationales

1. External controls and safety measures may be necessary until the child learns to exhibit self-control.

2. Using alternative coping skills helps prevent the outbreak of violent episodes and promotes improved social relationships and increased self-esteem.

3. Getting the child to recognize the causes and consequences of his violent behavior should encourage him to accept responsibility for his actions and the need for change.

4. Learning to solve problems fosters self-control and feelings of adequacy.

Documentation checklist

During the hospitalization, be sure to document the following:
___ the child's status and assessment findings upon admission
___ behavioral contracts
___ therapy and group involvement
___ family involvement
___ discharge planning guidelines.

Failure to Thrive

Introduction
Failure to thrive is a chronic, potentially life-threatening condition characterized by failure to maintain weight and sometimes height above the fifth percentile on age-appropriate growth charts (see Appendix C: Physical Growth Charts). Most children with this condition are diagnosed before age 2.

The condition, which can result from physical causes or emotional or psychological problems, may be classified as follows:
• organic—caused by a serious illness, such as gastroesophageal reflux, malabsorption syndrome, congenital heart defects, or cystic fibrosis
• inorganic—the most common type, caused by psychosocial problems between the child and primary caregiver (usually the mother), such as failure to bond
• mixed—results from a combination of organic and inorganic causes.

Treatment may include dietary therapy, total parenteral nutrition, family therapy, and a structured environment. Potential complications include impairment of the child-parent relationship, impaired or delayed physical and psychosocial growth, and mental retardation.

Assessment
Psychosocial
• maternal deprivation resulting from child's low birth weight, sex, or appearance
• factors affecting the parents' (mother's) ability to bond with child, including:
  □ marital discord (spouse may be unsupportive, frequently absent, or a substance abuser)
  □ inadequate income
  □ unwanted pregnancy
  □ maternal age (under age 16)
  □ neglect or lack of attention as a child
  □ poor self-esteem
  □ limited ability to perceive the needs of others
  □ limited capacity for concern
  □ depression or other psychological problems

Cardiovascular
• tetralogy of Fallot
• transposition of the great vessels

Neurologic
• cerebral palsy

Gastrointestinal
• malabsorption syndrome
• chronic diarrhea
• pernicious vomiting

Musculoskeletal
• muscular dystrophy

Nursing diagnosis: *Altered growth and development related to inadequate weight gain*

GOAL: The child will demonstrate improved growth and development as evidenced by maintaining body weight while hospitalized.

Interventions

1. Weigh the child upon admission.

2. Assess the child's growth and development using age-appropriate growth charts and developmental screening tests (such as the Denver Developmental Screening Test).

3. Observe the interaction between the parents (particularly the mother) and child, including the establishment of eye-to-eye contact and the parents' handling of and communication with the child.

Rationales

1. A baseline weight is needed to assess the infant's progress throughout the hospitalization.

2. Such assessments are necessary to determine the child's developmental level compared to other children of the same age-group.

3. Failure to interact appropriately with the child may signal the parents' inability to form an emotional attachment to the child, which may be the cause of the child's failure to thrive.

Interventions

4. Assess the child's neurologic and cardiovascular status.

5. Provide ongoing assessments of the child's feeding and elimination patterns by:
• assigning one nurse for feeding
• establishing a routine feeding time
• providing a calm environment
• holding the child when feeding.

6. Weigh the child daily, and carefully monitor his intake and output.

7. Provide the infant with visual and auditory stimulation by exposing him to bright colors, different shapes, and music. Provide the older child with age-appropriate stimulation, including books, games, and toys.

8. Place the infant on the floor to encourage crawling and head raising.

Rationales

4. Such assessment is necessary to help to determine whether the child's failure to thrive is based on physiologic causes.

5. Ongoing assessments help to determine if the child has any feeding difficulties, vomiting, pain, constipation, cramping, diarrhea, or any other problems that might indicate his failure to thrive. By establishing consistent feeding patterns and a nurturing environment, the nurse can help the child to begin forming normal attachments and trusting relationships, thereby helping to correct the failure to thrive.

6. Daily monitoring of the child's weight and intake and output allows for direct evaluation of his nutritional status and developmental progress.

7. Visual and auditory stimulation helps with normal sensory development but may lead to hyperactivity in some children.

8. This helps to stimulate development of the large muscles.

Nursing diagnosis: *Altered parenting related to inability to form normal maternal attachment to child*

GOAL: The parents will demonstrate improved parenting skills as evidenced by asking appropriate questions about the child's condition and participating in the child's care.

Interventions

1. Teach the parents (especially the mother) normal parenting skills by demonstrating proper holding, stroking, and feeding techniques and by communicating with the child using age-appropriate words and gestures.

2. Help the parents to develop organizational skills.

3. Provide counseling, as necessary, to help the parents overcome feelings of mistrust or neglect resulting from personal childhood experiences.

4. Monitor the parents' progress and provide reinforcement, when necessary.

Rationales

1. Parenting is a learned response, usually based on skills demonstrated by other parents or role models.

2. Parenting requires increased energy and effective planning to adequately meet the child's needs.

3. The parents may be responding to the child based on the way they were treated as children. Counseling can help to make them aware of the cause of the child's failure to thrive, thereby helping to promote improved parenting skills.

4. Continued monitoring and reinforcement promotes compliance with learned parenting skills and alerts the nurse to deficiencies that require further therapy.

Nursing diagnosis: *Knowledge deficit related to home care*

GOAL: The parents will demonstrate an understanding of home care instructions.

Interventions

1. Instruct the parents on the child's achievement of age-appropriate growth and development milestones (see Appendix A: Normal Growth and Development).

Rationales

1. Such instruction is necessary, as the parents may have unrealistic expectations of what the child may or may not be able to do.

Interventions	Rationales
2. Demonstrate appropriate feeding techniques, including details on how to hold the child, how long to feed him, and which specific foods to provide.	2. Such instruction is necessary, particularly if the child's failure to thrive stemmed from inorganic causes, such as the parents' inability to form normal attachments to the child. Also, stressing the importance of proper nutrition and feeding techniques encourages the parents to comply with therapeutic measures begun during the child's hospitalization.
3. Encourage the parents to remain in the hospital with the child for 2 to 3 days to provide any necessary teaching and reinforcement.	3. This enables the nursing staff to observe the parents' behavior and to provide further teaching, when necessary.

Documentation checklist

During the hospitalization, be sure to document the following:
___ the child's status and assessment findings upon admission
___ fluid intake and output
___ nutritional intake
___ the child's or infant's response to treatment
___ family therapy
___ discharge planning guidelines.

Suicidal Behavior

Introduction

Suicidal behavior refers to the conscious decision or deliberate attempt to cause self-inflicted harm that will result in death. Suicidal tendencies are most prevalent among adolescents (suicide is the third leading cause of death in children age 15 to 18), usually stemming from overwhelming feelings of hopelessness, powerlessness, and the inability to meet increased demands and expectations. Often, the adolescent blames himself for problems that are out of his control but cannot bring himself to ask for help. Such problems as depression, illness, family conflicts, and substance abuse often are involved. Usual treatment includes psychotherapy and the use of antidepressant medications.

Assessment

Psychosocial
• dispersal of personal items
• possible precipitating crisis
• possible previous suicidal threats

Neurologic
• depression
• withdrawal

Nursing diagnosis: *Potential for violence: self-directed related to loss of self-esteem*

GOAL: The child will demonstrate no further suicide attempts and will verbalize feelings of increased self-esteem and hope for the future.

Interventions

1. Ensure the child's safety by removing all potentially harmful objects from the room. Also, remove the child's clothing so that he cannot leave the hospital. Frequently observe the child's behavior—at least every 15 minutes if he is not under constant supervision.

2. Explain to the child that all procedures and restrictions are necessary to protect him and to help him with sorting out his feelings and thoughts.

3. Provide a warm, accepting, supportive environment, and identify and reinforce the child's strengths.

4. Teach the child appropriate social skills (such as communication skills, hygiene, and appropriate dress) and role behaviors (family and societal).

5. Discuss with the child his feelings of depression, shame, guilt, and loss.

6. Identify the child's maladaptive coping mechanisms and suggest alternative ways of dealing with negative feelings.

7. Assess the child's behavioral responses to therapy.

Rationales

1. Such measures are necessary to ensure the child's safety and to provide a sense of control until the child can maintain self-control.

2. Offering such explanations promotes a sense of trust that is basic to a therapeutic relationship.

3. Such support affirms the child's sense of self-worth and encourages him to concentrate on positive thoughts.

4. Learning appropriate social skills and role behaviors should help the child to establish successful interpersonal relationships, thereby helping to increase his self-esteem.

5. Discussing these feelings with the child may reveal the reason for his attempted suicide. Getting the child to accept these feelings and to forgive himself is crucial to building self-esteem.

6. Because the child has demonstrated an inability to cope with problems, he needs to learn to use alternative ways to manage his negative feelings and build his self-esteem.

7. Such assessment is necessary to determine the effectiveness of therapy and the need for further intervention.

Documentation checklist

During the hospitalization, be sure to document the following:

___ the child's status and assessment findings upon admission

___ the child's feelings about suicide

___ observations of the child's activities

___ family involvement

___ group and individual therapy

___ discharge planning guidelines.

SECTION II

PERIOPERATIVE CARE

Anesthesia (Induction Phase)

Introduction

The perioperative period, especially anesthesia induction and surgery itself, can be particularly frightening to a child. I.V. anesthetic agents are sometimes painful. Inhalational agents administered by a mask often have an unpleasant odor and cause much alarm.

Depending on the child's age, anesthesia-related anxieties may range from mild agitation to a fear of death. Infants may become irritable and fretful in response to parental anxieties over anesthesia induction. Toddlers usually fear separation from their parents at this time. Children under age 5 usually worry about what will happen when they wake up after surgery. School-age children often associate anesthesia with being "put to sleep," fearing that they will never awaken. Adolescents usually fear loss of control and worry what they might say or do while under anesthesia.

Potential complications resulting from anesthesia include respiratory distress, coma, and death.

Assessment

Psychosocial
- crying
- withdrawal
- fear (stated verbally or implied through facial expressions)

Nursing diagnosis: *Anxiety related to the induction of anesthesia*

GOAL: The child will experience minimal anxiety as evidenced by minimal crying and screaming.

Interventions

1. Use age-appropriate relaxation techniques, such as distraction, guided imagery, medical play, storytelling, and music, to calm the child.

2. When administering an anesthetic by mask, be sure to use a clear mask. Introduce the mask slowly, and avoid using such negative expressions as "smelly gas." Try to make the child think of it as a game.

3. Avoid undressing the child until after he is asleep.

4. When addressing the child, be sure to speak in a soft, calm monotonous voice and use slow movements.

5. Start all I.V. lines after the child is asleep, unless otherwise instructed.

6. Place a pleasant strong-smelling extract, such as chocolate, lemon, or vanilla, on the mask when administering the anesthetic.

7. Encourage the adolescent to participate in the anesthesia-induction process by allowing him to select the type of anesthetic (gas versus I.V.) and to hold the mask or select the I.V. site.

Rationales

1. Relaxation techniques allow the child to focus on something other than his fears, thereby reducing his anxieties and fears.

2. Clear masks are less frightening to a child than the older type black masks. Introducing the mask slowly and as a game decreases the child's anxiety and prevents him from fighting anesthesia.

3. Often, the act of removing the child's clothes is more frightening to a child than the surgery itself.

4. A soft voice, coupled with slow movements, promotes a more relaxing atmosphere.

5. I.V. administration often is a painful and frightening invasive procedure that is best begun after the child is asleep.

6. Strong-smelling extracts can mask the noxious smell of most anesthetic agents, thereby helping to decrease anxiety.

7. Being allowed to make such decisions fosters a feeling of self-control (adolescents typically fear losing self-control while under anesthesia).

Nursing diagnosis: *Ineffective breathing pattern related to anesthesia induction*

GOAL: The child will have no signs of respiratory compromise as evidenced by maintaining a respiratory rate of 16 to 30 breaths/minute and exhibiting no signs of respiratory distress.

Interventions

1. Closely monitor the child's respirations and assess his skin color during the induction phase.

2. Closely observe the child for vomiting until the airway is protected by the insertion of an endotracheal tube.

3. Be prepared to apply cricoid pressure if instructed to do so by the anesthesiologist.

Rationales

1. The induction phase is the most dangerous period of anesthesia. Monitoring the respirations and skin color during this phase helps ensure the early detection and prompt treatment of such potential complications as respiratory distress, cardiac arrest, and anaphylactic shock.

2. The child is at risk for aspiration until intubated.

3. Cricoid pressure occludes the esophagus and prevents passive regurgitation.

Nursing diagnosis: *Potential for injury related to anesthesia induction*

GOAL: The child will suffer no injury or trauma during the induction phase.

Interventions

1. Be prepared to restrain the child with soft arm or leg restraints during the induction phase.

2. Secure the child to the operating table, as necessary, by placing a strap across his abdomen or chest until the induction phase is complete.

Rationales

1. Most children experience an excitement phase before losing consciousness during the induction of general anesthesia. Restraints may be necessary to prevent the child from injuring himself at this time.

2. Securing the child in this manner ensures that he does not fall off the table.

Documentation checklist

During the perioperative period, be sure to document the following:
___ the child's status upon admission to the operating room
___ vital signs
___ nothing-by-mouth status
___ preoperative medications
___ preoperative teaching.

Anxiety (Preoperative)

Introduction

Because of the strangeness of the hospital environment and the upcoming surgery, most children experience some degree of anxiety during the preoperative period. For this reason, pediatric patients should become oriented to the operating room, surgical procedure, postanesthesia unit, intensive care unit (if applicable), and postoperative care procedures during the preoperative period.

Teaching, which is based on the child's developmental level, should include age-appropriate explanations and demonstrations using illustrations, videotapes, and sample equipment, when available. It also should include a tour of the operating room and adjunct facilities and, for the younger child, play demonstrations of the actual surgical procedure using dolls or puppets.

Assessment
Psychosocial
- hyperactivity
- crying
- withdrawal
- acting out
- regression
- expressions of fear of death

Nursing diagnosis: *Anxiety (child) related to surgery*

GOAL: The child will demonstrate little anxiety as evidenced by continuing to interact with parents and significant others.

Interventions

1. Explain to the child the perioperative events surrounding surgery, using simple, age-appropriate terms and illustrations, dolls, puppets, and sample equipment (when available).

2. Provide age-appropriate emotional support when the child enters the operating room environment. Such support may include cuddling the infant, providing familiar toys for the small child, or conversing superficially with the older child about topics of interest.

3. Allow the parents to accompany the child to the entrance of the operating room, and involve them in the recovery process as early as possible.

4. Help the parents to cope with their own anxieties by providing preoperative teaching, counseling, and a therapeutic environment.

5. Use such relaxation techniques as deep breathing, distraction and redirection, or focusing and guided imagery (alone or in combination) to help reduce the child's and parents' anxieties.

Rationales

1. Offering such explanations allows the child to anticipate the preoperative and postoperative events, thereby helping to reduce his anxiety.

2. Because the child is at risk for emotional scarring and fear, meeting his emotional needs is essential to ensure a positive surgical experience.

3. Parents represent a familiar, stabilizing force to the child. Their presence immediately before and after surgery is important to foster the child's emotional well-being.

4. Parental anxiety has a direct effect on the degree of anxiety experienced by a child. Reducing the parents' anxiety should consequently reduce the child's anxiety.

5. Relaxation techniques enable the child and parents to concentrate their thoughts and attention on other, pleasant matters, thereby helping to reduce their anxieties and fears.

Documentation checklist

During the perioperative period, be sure to document the following:
___ the child's status upon admission to the operating room
___ any questions the child may ask
___ the child's expressions of fear or anxiety
___ the child's understanding of the surgical procedure.

Hypothermia

Introduction

Hypothermia refers to a low body temperature usually resulting from exposure of skin surface areas to cool temperatures or solutions. During the perioperative period, infants are at greater risk than older children for developing hypothermia because of their larger body surface area.

Hypothermia usually is accompanied by increased heart and respiratory rates and decreased glucose levels. Usual treatment involves covering as much of the body surface as possible, using head caps, blankets, and warming pads.

Assessment

Integumentary
• decreased temperature
• cyanosis

Cardiovascular
• tachycardia

Respiratory
• increased respiratory rate

Nursing diagnosis: *Ineffective thermoregulation related to surgery*

GOAL: The child will maintain normal thermoregulation as evidenced by maintaining an axillary temperature of 97.7° to 99° F. (36.5° to 37.2° C.).

Interventions

1. Ensure that the operating room temperature is set at 96.8° to 98.6° F. (36° to 37° C.) 30 minutes before the child's arrival.

2. Keep an aquamatic K-pad set at 101.3° F. (38.5° C.) on the operating table. Remove the pad before placing the child on the table.

3. Provide the child with warm blankets upon his arrival in the operating room.

4. Avoid any unnecessary or prolonged exposure of the child's skin during the preoperative period and the induction and emergence phases of anesthesia.

5. Monitor and document the child's temperature continually during the procedure.

6. Use thermal heat lamps, as necessary, during the induction and emergence phases of anesthesia.

7. Warm all solutions to be used on the operative field in normal saline solution or sterile water.

8. Cover the child's extremities with plastic bags.

9. After the surgical procedure is completed, dry the child thoroughly.

10. If an Isolette is to be used for transportation, pre-warm the unit 45 minutes before transferring the child.

Rationales

1. Maintaining the room temperature at this setting decreases the risk of hypothermia from environmental causes.

2. An aquamatic pad warms the operating table to help maintain normal body temperature and reduce the risk of heat loss through conduction during the surgical procedure.

3. Warm blankets reduce the risk of heat loss through conduction.

4. Prolonged skin exposure leads to decreased body temperature and increased metabolic activity.

5. Frequent monitoring is essential for the early detection and prompt treatment of significant fluctuations in the child's body temperature.

6. Thermal lamps provide radiant heat and help to maintain body temperature.

7. Using warm solutions is necessary, as cold solutions can decrease body temperature, including the internal temperature if the solution is used as a flush.

8. Plastic bags provide extra insulation.

9. Drying prevents chilling by evaporation.

10. Warming the Isolette prevents heat loss by convection and conduction.

Documentation checklist

During the perioperative period, be sure to document the following:

___ the child's vital signs

___ preoperative teaching

___ the child's and parents' response to teaching.

Hypovolemia

Introduction

A decrease in the extracellular fluid (plasma) volume, hypovolemia can result in lowered blood pressure and poor perfusion to vital organs. During the perioperative period, this may occur as a result of the child's nothing-by-mouth (NPO) status (withholding of fluids), the surgical procedure itself, or third-space fluid shifting. Other possible causes include fluid loss from diarrhea, fever, vomiting, systemic infection, and impaired ability to concentrate urine.

Assessment

Cardiovascular
• decreased blood pressure
• increased pulse rate
• decreased central venous pressure
• decreased capillary refill time
• little or no neck distention (when placed in supine position)

Genitourinary
• decreased urine output

Integumentary
• skin tenting
• flushing
• dry skin
• cool extremities

Nursing diagnosis: *Fluid volume deficit related to surgery*

GOAL: The child will maintain adequate hydration as evidenced by good skin turgor and a capillary refill time of 3 to 5 seconds.

Interventions

1. Monitor the child's vital signs throughout the perioperative period, noting any changes in the pulse rate and blood pressure. Also assess the child's skin for dryness and coolness.

2. Monitor the amount of blood lost during surgery.

3. Monitor the child's hemoglobin and hematocrit levels and capillary refill time preoperatively.

4. Administer I.V. fluids, as ordered, and document the amount administered.

5. Evaluate for additional fluid loss resulting from:

• NPO status

• vomiting or diarrhea

• nasogastric suctioning

• diuretic usage

Rationales

1. Increased pulse rate, decreased blood pressure, and dry, cool skin indicate a fluid deficit, which requires the administration of replacement fluids.

2. Such monitoring is essential to determine whether the child is becoming hypovolemic during the course of the surgery. (Children undergoing surgery can lose between 10% and 20% of their total blood volume during this time.)

3. Preoperative blood values help in determining the need for blood or fluid replacement. Capillary refill time normally is delayed with hypovolemia.

4. Careful documentation of all I.V. fluids administered during the perioperative period helps in determining the child's overall fluid status.

5. The child may experience hypovolemia as a result of any of these conditions or procedures during the perioperative period.

• Maintaining the child on NPO status increases the amount of fluid lost through the skin, lungs, and bowel.

• Vomiting and diarrhea increase the amount of fluid lost through the alimentary tract and bowel.

• Nasogastric suctioning removes gastric contents from the stomach, thereby increasing the amount of fluid loss.

• Diuretics help to increase the total urine output, thereby contributing to the total fluid loss.

Interventions

• third-space fluid shifts

• elevated temperature

• mechanical ventilation.

Rationales

• Third-space fluid shifting results from internal mechanisms in which fluid is shifted to inflammatory sites, causing a general reduction in the overall circulation.

• Elevated temperature increases the amount of fluid lost through the skin and lungs.

• Mechanical ventilation with warm, humidified air usually decreases the drying of mucous membranes and the amount of fluid lost through the lungs. Careful monitoring is essential to ensure that the ventilator is functioning properly and that the child's ventilatory readings are within normal ranges.

Documentation checklist

During the perioperative period, be sure to document the following:

___ the child's status and assessment findings upon admission to the operating room

___ vital signs

___ NPO status

___ medications administered

___ skin turgor and capillary refill time

___ amount and dosage of I.V. fluids administered.

PERIOPERATIVE CARE

Pain (Postoperative)

Introduction

Postoperative pain is caused by the disruption of tissue and nerve endings, usually from an incision. Children tend to respond differently to pain, depending on their age and individual pain threshold.

Infants generally respond to pain by crying and flailing their arms and legs. However, how an infant perceives pain and how much he can remember of the experience remains controversial. Toddlers usually are influenced by their previous experiences and may react violently to pain or attempt to escape painful situations. Often, they are difficult to control. Preschoolers usually react similarly to toddlers during their early years. However, as they grow older, children develop increasingly personalized ways of dealing with pain, such as self-control measures. School-age children use various methods of dealing with pain, including deep breathing, counting out loud to 10, and yelling "ouch." Adolescents tend to be more reserved and usually do not verbalize feelings of anxiety or pain, fearing loss of self-control.

Assessment

Neurologic
• crying
• guarding
• verbalization of pain
• withdrawal

Cardiovascular
• increased blood pressure
• increased heart rate

Respiratory
• increased respiratory rate

Nursing diagnosis: *Altered comfort: pain related to surgery*

GOAL: The child will have minimal postoperative pain as evidenced by decreased restlessness and irritability and by normal blood pressure, pulse rate, and respiratory rate.

Interventions

1. Take the following measures to assess the child's pain:

• Ask the child if he is comfortable. If he indicates that he is uncomfortable, ask him to describe the pain by using a face interval scale, numerical rating scale, or pain color scale (depending on the child's developmental level).

• Observe the child for guarding, rigidity, restlessness, or crying.

• Evaluate the child's autonomic responses for increased heart rate and blood pressure.

2. Administer narcotics along with other pain medication, as ordered, carefully observing and documenting the child's response.

3. Involve the parents in managing the child's pain as early as possible after surgery.

Rationales

1. Depending on the child's age and usual response to pain, the nurse may need to rely on certain measures to confirm the child's pain.

• Because children are easily influenced by negatively phrased questions, asking whether the child is comfortable rather than whether he is in pain allows him to respond more objectively. A pain-rating scale may be necessary, especially if the child is too young to describe the severity of his pain in words.

• Some children may be too young or feel too embarrassed to verbalize their pain. In such cases, nonverbal cues, such as guarding, rigidity, restlessness, or crying, may signal that the child is experiencing increased discomfort.

• The body's autonomic responses of increased heart rate and blood pressure may indicate that the child is experiencing pain.

2. During the immediate postoperative phase, narcotic administration requires careful evaluation because of the potential residual effects of anesthetic agents, such as respiratory depression and hypotension.

3. Parents are most familiar with the child's normal response to pain and know which techniques have worked in the past to help control his pain.

Interventions

4. Reposition the child, as needed, to maximize his comfort.

5. Speak to the child in a soothing voice, and provide a quiet, nonstimulating environment.

6. Use other techniques, such as distraction and imagery, to help control the child's pain.

Rationales

4. Repositioning can help to decrease skin pressure and muscle cramping.

5. A calm, soothing voice combined with quiet surroundings can effectively calm the child, reducing his tension and thereby reducing his pain.

6. The use of toys, stories, imagery, and other distractions may help the child to focus his attention on something other than his pain, thereby helping to decrease the pain.

Documentation checklist

During the perioperative period, be sure to document the following:

___ the child's status and ongoing assessment
___ vital signs
___ medications administered
___ responses to pain.

PERIOPERATIVE CARE

Respiratory Compromise (Postoperative)

Introduction

During the postanesthesia recovery period, children are at risk for respiratory compromise because of the residual effects of anesthetics and irritation from the endotracheal tube. Infants are at particular risk because they are obligatory nose and diaphragmatic breathers. Treatment for this condition includes the administration of oxygen and reintubation, when necessary.

Assessment

Respiratory
• increased respiratory rate
• sternal retractions
• decreased tidal volume

Integumentary
• cyanosis

Nursing diagnosis: *Ineffective breathing pattern related to anesthetic administration*

GOAL: The child will maintain effective breathing patterns and an adequate level of oxygenation as evidenced by maintaining a pinkish skin color and nonlabored respirations (from 16 to 30 breaths/minute).

Interventions

1. Administer up to 40% humidified oxygen at a rate of 2 to 3 liters/hour by face mask until the child is awake and responsive.

2. Monitor the oxygen saturation rate with a pulse oximeter until the child is awake and stable.

3. Place the child in a semiprone or lateral position unless contraindicated by the surgical procedure.

4. Carefully assess the child's respirations (noting rate, depth, and effort) and skin color every 15 minutes. Be sure to note the anesthetic agent used during surgery when making evaluations.

5. Assess the child every 15 minutes for signs of airway obstruction, including croup-like cough, hoarseness, inspiratory stridor, and cyanosis.

6. Administer 100% oxygen by Ambu bag or face mask if the child has signs and symptoms of airway obstruction.

7. Carefully suction the child's mouth when airway obstruction becomes evident, avoiding contact with the surgical site.

Rationales

1. Administering oxygen during the postanesthesia recovery period increases the total oxygen concentration in circulation until the child's respiratory rate is fully established. Humidified air helps keep the mucous membranes moist. Administering humidified oxygen at levels higher than 40% places the child at risk for retrolental fibroplasia.

2. Monitoring the oxygen saturation is important because the child's respiratory control center is easily fatigued after surgery. (Saturation levels should be above 90%, preferably above 95%.) This is especially important for infants, who sometimes breathe irregularly.

3. Placing the child in this postion maintains airway patency and provides easy access for suctioning. It also lessens the risk of the child's tongue obstructing the airway as sometimes occurs in the supine position.

4. Respiratory depression (marked by decreased respiratory rate, cyanosis, and decreased oxygen saturation rate) occurs more often when muscle relaxants (common anesthetic agents used in pediatric surgery) are used.

5. Postintubation croup may occur because of edema caused by the tube's irritating effects on the child's small airway.

6. High levels of oxygen reduce the risk of hypoxia when the airway is compromised.

7. The pooling of secretions near the obstructed airway can cause laryngospasm.

Interventions

8. Take necessary measures to open the child's airway, such as inserting an oral or nasal airway, using the jaw-thrust maneuver, or inserting an endotracheal tube.

Rationales

8. Such measures may be necessary to ensure a patent airway if airway blockage should occur.

Documentation checklist

During the perioperative period, be sure to document the following:

___ the child's ongoing status
___ vital signs
___ signs and symptoms of respiratory distress
___ oxygen saturation rate
___ amount and dosage of oxygen administered.

SECTION III

DIAGNOSTIC STUDIES

DIAGNOSTIC STUDIES

Arteriography

Introduction

Arteriography refers to the fluoroscopic and radiographic examination of the vascular system to evaluate the arteries of the extremities, cerebrum, and abdomen. This procedure involves the injection of a contrast medium for visualization of the arteries and, depending on the child's age, the use of a sedative or general anesthetic to ensure cooperation.

Indications for testing

Any of the following conditions may indicate a need for arteriography:
• embolism
• aneurysm
• neoplasm
• hemorrhage
• fistula
• atrioventricular malformation
• arterial stenosis.

Nursing diagnosis: *Knowledge deficit related to procedure*

GOAL: The parents and child will verbalize an understanding of the procedure.

Interventions

1. Explain to the parents and child the need for withholding all oral intake for at least 8 hours before the test.

2. Explain that the nurse will check the child's history for any allergy to iodine or iodine-containing products, such as seafood or povidone-iodine solution.

3. If the child is to remain awake during the procedure, make sure that he understands the following:

• He will feel sleepy from the premedication.

• The people in the room will be wearing surgical gowns and gloves.

• He will be positioned on his back and asked to lie still for the duration of the procedure (1 hour).

• If the femoral area is used, his groin area will be washed with povidone-iodine solution or a "yellowish brown soap" (be sure to show the child where the groin area is). After the site is cleansed, he may feel a stinging sensation in his leg or groin as the area is being anesthetized.

Rationales

1. Withholding oral intake is necessary to prevent aspiration should nausea and vomiting occur from a reaction to contrast medium.

2. The contrast medium used in this procedure contains iodine, which could cause an anaphylactic reaction if given to an iodine-sensitive child.

3. Explaining the procedure to the child in age-appropriate language enhances his cooperation and may help to decrease his anxiety.

• A narcotic agent having sedative effects is usually used if the child is to remain awake during the procedure.

• The child may become frightened by seeing health care workers in hospital gowns and gloves (required for this sterile procedure) if he has not been told to expect to see them.

• The supine position is used for easy access to the femoral area through which the contrast medium is injected. The child needs to lie as still as possible throughout the procedure, as any movement could distort the image or cause the catheter to become dislodged or kinked.

• Cleansing with povidone-iodine solution is necessary to prepare the site for anesthetic injection. Infiltration of local anesthetics, such as xylocaine, can be painful initially.

Interventions

• A small catheter or "tube" will be placed in his leg to infuse the contrast medium. Explain that this will not hurt, but that he may feel some pushing on his leg. However, while the contrast medium is being injected, he may feel warm and nauseated or have a slight burning sensation.

• After the procedure, the catheter will be removed and pressure will be applied to his leg for a few minutes; then, a dressing will be placed over the site.

Rationales

• The child may feel some pressure from the manipulation of the guide wire used to place the catheter. Once the guide wire is removed, the catheter remains in place for injection of the contrast medium. Feelings of warmth, nausea, or burning are caused by the forceful injection of the iodine contrast medium.

• Pressure applied to the artery for about 15 minutes helps to prevent bleeding and hematoma formation. A pressure dressing is applied to further prevent bleeding.

Nursing diagnosis: *Potential for injury related to allergic reaction secondary to administration of contrast medium*

GOAL: The child will exhibit no signs of allergic reaction as evidenced by the absence of a rash, an increased pulse rate, and a decreased blood pressure.

Interventions

1. Before administration of the contrast medium, be sure to check the child's history for hypersensitivity to iodine or iodine-containing foods (such as seafood) and for asthma or other severe allergies. If the child has such a history, notify the doctor.

2. Alert the radiology department about the potential for allergic reaction.

3. After injection of the contrast medium, observe the child for signs and symptoms of an allergic reaction, including skin rash, hives, urticaria, headache, vomiting, sneezing, flushing, respiratory distress, hoarseness, tachycardia, and palpitations. Institute emergency measures, as necessary.

Rationales

1. Checking the history is prerequisite to any procedure involving the administration of a contrast medium because of the risk of allergic reaction. If the child's history indicates a previous allergic reaction, antihistamines and steroids may be necessary to counteract the medium's adverse effects.

2. The radiology department should be alerted to the child's condition in case an emergency occurs. Emergency drugs, such as epinephrine and diphenhydramine, and other equipment should be on hand.

3. Any of these reactions might occur from the release of histamine, which causes capillary dilation, increased permeability of the blood vessels, smooth-muscle contractions, and stimulation of the mucus-secreting glands.

Nursing diagnosis: *Altered tissue perfusion: peripheral (postprocedural) related to catheterization*

GOAL: The child will maintain adequate tissue perfusion in the involved leg as evidenced by a capillary refill time of 3 to 5 seconds, normal pedal pulses, and warm extremities.

Interventions

1. Maintain the child in a supine position for 8 to 12 hours after the procedure, restraining the involved leg if necessary. Make sure he remains nonambulatory for 24 hours.

2. Assess the child's vital signs every 15 minutes for 1 hour, followed by every 30 minutes for 2 hours, then every hour for the first 24 hours.

3. Monitor the popliteal and dorsal pedal pulses in both legs.

4. Monitor the temperature and color of the affected leg.

Rationales

1. Maintaining the child in the supine position with his leg flat and not bent helps prevent thrombus dislodgment.

2. Frequent assessments are necessary to ensure the circulatory status of the involved leg. Hypotension may indicate bleeding at the catheterization site.

3. Monitoring the pulses in both legs helps to detect any deficits in the involved leg suggesting decreased perfusion.

4. Coolness, cyanosis, or blanching may indicate an obstruction in the catheterized vessel.

Nursing diagnosis: *Potential for injury (hemorrhage) related to catheterization*

GOAL: The child will exhibit no bleeding at the catheterization site.

Interventions

1. After the procedure, maintain a pressure dressing over the catheterization site.

2. Check for bleeding at the site every 30 minutes for 2 hours, then every hour for 4 hours.

3. If bleeding occurs, apply direct pressure to the site and notify the doctor immediately.

Rationales

1. Applying a pressure dressing to the site helps prevent bleeding and hematoma formation.

2. Frequent assessments help to detect any bleeding resulting from detachment of the thrombus from the catheterization site.

3. Direct pressure helps to stop the bleeding and to prevent hematoma formation.

Documentation checklist

After the procedure, be sure to document the following:
___ the child's status
___ vital signs
___ the color and pulse rate of the extremity used for catheterization
___ any allergic reactions.

Barium Enema

Introduction

Barium enema (lower gastrointestinal examination) involves the fluoroscopic and radiologic examination of the large intestine after the rectal instillation of barium sulfate (single-contrast technique) or barium sulfate and air (double-contrast technique). It is commonly indicated for children with altered bowel habits, lower abdominal pain, or the passage of blood, mucus, or pus in the stool.

This test should always precede the barium swallow and upper-GI and small-bowel series when a full GI series is ordered since ingested barium may cloud anatomic structures on X-rays.

Indications for testing

Any of the following conditions may indicate the need for barium enema:
• history of altered bowel habits, lower abdominal pain, or passage of blood, mucus, or pus in stool
• inflammatory bowel disease
• polyps
• diverticula
• structural deformities.

Nursing diagnosis: *Knowledge deficit related to procedure*

GOAL: The child (or parents) will verbalize an understanding of the procedure.

Interventions

1. Explain to the child that, before the test, he may be given castor oil (or another cathartic) and a cleansing enema to clear the bowel of any feces.

2. Tell the child that the procedure will be performed in the radiology department and that the technicians will be wearing lead aprons. Explain that he will need to wear a hospital gown and that he will be asked to lie on a hard table.

3. Explain the following procedural events to the child, using age-appropriate terms:
• A tube will be placed inside his rectum and taped in place to prevent its dislodgement and the leakage of barium. Reassure him that, as soon as the test is over, the tube will be removed.
• He will have an urge to defecate as the barium is instilled, but he must remain as still as possible.
• He may be turned in various positions on the table during the procedure. Reassure him that he will not fall.

4. Explain to the child that the technicians will help him to the bathroom once the procedure is over. Reassure him that, if he accidentally defecates before reaching the bathroom, he should not feel embarrassed or ashamed.

Rationales

1. Use of cathartics and cleansing enemas ensures the removal of any fecal matter that might interfere with the visualization of anatomic structures during testing.

2. Offering such explanations helps to prepare the child for the visual impact of the radiology room, which may be especially frightening to a younger child.

3. The child should be prepared for the actual procedure, as it can be a frightening experience, especially for a younger child.

4. Older children often feel embarrassed or ashamed in this situation and require reassurance that this is normal and expected.

Nursing diagnosis: *Altered bowel elimination: constipation related to the retention of barium*

GOAL: The child will have no signs of constipation as evidenced by maintaining normal (preprocedural) elimination habits.

Interventions

1. After confirming with the radiology department that all procedures have been completed, begin the child on his regular diet.

2. Assess the number and quality of stools passed during the first few days after the procedure (be sure to warn the child and parents that the stools will be white or light-colored during this period). Inform the doctor if the child is still constipated after 3 days.

3. Administer castor oil or milk of magnesia, as ordered.

4. Encourage the child to increase his fluid intake, if not contraindicated.

Rationales

1. A normal, well-balanced diet should help to ease the child's constipation.

2. Such assessments help to determine whether the child is constipated and in need of a cathartic.

3. Cathartic medications, such as castor oil and milk of magnesia, help to eliminate any remaining barium from the child's system.

4. Liberal fluid intake can help to promote the elimination of barium.

Documentation checklist

After the procedure, be sure to document the following:
___ the child's status
___ any abdominal pain
___ bowel sounds
___ bowel movements.

Barium Swallow

Introduction

Barium swallow (esophagography) involves the cineradiographic examination of the pharynx and the fluoroscopic examination of the esophagus after swallows of barium sulfate. Most commonly performed as part of an upper GI series, this test is indicated for children with dysphagia or regurgitation.

This test should always follow a barium enema when testing involves a full GI series, as ingested barium may cloud anatomic structures on X-rays.

Indications for testing

Any of the following conditions may indicate the need for barium swallow:
• gastroesophageal reflux
• stricture
• obstruction by a foreign body
• varices
• fistula
• atresia.

Nursing diagnosis: *Knowledge deficit related to procedure*

GOAL: The child (or parents) will verbalize an understanding of the procedure.

Interventions

1. Explain to the child (or parents) that he will be allowed nothing to eat or drink beginning at midnight on the day of testing (or beginning 3 hours before testing for children under age 2).

2. Explain to the child that the test will be done in the radiology department and that the technicians will be wearing lead aprons. Also explain that he will be asked to wear a hospital gown and to remove all metal objects (such as necklaces) that may interfere with the X-rays.

3. Explain the following procedural events to the child, using age-appropriate terms:
• He will be given some barium sulfate to swallow from a cup or a bottle (infants are given the barium from a bottle; young children may sip the liquid through a straw). Explain to the younger child that the barium is thick like a milkshake, but that it may not taste quite as good (some hospitals flavor the barium with strawberry or chocolate to improve the taste).
• He may be turned in various positions on a tilted table when the X-rays are being taken (reassure him that he will not fall).

Rationales

1. The child's stomach should be empty to allow for the complete digestion of barium. Fasting in children under age 2 should be limited to 3 hours to prevent hypoglycemia.

2. Offering such explanations helps to prepare the child for the visual impact of the radiology room, which can be especially frightening to a younger child.

3. The child should be prepared for the actual procedure, as this can be especially frightening to a younger child.

Nursing diagnosis: *Ineffective breathing pattern related to procedure*

GOAL: The child will maintain normal breathing patterns during and after the procedure as evidenced by having no signs or symptoms of respiratory distress.

Interventions

1. Alert the radiology technicians if a child is prone to reflux or vomiting.

Rationales

1. Because the procedure is performed using various positions, the child may be at risk for gastroesophageal reflux or vomiting, possibly leading to respiratory distress. Suction equipment should be on hand in case of an emergency.

Interventions

2. Maintain the child in an upright position after the test (infants can be positioned in an infant seat).

Rationales

2. An upright position helps prevent the reflux of barium and the risk of aspiration, thereby preventing respiratory distress.

Nursing diagnosis: *Altered bowel elimination: constipation related to the retention of barium*

GOAL: The child will maintain normal bowel elimination patterns as evidenced by having a normal bowel movement within 24 hours after the procedure.

Interventions

1. Notify the doctor before the test if the child is taking anticholinergics or narcotics. Administer laxatives, as ordered.

2. After confirming with the radiology department that all tests have been completed, begin the child on a regular diet.

3. Assess the quantity and quality of the child's stools for the first few days after the procedure (warn the child and parents that the stools will be white or light-colored [possibly pink if a strawberry flavoring was used] during this time).

4. Administer castor oil or milk of magnesia, as ordered.

5. Inform the doctor if the child has not expelled all of the barium within 3 days.

6. If appropriate, encourage the child to increase his fluid intake.

Rationales

1. Anticholinergics and narcotics may decrease peristalsis and impede the elimination of barium from the GI tract, possibly leading to constipation.

2. A normal, well-balanced diet can help to prevent constipation.

3. Such assessments are necessary to determine whether the child is constipated and in need of a cathartic.

4. Cathartics, such as castor oil or milk of magnesia, may be given to help eliminate any remaining barium from the child's system.

5. Barium may absorb fecal water and solidify in the colon, causing constipation and impaction.

6. Liberal fluid intake can help promote the elimination of barium from the child's system.

Documentation checklist

After the procedure, be sure to document the following:
___ the child's status
___ any abdominal distention
___ vomiting
___ bowel sounds
___ bowel movements.

DIAGNOSTIC STUDIES

Computed Tomography

Introduction

In computed tomography (CT), multiple X-rays pass through a specified body area and are measured while detectors record differences in tissue attenuation. A computer is used to reconstruct this data as a three-dimensional image on an oscilloscope screen. Attenuation varies with tissue density and appears as shades of gray on the screen. Contrast medium may be used to accentuate the density.

Indications for testing

Any of the following conditions may indicate the need for CT scanning:
• abscesses
• cysts
• cerebral hematomas
• intracranial hemorrhages
• cerebral edema
• tumors
• hydrocephalus
• liver disease
• renal calculi.

Nursing diagnosis: *Knowledge deficit related to procedure*

GOAL: The child and parents will verbalize an understanding of the procedure.

Interventions

1. Explain to the child and parents the purpose of the test. Also explain that the test will be performed in the radiology department and that the radiologist will determine whether the parents can remain in the room while the test is performed. Indicate that, depending on the type of X-rays required, the test should take from 30 to 60 minutes.

2. Describe the equipment to the child in age-appropriate terms. Tell him that he will be placed on a table that slides in and out of a scanner (tell the younger child that the scanner looks like a big donut and that the table will slide in and out of the hole). Show him a picture of the scanner, if one is available.

3. Explain that the child will need to remove all metallic objects, such as barrettes, jewelry, or eyeglasses, before the test.

4. Explain that, while the X-rays are being taken, the child will hear loud clicking noises.

5. Explain to the child that he will need to lie very still while the X-rays are being taken and that restraints (such as straps or body wraps) may be necessary to ensure that he does not move. If chest or abdominal scans are required, explain that he may be asked to hold his breath for a short while.

Rationales

1. Offering such explanations helps to alleviate any fears or anxieties and helps ensure the child's cooperation with the test.

2. The CT scanner can appear ominous and frightening, especially to a younger child. Describing the equipment to the child or showing him a picture of the scanner should prepare him for the visual impact of the machine, thereby helping to ensure his cooperation at the time of testing.

3. The high density of metallic objects can cause images to appear darker on the screen, thereby interfering with test results.

4. Such noises, caused by the X-ray tube rotating within the cylinder, can be alarming if the child is unprepared for them.

5. Any movement, including respirations, during the filming of X-rays can result in blurred images on the screen.

Interventions	Rationales
6. If the test involves use of a contrast medium, offer the following information, using age-appropriate terms as necessary: • The child will not be allowed to eat or drink for 4 to 6 hours before the test to prevent the risk of vomiting and aspiration from use of the contrast medium. • Contrast medium is used to enhance the image of body parts so that they are more visible on the screen. • If the child does not already have an I.V. line in place, the contrast medium will be injected through a small needle placed under his skin (reassure the child that the needle will be removed once the injection is complete). • The contrast medium may cause a burning or stinging sensation at the injection site, warmth, nausea, or a salty or metallic taste (reassure the child that these effects will last only a few minutes).	6. The child should be adequately prepared for the use of contrast medium, as the injection and adverse effects can be stressful and frightening if the child is unprepared. (*Note:* Avoid using the word "dye" to refer to contrast medium, as the child may misinterpret the word to mean "die.")

Nursing diagnosis: *Potential for injury related to sedatives used for the procedure*

GOAL: The child will suffer no adverse effects from the sedatives.

Interventions	Rationales
1. If you think the child will not lie still during the procedure, consult the doctor about administering a sedative-hypnotic, such as chloral hydrate or pentobarbital. Withhold food and fluids for 6 hours before administering the medication.	1. A child under age 5 may have a hard time lying still for the procedure. Administering a sedative-hypnotic 20 to 30 minutes before the study usually keeps the child sedated for the time required. Withholding food and fluids for 6 hours empties the stomach, which helps prevent vomiting and aspiration of gastric contents.
2. Observe the child closely during the procedure to ensure adequate breathing.	2. Sedatives can depress the respiratory drive and result in apnea.
3. Assess the child's vital signs when he is fully awake.	3. Such assessment can identify adverse effects from the sedative, such as respiratory depression.

Nursing diagnosis: *Potential for injury (allergic reaction) related to the use of contrast medium during procedure*

GOAL: The child will exhibit no signs of allergic reaction to the contrast agent.

Interventions	Rationales
1. Check the child's record for a history of hypersensitivity to iodine-containing contrast medium or for a history of asthma or other severe allergies. Ask the parents if the child has ever had a reaction to iodine or iodine-containing foods (such as seafood). Alert the doctor to any positive findings.	1. The iodine contained in the contrast medium may cause the child to have an allergic reaction, especially if he has a history of such allergy or a history of asthma. If use of contrast medium is essential to the test, the doctor may order the administration of antihistamines or steroids to prevent an allergic reaction.
2. Alert the radiology department to the child's potential for allergic reaction, and ensure that emergency drugs (precalculated to the child's weight) and equipment are on hand.	2. Emergency drugs, such as epinephrine and diphenhydramine hydrochloride, and emergency equipment should be readily available in case of an allergic reaction.
3. Observe the child for signs and symptoms of allergic reaction (including skin rash, hives, urticaria, headache, vomiting, sneezing, flushing, respiratory distress, hoarseness, tachycardia, and palpitations). If necessary, administer diphenhydramine for a mild reaction or epinephrine for a severe reaction.	3. The release of histamine causes capillary dilation, increased permeability of the blood vessels, contraction of smooth muscle, and stimulation of mucus-secreting glands.

Interventions

4. Instruct the parents on the signs and symptoms of a delayed allergic reaction, including headache, urticaria (itching), skin rash, nausea, and vomiting. Advise them to call the doctor immediately if such a reaction occurs.

Rationales

4. The child may experience a delayed reaction after leaving the radiology department and going home. Immediate medical attention is necessary if the reaction is severe. The doctor may order an oral antihistamine if the reaction is mild.

Documentation checklist

After the procedure, be sure to document the following:
___ the child's status
___ vital signs
___ any allergic reaction
___ level of consciousness.

DIAGNOSTIC STUDIES

Intravenous Pyelography

Introduction

Intravenous pyelography (IVP), also called excretory urography, is the radiographic examination of the kidneys, ureters, and bladder after injection of a contrast medium. The contrast is excreted through the kidneys, allowing visualization of the urinary tract. Several X-rays are taken to identify suspected renal or urinary tract disease, space-occupying lesions, congenital anomalies, or trauma to the urinary system.

Indications for testing

Any of the following conditions may indicate the need for IVP:
• polycystic kidney
• renal calculi
• tumors.

Nursing diagnosis: *Knowledge deficit related to IVP*

GOAL: The child and parents will verbalize an understanding of the procedure.

Interventions

1. Explain to the child and parents that food and fluids may be restricted at midnight before the procedure. Tell them a suppository will be administered the evening before and morning of the procedure and a Fleet enema may be ordered, if necessary. If the patient is a young child, briefly describe suppository and enema administration in age-appropriate terms.

2. Tell the parents they will have to sign a consent form.

3. Explain to the child that he will go to the radiology department for the procedure, and let the parents know whether they can accompany the child.

4. Tell the child he will wear a hospital gown and to remove all metal objects.

5. Explain the X-ray equipment to be used, and show the equipment to the child and parents before the study, if possible. Use age-appropriate terms in your descriptions. For example, if the patient is a young child, describe the equipment as a special camera that will take his picture. Explain that the machine will be placed close to his body but will not touch him.

6. Tell the child he will be asked to void just before the test and then asked to lie flat on the X-ray table while one picture of his stomach is taken.

7. Explain that a small needle will be placed under the child's skin to inject the contrast medium and will be removed when the injection is complete. Tell him the contrast medium may cause a burning, stinging, or warm sensation; nausea; and a salty or metallic taste for a few minutes.

Rationales

1. Fluid restrictions facilitate concentration of the contrast medium. Food restrictions, suppositories, and enemas help clean the bowel of feces to permit visualization of the kidney. A young child may feel less threatened by unfamiliar experiences if he is given clear explanations to prepare him. (*Note:* Diet restrictions, suppositories, and enemas may be contraindicated in children under age 2.)

2. Because the contrast medium is injected, intravenous pyelography is considered an invasive procedure.

3. Such factors as limited space, physical constraints, or the mother's pregnancy may prevent the parents from accompanying the child.

4. Metal objects (such as jewelry or diaper pins) can obscure the anatomical view because X-rays cannot penetrate them.

5. A clear explanation helps ease the family's fears, particularly those of a young child, who may fantasize that the X-ray machine looks like a monster.

6. Retained urine dilutes the contrast medium and impairs visualization of the bladder. A scout film is taken to detect gross abnormalities of the urinary system before the contrast medium is injected.

7. Preparing the family for the test by providing clear explanations can enhance their cooperation and may alleviate some of their anxiety.

Interventions	**Rationales**
8. Tell the child he may be asked to drink a carbonated beverage during the test.	8. Carbonation produces gas in the stomach, which enhances visualization of the kidneys.
9. Caution the child that the X-ray technician may press on his abdomen with a compression board (a board with half of a ball attached to it). Assure the child it will not hurt.	9. The round part of the ball is pressed into the abdomen to promote better visualization of the kidneys or renal pelvis.
10. Tell the child that he must lie still while the pictures are being taken, that he will be allowed to move between pictures, and that the test lasts about 30 minutes. Assure a young child that he will not be left alone.	10. Movement while X-rays are being taken distorts the image. Because the time between pictures can seem like an eternity to a young child, support should be provided during the waiting period.

Nursing diagnosis: *Potential for injury related to the contrast medium*

GOAL: The child will exhibit no signs of allergic reaction to the contrast medium.

Interventions	**Rationales**
1. Check the child's history for hypersensitivity to iodine or to food (such as shellfish) or contrast media that contain iodine. Also check for a history of asthma or other severe allergies.	1. These conditions may cause a hypersensitive reaction to the contrast medium.
2. Notify the doctor if the child's history is positive for any of the above conditions.	2. Antihistamines or steroids may be administered before the test if the study must be done.
3. Alert the radiology department of the potential for an allergic reaction.	3. Emergency equipment and drugs (such as epinephrine and diphenhydramine) should be available in case of a reaction.

Documentation checklist

After the procedure, be sure to document the following:
__ the child's status
__ the insertion site used for administering contrast medium
__ any allergic reaction
__ vital signs.

Magnetic Resonance Imaging

Introduction

Magnetic resonance imaging (MRI, also called nuclear magnetic resonance) is a noninvasive procedure used for neurologic diagnosis of such conditions as cerebral infarction, tumors, abscesses, edema, and hemorrhage. Like computed tomography (CT), MRI produces cross-sectional images of the brain and spinal cord in multiple layers without bone interference. Unlike CT, however, MRI does not rely on ionizing radiation or injected contrast media to produce the images. The child is placed in a supine position on a narrow table in the MRI scanner, which uses a strong magnetic field and short bursts of energy in the form of radio waves. Radio receivers detect the energy released from hydrogen ions exposed to the radio waves. The MRI computer processes the signals and displays the high-resolution images on a video monitor. The test is painless, and no harmful effects have been documented.

Indications for testing

Any of the following conditions may indicate the need for MRI:
• hemorrhage
• neoplasm
• cystic lesion
• hydrocephalus
• head trauma
• cerebrovascular accident
• atrophy
• birth defects
• tethered cord
• hydromyelia
• vascular and structural abnormalities.

Nursing diagnosis: *Knowledge deficit related to MRI*

GOAL: The child and parents will verbalize an understanding of the procedure

Interventions

1. Explain MRI and its purpose to the parents and child. Tell them that the procedure is a way to detect and examine abnormalities in the head and body. Use age-appropriate terms in your descriptions. For example, if the patient is a young child, describe the scanner as a long tunnel open at both ends and the radio frequency coil as a hard shell or space helmet. If possible, show the family a picture of the scanner to help them visualize it. Tell them the procedure will take 30 to 60 minutes, depending on the body area being examined.

2. Remove any jewelry, ECG pads, or diaper pins from the child, and have him wear pajamas without metal snaps. If the parents want to accompany the child, tell them to remove credit cards, watches, beepers, loose jewelry, belts with metal buckles, keys, or other metal objects.

3. Tell the child he must lie still during the procedure. Explain that he will hear repetitive knocking sounds at different pitches; consider giving him earplugs if necessary.

Rationales

1. Clearly explaining the procedure and equipment can enhance the family's cooperation and may alleviate some of their anxiety.

2. Metal objects should not be brought into the magnetic field. Loose objects, such as jewelry or keys, would be propelled toward the magnet, creating a hazard. The powerful magnetic field also can damage credit cards, watches, and beepers.

3. The slightest movement can cause the images to be distorted. The sounds heard during the procedure (caused by the radio frequencies) may disturb the child and make him restless (although the monotony sometimes lulls younger children to sleep).

Nursing diagnosis: *Potential for injury related to MRI*

GOAL: The child will be free of discomfort and injury.

Interventions

1. Assess the child to determine his suitability for MRI. Contact the radiology department if the child has:
• a winged needle device for I.V. access

• an infusion pump

• spring-action cassettes in I.V. tubing

• a stainless steel porta-cath

• implanted metal objects, such as intracranial surgical clips, aneurysm clips, artificial heart valves, or rods

• a history of foreign bodies in the eyes
• claustrophobia

• a history of nausea or headaches

• mechanical ventilation

• a critical illness

2. If you think the child will not lie still during the procedure, consult the doctor about administering a sedative-hypnotic, such as chloral hydrate or pentobarbital. Give the child nothing by mouth for 6 hours before administering the medication.

3. Observe the child closely during the procedure to ensure adequate breathing. Use a cardiac output monitor or a pulse oximeter designed for use with MRI, if your hospital has one.

4. Assess the child's vital signs when he is fully awake.

Rationales

1. Various factors may prevent a child from undergoing MRI.
• The magnetic field can cause the needle to dislodge.
• The magnetic field can cause mechanical failure of equipment.
• Tubing with stainless steel springs may inhibit fluid flow.
• The magnetic field may pull on a stainless steel porta-cath within the chest wall. (*Note:* Plastic porta-caths have been developed for use in MRI. Porta-caths in place for over 3 months pose little safety hazard but may degrade image quality.)
• Magnetic pull on implanted objects can cause tissue damage. Certain rods and clips may not be contraindicated if they have been in place longer than 3 months and adhesions have developed.
• Movement of objects can result in tissue damage.
• A child with claustrophobia may have a difficult time because of the scanner's narrow diameter.
• The sounds generated during MRI may exacerbate nausea or headaches.
• Mechanical ventilators cannot be taken into the magnetic field. Manual ventilation would be required.
• Poor access and the metal components of most resuscitative equipment make resuscitating a critically ill child difficult—and potentially dangerous for the child and staff.

2. A child under age 5 may have a hard time lying still for the procedure. Administering a sedative-hypnotic 20 to 30 minutes before the study usually keeps the child sedated for the time required. Withholding food and fluids for 6 hours empties the stomach, which helps prevent vomiting and aspiration of gastric contents.

3. Sedatives can depress the respiratory drive and result in apnea. Monitoring a child inside the scanner is difficult. Visibility is not ideal, and cardiac or apnea monitors cannot be used because of metallic components and interference from radio waves.

4. Such assessment can identify adverse effects from the sedative.

Documentation checklist

After the procedure, be sure to document the following:
___ the child's status
___ the results of the test.

Myelography

Introduction

Myelography is the fluoroscopic and radiographic examination of the spinal subarachnoid space after injection of a contrast medium. The fluoroscope permits visualization of the flow of the contrast medium and the outline of the subarachnoid space. Radiographs are taken for a permanent record. The study is done to demonstrate lesions, such as tumors and herniated intervertebral disks, that partially or completely block the flow of cerebrospinal fluid (CSF) in the subarachnoid space or to detect arachnoiditis, spinal nerve root injury, or tumors in the posterior fossa of the skull. A water-soluble contrast medium, such as metrizamide, is usually used because oil-based media must be removed after the procedure. An infant or young child usually requires general anesthesia. An older child who can cooperate during the procedure may be given a sedative.

Indications for testing

Any of the following conditions may indicate the need for myelography:
- masses
- tumors
- cysts
- tethered cord
- fractures
- dislocations
- hydromyelia.

Nursing diagnosis: *Knowledge deficit related to myelography*

GOAL: The child and parents will verbalize an understanding of the procedure

Interventions

1. Explain to the child and parents that the child cannot eat or drink for 8 hours before the study.

2. Ask the parents if the child is allergic to iodine or iodine-containing products, such as shellfish.

3. Tell the child and parents that X-rays will be taken during the procedure. Describe radiologic equipment in age-appropriate terms; for example, if the patient is a young child, tell him an X-ray is a picture taken with a large camera. Explain that the machine will be placed close to his body but that it will not touch him. If possible, show the equipment to the child before the procedure.

4. Explain that the child will wear a hospital gown during the procedure and must be free of any metal objects, such as diaper pins, or jewelry.

5. If the child will be awake during the procedure, tell him that he will experience drowsiness from the sedative, a stinging or burning sensation in his back as the contrast medium is injected, and pressure at the injection site as the needle is removed. Explain that he will be placed on his side, with his knees drawn up to his abdomen and his chin touching his chest. Use age-appropriate terms (such as telling a young child he will be arching his back like a cat or curling up in a ball). Explain that he may be tilted in several positions during the procedure to allow the contrast agent to flow through his spinal cord, but assure him that he will not be allowed to fall.

Rationales

1. The contrast medium may cause nausea and vomiting. Restricting food and fluids helps prevent aspiration of gastric contents.

2. The contrast medium contains iodine; a child who is hypersensitive to iodine may experience an anaphylactic reaction.

3. A young child is prone to fantasy and may imagine the X-ray machine is a monster. A clear explanation of medical terms and demonstration of equipment can ease the child's fears.

4. Metal objects would distort the image because X-rays cannot penetrate them.

5. Myelography, an uncomfortable experience for any patient, can be especially unsettling for a child who has been ill-prepared for the procedure. Explaining key steps in clear terms—and in a calm, reassuring manner—can help alleviate the child's anxiety.

Interventions	Rationales
6. Tell the child and parents that the procedure will take about 2 hours. Briefly describe postmyelography precautions, such as elevating the head of the bed 30 degrees, maintaining a quiet environment, and encouraging fluids as ordered.	6. A brief explanation of precautions can help parents to begin planning how they will care for the child after the procedure. More detailed care instructions are given at that time.
7. Prepare the child and parents for symptoms the child may exhibit after the procedure, such as nausea, vomiting, and headache.	7. Advance preparation assures the parents that these symptoms are not unusual and may help the child cope with the symptoms more effectively if he experiences them.

Nursing diagnosis: *Altered comfort: pain, related to the contrast medium*

GOAL: The child will be free of pain.

Interventions	Rationales
1. Move the child slowly and have him remain completely passive during transfers, such as from the stretcher to the bed. Advise the child and parents to avoid unnecessary movement. Provide a quiet environment free of excessive stimuli.	1. Avoiding sudden and unnecessary movement and maintaining a quiet environment can help prevent or minimize headache.
2. If a water-soluble contrast medium was used, elevate the head of the bed 30 degrees for 24 hours. Observe the child for irritability, stiff neck, or photophobia, and document his tolerance of the procedure.	2. The contrast medium can cause chemical meningitis; elevation reduces the amount of contrast reaching the cerebral area. Irritability, a stiff neck, or photophobia may indicate meningeal irritation.

Nursing diagnosis: *Potential for injury related to seizures resulting from contrast medium injection*

GOAL: The child will not be injured as a result of seizure activity.

Interventions	Rationales
1. Assess the child every 2 hours for 12 hours. Monitor and record vital signs, neurologic status, and movement of extremities.	1. Frequent assessment can detect changes in the child's health status and decreased CNS activity that can lead to seizure.
2. Institute seizure precautions for 24 hours. Keep suctioning equipment, an oral airway, and an Ambu bag at the bedside.	2. Suctioning may be needed if the child salivates excessively during a seizure; an oral airway, if the child's airway becomes obstructed; and an Ambu bag, if respiratory arrest occurs.

Nursing diagnosis: *Potential fluid volume deficit related to vomiting*

GOAL: The child will remain adequately hydrated as evidenced by moist mucous membranes, normal urine output, and good skin turgor.

Interventions	Rationales
1. Encourage fluid intake unless contraindicated.	1. Adequate fluid intake promotes rehydration, replaces CSF, and dilutes the contrast medium.
2. Monitor and document the child's fluid intake and output.	2. The child should void within 8 hours of the procedure. The contrast agent is excreted by the kidney. Documenting intake and output provides information on the child's hydration status.
3. Request I.V. therapy if prolonged vomiting occurs.	3. I.V. therapy promotes rehydration.

Nursing diagnosis: *Knowledge deficit related to home care after myelography*

GOAL: The child and parents will verbalize specific discharge instructions

Interventions

1. Instruct the parents to call the doctor if the child experiences nausea or vomiting at home.

2. Teach the parents the signs and symptoms of dehydration, such as poor skin turgor, dry mucous membranes, and decreased urine output.

3. Encourage rest periods at home.

4. Tell the parents when the child can return to school, according to doctor's orders (usually within 4 days).

Rationales

1. Continual nausea and vomiting can lead to dehydration.

2. Rapid fluid loss can occur with vomiting. Knowing how to recognize signs and symptoms of dehydration facilitates prompt intervention and treatment.

3. Frequent resting helps prevent headaches.

4. The child may experience residual adverse effects of the contrast medium for up to 4 days after the procedure.

Documentation checklist

After the procedure, be sure to document the following:
___ the child's status
___ vital signs
___ headaches.

DIAGNOSTIC STUDIES

Nuclear Medicine

Introduction

Nuclear medicine studies use radioactive isotopes to image tumors, abscesses, or other abnormalities in the bones, thyroid, kidney, liver, heart, brain, or lung. Usually, the radioisotope is administered intravenously and concentrates in certain body organs based on the radiopharmaceutical used. Gamma camera detectors record the radiation emitted from the organ. Nuclear medicine scans involve very low radiation doses and pose minimal risk to the patient and staff.

Indications for testing

Any of the following conditions may indicate the need for nuclear medicine studies:

Cardiovascular disorders
• structural defects
• cardiomegaly

Neurologic disorders
• brain tumors

Respiratory disorders
• lung tumors

Musculoskeletal disorders
• osteomyelitis
• metastatic neoplasms
• degenerative processes
• fractures

Thyroid disorders
• goiters
• nodules
• substernal masses
• hyperthyroidism
• hypothyroidism
• thyroid cancer
• metastases

Genitourinary disorders
• trauma
• acute or chronic renal failure
• cysts
• transplant rejection
• impaired renal function.

Nursing diagnosis: *Knowledge deficit related to nuclear medicine*

GOAL: The child and parents will verbalize an understanding of the procedure.

Interventions

1. Briefly explain the procedure and its purpose to the child and parents. Use age-appropriate terms the child can understand. Tell them a needle will be placed under the child's skin to inject the contrast medium. Assure them that the injection will hurt for just a minute and that the needle will be removed once the contrast medium has been injected.

2. Avoid using the word "dye" to describe the contrast medium.

3. Tell the child he will be asked to void before the study. (*Note:* If the patient is an infant, his diapers may need changing during the procedure.)

4. Explain that the camera will be brought close to the child's body but will not touch it. Assure the child that the camera will not fall on him.

5. Tell the child he may be asked to change positions during the test but that he must try to lie still while the camera is taking pictures. Assure him that he will be allowed to move between pictures.

Rationales

1. Clearly explaining the procedure helps the family prepare for what will happen to the child, can improve their cooperation, and may alleviate some of their anxiety.

2. The child may misinterpret the word "dye" for "die."

3. The kidneys usually excrete the isotope. Voiding diminishes bladder activity seen on the pictures. Wet diapers may also result in artifact.

4. The gamma camera detector is a large, round cylinder placed over the organ being imaged. Preparing the child for the experience can prevent him from becoming afraid.

5. Movement causes a distorted image. The time required for each picture may vary. Changing positions is required if different angles of an organ must be imaged.

Interventions

6. Explain to the parents that the amount of radiation received is less than that from X-rays.

7. Tell the child to remove metal objects, such as jewelry, before the procedure.

Rationales

6. This information can allay the concerns of parents worried by the terms "nuclear" and "radiation."

7. Metal objects obstruct the view of organs.

Nursing diagnosis: *Potential for injury related to sedatives used for the procedure*

GOAL: The child will suffer no adverse effects from the sedatives.

Interventions

1. If you think the child will not lie still during the procedure, consult the doctor about administering a sedative-hypnotic, such as chloral hydrate or pentobarbital. Withhold food and fluids for 6 hours before administering the medication.

2. Observe the child closely during the procedure to ensure adequate breathing.

3. Assess the child's vital signs when he is fully awake.

Rationales

1. A child under age 5 may have a hard time lying still for the procedure. Administering a sedative-hypnotic 20 to 30 minutes before the study usually keeps the child sedated for the time required. Withholding food and fluids for 6 hours empties the stomach, which helps prevent vomiting and aspiration of gastric contents.

2. Sedatives can depress the respiratory drive and result in apnea.

3. Such assessment can identify adverse effects from the sedative.

Nursing diagnosis: *Potential for injury related to radiation exposure*

GOAL: Radiation exposure to the child, parents, staff, and other patients will be minimal.

Interventions

1. Wear gloves when coming in contact with the child's body fluids, and dispose of urine and other excretions in the toilet. Wash hands thoroughly.

2. If the child has an indwelling catheter, empty the collection bag every hour for 24 hours.

3. Double-bag linens before putting them in the hospital laundry. Double-bag disposable waste, especially soiled diapers, before discarding in the trash.

4. If you are pregnant or must hold the child for longer than 1 hour, wear a lead apron. Caution the parents to do likewise.

Rationales

1. Most radioisotopes are excreted in the urine, which can be disposed of in the toilet without harm to the sanitation system.

2. Radioactive substances in the urine consolidate in a collection bag if the bag is not emptied each hour.

3. Double bagging helps prevent contamination of laundry bins and trash receptacles.

4. Although radiation emission is minimal, prolonged exposure may be harmful.

Documentation checklist

After the procedure, be sure to document the following:
___ the child's status
___ vital signs.

DIAGNOSTIC STUDIES

Upper GI and Small Bowel Series

Introduction

Upper GI and small bowel series involves the fluoroscopic examination of the esophagus, stomach, and small intestine after the ingestion of barium sulfate (barium swallow). This test is indicated for children with upper GI symptoms (swallowing difficulty, regurgitation, and burning or gnawing epigastric pain), signs of small bowel disease (diarrhea and weight loss), and signs of GI bleeding (hematemesis and melena).

When performing a complete GI series, barium enema should always precede this test because retained barium may cloud anatomic structures on X-rays.

Indications for testing

Any of the following conditions may indicate the need for an upper GI and small bowel series:

Upper GI
• pyloric stenosis
• ulcers

• abdominal pain
• diarrhea

Small bowel follow-through
• malabsorption syndrome
• small-bowel strictures.

Nursing diagnosis: *Knowledge deficit related to the procedure*

GOAL: The child (or parents) will verbalize an understanding of the procedure.

Interventions

1. Explain to the child that he will be allowed nothing to eat or drink beginning at midnight on the day of testing (beginning 3 hours before testing for children under age 2).

2. Explain that, if the child has undergone other diagnostic testing involving the use of barium sulfate (such as barium enema or barium swallow) within the last few days, he may require laxatives or enemas.

3. Explain to the child that the test will be performed in the radiology department and that the technicians will be wearing lead aprons. Tell him that he will need to wear a hospital gown and to remove all metal objects, such as necklaces, that might interfere with the X-rays.

4. Explain the following procedural events to the child, using age-appropriate terms:
• He will be given some barium sulfate to swallow from a cup or a bottle (infants are given the barium from a bottle; young children may sip the liquid through a straw). Explain to the younger child that the barium is thick like a milkshake, but that it may not taste quite as good (some hospitals flavor the barium with strawberry or chocolate to improve the taste).

Rationales

1. Withholding food and drink allows for the complete digestion of barium. Fasting in infants should be limited to 3 hours before testing to prevent hypoglycemia.

2. Laxatives and enemas are prescribed in this situation to clear the digestive tract of any residual barium. However, they are contraindicated in children with inflammatory bowel disease, ulcerative colitis, or Crohn's disease because of their irritating effects on the GI system.

3. Offering such explanations helps to prepare the child for the visual impact of the radiology room, which can be particularly frightening to a younger child.

4. Because this can be a frightening experience (especially for a younger child), the child should receive detailed explanations so that he is adequately prepared for the actual procedure.

Interventions

• He may be turned in various positions on a tilted table when the X-rays are being taken (reassure him that he will not fall).
• Depending on the child's condition, he may require the insertion of a nasogastric tube so that the remainder of the barium can be instilled directly into his stomach. Also explain that the radiologist, wearing a lead-lined glove, may compress his stomach to ensure that the gastric mucosa is adequately coated with barium.
• He should be prepared to wait between X-rays and can expect to be in the radiology room for 2 to 4 hours before the small-bowel series is completed (reassure the younger child that his parents or a nurse will be with him throughout this period).

Rationales

Nursing diagnosis: *Altered bowel elimination: constipation related to the retention of barium*

GOAL: The child will maintain normal bowel elimination patterns as evidenced by having a normal bowel movement within 24 hours after the procedure.

Interventions

1. Notify the doctor before the test if the child is taking anticholinergics or narcotics. Administer laxatives, as ordered.

2. After confirming with the radiology department that all tests have been completed, begin the child on a regular diet.

3. Assess the quantity and quality of the child's stools for the first few days after the procedure (warn the child and parents that the stools will be white or light-colored [possibly pink if a strawberry flavoring was used] during this time).

4. Administer castor oil or milk of magnesia, as ordered.

5. Inform the doctor if the child has not expelled all of the barium within 3 days.

6. If appropriate, encourage the child to increase his fluid intake.

Rationales

1. Anticholinergics and narcotics may decrease peristalsis and impede the elimination of barium from the GI tract, possibly leading to constipation.

2. A normal, well-balanced diet can help to prevent constipation.

3. Such assessments are necessary to determine whether the child is constipated and in need of a cathartic.

4. Cathartics, such as castor oil or milk of magnesia, may be given to help eliminate any remaining barium from the child's system.

5. Barium may absorb fecal water and solidify in the colon, causing constipation and impaction.

6. Liberal fluid intake can help promote the elimination of barium from the child's system.

Documentation checklist

After the procedure, be sure to document the following:
___ the child's status
___ bowel sounds
___ bowel movements.

X-Ray Studies

Introduction

X-ray studies involve radiographic examination of one or more body areas, depending on the specific study ordered. The four densities of the body—air, water, fat, and bone—absorb varying degrees of radiation. For instance, air has the least density and results in dark images on the film. Bone causes light images or white structures on film (the calcium in bone absorbs much of the radiation, thereby preventing radiation from striking the X-ray film). Abnormalities can then be detected using these principles; for example, white areas in a normally dark lung field might indicate pneumonia.

Indications for testing

Any of the following conditions may indicate the need for X-ray studies:

Chest
• atelectasis
• pneumonia
• lung abscess
• tumor
• pneumothorax
• scoliosis
• kyphosis
• cardiomegaly
• vessel anomalies

Abdomen
• masses
• small bowel obstruction
• ascites
• tissue trauma

Kidney, ureter, bladder
• abnormal size and structure
• renal calculi
• kidney or bladder masses

Skull
• trauma
• fracture
• congenital anomalies
• bone defects.

Nursing diagnosis: *Knowledge deficit related to X-ray studies*

GOAL: The child and parents will verbalize an understanding of the specific X-ray study ordered.

Interventions

1. Explain food or fluid restrictions, if applicable.

2. Tell the child and parents that the study will be done in the radiology department unless a portable X-ray has been ordered. Let the parents know whether they can accompany the child.

3. Tell the child he will wear a hospital gown and must remove all metal objects.

4. Explain the X-ray equipment to be used, and show the equipment to the child and parents before the study, if possible. Use age-appropriate terms in your descriptions. For example, if the patient is a young child, describe the equipment as a special camera that will take his picture. Explain that the machine will be placed close to the child's body but will not touch him. Tell them the study usually takes 10 to 15 minutes.

Rationales

1. Usually, X-ray studies do not require food or fluid restrictions, although the child may be given a restricted diet to conform with other tests administered after general X-rays.

2. Portable films are inferior in quality to those taken in the radiology department but may be indicated if the child is acutely ill or immobilized. Such factors as limited space, physical constraints, or the mother's pregnancy may prevent the parents from accompanying the child.

3. Metal objects (such as jewelry, diaper pins, snaps, or belt buckles) can obscure the anatomical view because X-rays cannot penetrate them.

4. A clear explanation helps ease the family's fears, particularly those of a young child, who may fantasize that the X-ray machine looks like a monster.

Interventions

5. Explain that the child may be asked to stand, sit, or lie down during the study. Remind the child that he must remain still while the picture is taken, and assure him that he can move between pictures.

6. Tell the child he may be asked to take a deep breath and hold it while the picture is being taken. If the patient is a young child, demonstrate the task, have him practice it, and provide feedback on how well he did.

Rationales

5. Various positions may be required, depending on the study, the body area involved, or the angle desired. For example, the child usually stands for posteroanterior chest films and may sit or lie down for anteroposterior views. Movement while the X-ray is being taken will distort the image.

6. For a chest X-ray, holding a deep breath enhances full visualization of lung expansion. Practice and feedback can help a young child master an unfamiliar task and lessen his fear of the procedure.

Documentation checklist

After the procedure, be sure to document the following:
___ the child's status
___ results of the test.

SECTION IV

HOME HEALTH CARE

Antibacterial or Antifungal Therapy

Introduction

Long-term home antibacterial or antifungal therapy is sometimes necessary to treat infection (such as respiratory syncytial virus, histoplasmosis, and cryptococcosis), even after a prolonged hospital stay. This care plan focuses on the care required for children on home I.M. or I.V. therapy. Such care may be provided by the parents or another caregiver, such as a home health nurse.

Assessment

The following findings indicate complications associated with home therapy:

Respiratory
• wheezing
• dyspnea

Integumentary
• rash
• hives
• urticaria
• elevated temperature.

Nursing diagnosis: *Impaired tissue integrity related to bacterial or fungal infection*

GOAL: The child will maintain tissue integrity as evidenced by decreases in temperature, white blood cell count, heart rate, and (if the infection is localized) purulent drainage and odor.

Interventions

1. If appropriate, instruct the parents to administer medications I.V. (through an I.V. access by continuous infusion or intermittent infusion with a heparin lock) rather than I.M. during the course of therapy.

2. Make sure the parents know to administer medications around the clock, as indicated.

3. Inform the parents that the home health nurse will routinely monitor the child's blood work (including the complete blood count, erythrocyte sedimentation rate, and any necessary bacterial or fungal cultures) and assess vital signs and affected body systems daily or every 2 days, as indicated.

Rationales

1. Using the I.V. route, when appropriate, alleviates the trauma, anxiety, and pain sometimes associated with I.M. administration.

2. Administering medications around the clock helps maintain appropriate blood levels, thereby ensuring optimal bacteriostatic or fungistatic action.

3. Routine monitoring and assessment help determine the need for dosage adjustments or the discontinuation of therapy.

Nursing diagnosis: *Knowledge deficit related to home care*

GOAL: The parents will verbalize an understanding of home care instructions.

Interventions

1. Instruct the parents on the following:
• flushing a heparin lock
• priming and administering medications with or without an infusion pump
• caring for an I.V. dressing
• caring for injection sites (if antibiotics are to be given I.M.)
• administering I.M. injections.

Rationales

1. The parents need to know how to perform these tasks to provide proper home care, especially if the child requires daily medication administration and a home health nurse is unavailable.

Interventions

2. Instruct the parents on the importance of the following:
• gathering all supplies ahead of time
• inspecting the I.V. access device for patency
• double-checking all medications for correct dosage
• checking for any unusual color or precipitates in solutions
• preparing the administration set
• setting the infusion pump for the desired rate (if applicable)
• if using a heparin lock system, swabbing the cap with alcohol or iodine, inserting the needle into the cap, and securing the needle with tape.

3. Review with the parents the potential adverse effects of each prescribed medication

Rationales

2. Gathering supplies ahead of time and taking the time to prepare for the administration procedure help to prevent mistakes that can result in adverse reactions.

3. Knowing the potential adverse effects should prompt the parents to seek medical advice and attention, when necessary.

Documentation checklist

During the home care session, be sure to document the following:
___ the child's status
___ the child's response to antibiotic therapy
___ adverse reactions to antibiotics
___ I.V. or I.M. site used.

Colostomy, Ileostomy

Introduction

Colostomy refers to the surgical creation of an opening between the colon and the outside surface of the body. Ileostomy refers to the surgical creation of an opening into the ileum.

Children usually require ostomies for various reasons, including congenital anomalies (such as imperforate anus, intestinal atresia, or Hirschsprung's disease) or some other disease or condition (such as necrotizing enterocolitis, ulcerative colitis, or trauma from an automobile accident).

Assessment

The following findings indicate normal functioning of the colostomy or ileostomy:

Gastrointestinal
• brown or brownish green stool
• normal stool consistency (loose stools with an ileostomy; formed stools with a colostomy)

Integumentary
• pinkish or pale red skin at the stoma site
• moist mucous membranes forming the stoma
• clear, intact skin around the stoma site.

Nursing diagnosis: *Impaired skin integrity related to exposure of skin to stool*

GOAL: The child will have no signs of impaired skin integrity as evidenced by intact periostomal skin.

Interventions

1. Tell the parents (and child, if age-appropriate) to use a properly fitting ostomy bag and to secure it to the skin with a skin barrier (such as Hollihesive, Stomahesive, or Comfed) to prevent leakage from the bag. If the child is an infant, instruct the parents to always apply a bag before diapering the child.

2. Instruct the parents to check the ostomy bag for leakage every 2 hours and to change the bag as soon as leakage occurs or is suspected.

3. Instruct the parents on the importance of emptying the ostomy bag when it is one-fourth to one-third full.

4. Tell the parents to change the ostomy bag at least every 24 hours until the skin is healed (usually within 1 to 3 days).

5. Teach the parents how to cleanse the skin around the stoma using water or a normal saline solution.

6. If skin breakdown (marked by redness or excoriated skin) occurs, instruct the parents to treat the skin using the method and medications ordered by the doctor, enterostomal therapist, and ostomy nurse.

Rationales

1. Using a properly fitting bag and an effective skin barrier protects the skin from the caustic effects of stool. Diapering without a bag usually results in skin breakdown.

2. Prolonged contact of stool on skin increases the risk of skin breakdown.

3. Allowing the bag to fill up increases the risk of leakage as the weight of the stool pulls against the seal, causing the seal to break.

4. Daily changing allows for frequent observation and treatment, when necessary.

5. Cleansing removes stool from the skin surface and prevents irritation.

6. The degree of skin breakdown will determine the specific treatment required.

Nursing diagnosis: *Potential for infection (postoperative incisional wound) related to contamination with stool*

GOAL: The child will remain free of infection as evidenced by maintaining a normal temperature and having no signs of erythema, induration, or drainage from the incision site.

Interventions	**Rationales**
1. Instruct the parents (and child, if age-appropriate) to change the ostomy bag daily until the incision is healed (if the incision is covered by a bag). Also, tell them to change the ostomy bag immediately if leakage occurs or is suspected. (This is especially important if the skin barrier and bag partially or completely cover the incision.)	1. Daily changing allows for frequent observation of the incision for signs of contamination and infection. Leakage can lead to skin breakdown and infection from prolonged contact of stool with skin.
2. Make sure the parents understand that, whenever the bag needs to be changed, the incision should be assessed for signs of infection, including redness, skin breakdown, purulent drainage, and elevated body temperature.	2. This allows for early detection and prompt treatment with antibiotics in case infection occurs.

Nursing diagnosis: *Altered nutrition: less than body requirements related to colostomy or ileostomy*

GOAL: The child will maintain adequate nutritional intake as evidenced by eating 80% of all meals.

Interventions	**Rationales**
1. Instruct the parents to serve the child small, frequent meals.	1. Serving the child small, frequent meals ensures that he receives adequate nutrition without overfilling his stomach.
2. Stress the importance of limiting or eliminating foods from the child's diet that cause gas or diarrhea, including cabbage, spicy foods, beans, brussels sprouts, and fruits or fruit juices.	2. Limiting or eliminating these foods helps prevent gas, which can cause distention and disinterest in eating.

Nursing diagnosis: *Altered bowel elimination: constipation related to colostomy requiring irrigation*

GOAL: The child will have normal bowel elimination and no constipation as evidenced by softened bowel movements and lack of pain during elimination.

Interventions	**Rationales**
1. Tell the parents (and child, if age-appropriate) to irrigate the colostomy or ileostomy early in the morning (see *Colostomy irrigation,* page 252).	1. Irrigation early in the morning empties the bowel and helps prevent stool formation that could lead to constipation later in the day.
2. Provide a high-fiber diet.	2. A high-fiber diet helps to increase the bulk of stool, thereby preventing constipation.
3. Increase the child's fluid intake, as ordered.	3. An increased fluid intake increases the water content of stools, thereby helping to prevent constipation.

COLOSTOMY IRRIGATION

When irrigating an ostomy, be sure to perform the irrigation at the same time each day, allowing an hour for the entire procedure. Proceed as follows:
• Fill the irrigation bag with warm water or another solution as instructed by the doctor or enterostomal therapist. Be sure to use warm rather than cold water to decrease the risk of cramping.
• Fasten an irrigation sleeve around the stoma, and place the end of the sleeve in the toilet. This allows the irrigation solution to drain directly into the toilet.
• Insert a plastic irrigation tube 1⅛" to 1⅝" (3 to 4 cm) into the stoma. Avoid forcing the tube into the stoma by first dilating the stomal opening with a lubricated, gloved finger, as any forced movement could perforate the bowel. Be sure to apply lubricant to the tube as well.

• After the tube is in place, begin instilling the solution. Slow down the rate if cramping occurs. Hold the irrigation cone against the stomal opening to prevent the water from flowing back into the irrigation bag.
• Allow most of the fluid to drain into the toilet (this usually takes about 10 to 15 minutes). After draining, close the end of the sleeve and instruct the child to wear the bag for another hour. Tell him to move around during this time to help the rest of the solution to drain into the bag.
• After the colostomy has completely drained, reapply a regular ostomy bag and skin barrier to contain any feces produced later in the day.

Nursing diagnosis: *Disturbance in self-concept: body image related to colostomy or ileostomy*

GOAL: The child will demonstrate an improved self-concept as evidenced by verbalizing about the colostomy or ileostomy, changing the bag, and showing increased interest in self-care.

Interventions

1. Encourage the child to participate in self-care. Advise him to change or rinse the ostomy bag at least daily to prevent odor.

2. Encourage the child to express his feelings.

3. Encourage the child to join a local, age-appropriate ostomy support group.

Rationales

1. Such encouragement promotes continued interest in hygiene and appearances, thereby helping to improve the child's self-concept. Changing or rinsing the bag on a daily basis helps prevent foul-smelling odors that can make the child feel self-conscious.

2. Getting the child to express his feelings enables him to face his altered body image without fear of rejection.

3. Group support promotes a feeling of acceptance and allows the child to share experiences with others in similar situations.

Documentation checklist

During the home care session, be sure to document the following:
___ condition of the stoma site
___ elimination pattern
___ nutritional intake
___ fluid intake and output
___ any comments by the child or family.

Mechanical Ventilation

Introduction

Mechanical ventilation—a means of artificially controlling or assisting respiration—usually involves ventilation with a volume-cycled or pressure-cycled ventilator that is somewhat modified for home use. Conditions that require ventilatory assistance include bronchopulmonary dysplasia, coma, and musculoskeletal disorders.

Assessment

The following findings indicate normal ventilator functioning:

Respiratory
- normal respiratory rate and rhythm
- clear breath sounds
- absence of crackles or rhonchi

Cardiovascular
- normal heart rate and rhythm

Neurologic
- quietness
- level of consciousness (depending on diagnosis): opens eyes, moves to commands, blinks eyes on command.

Integumentary
- pale pink color
- brisk capillary refill time

Nursing diagnosis: *Ineffective breathing pattern related to possible airway obstruction*

GOAL: The child will maintain effective breathing as evidenced by the absence of respiratory distress.

Interventions

1. Explain that the parents need to provide humidified oxygen for ventilation.

2. Instruct the parents to preoxygenate and hyperventilate the child with 100% oxygen for 30 to 60 minutes before suctioning.

3. Instruct the parents to instill 0.5 ml of normal saline solution into the endotracheal tube before suctioning.

4. Explain that the child should be suctioned, as needed, only if he is dyspneic or gurgling or if he has a high intracranial pressure.

5. When suctioning the child, have the parents monitor his heart rate (using a stethoscope or home cardiac monitor) and assess his color.

6. Instruct the parents to change the child's tracheostomy tube, as ordered (usually once weekly) or whenever plugging occurs. Tell them to keep two or three extra tubes on hand at all times.

7. Instruct the parents to administer aerosol bronchodilators and perform chest physiotherapy, as ordered.

8. Teach the parents to assess the child's respiratory status every 4 to 8 hours.

Rationales

1. Moist, warm air prevents the impairment of mucus secretions.

2. Preoxygenation may combat the hypoxia associated with suctioning. Hyperventilation opens the alveoli and decreases the risk of atelectasis.

3. Instilling saline solution may help to liquefy thickened secretions.

4. Suctioning may result in such complications as bleeding, decreased oxygen saturation rate, and intracranial pressure and should be done only when necessary.

5. Such monitoring and assessment may reveal dysrhythmias or hypoxemia, which are potential complications of suctioning.

6. Weekly tube changes help decrease the risk of plugging. Dyspnea that does not improve with suctioning indicates the need for emergency tube replacement.

7. Bronchodilators help relieve bronchospasms. Chest physiotherapy helps to loosen and mobilize mucus secretions.

8. Frequent assessments are necessary to evaluate the effectiveness of care.

Nursing diagnosis: *Potential for injury (tracheal trauma) related to tracheostomy tube movement and suctioning*

GOAL: The child will suffer minimal tracheal trauma as evidenced by the lack of stenotic tissue and the lack of bleeding during suctioning.

Interventions

1. Tell the parents to secure the ventilator circuit to the tracheostomy tube by tying it in place and to clip the circuit to the child's clothing.

2. Instruct the parents to hold the tracheostomy tube in place when changing tracheostomy ties.

Rationales

1. Securing the circuit avoids unnecesary manipulation of the tracheostomy and decreases any tension on the tube that could lead to dislodgment.

2. Maintaining the tracheostomy tube in place during tie changes helps to prevent or minimize trauma to the area.

Nursing diagnosis: *Potential for impaired skin integrity related to moisture and tube manipulation*

GOAL: The child will maintain normal skin integrity as evidenced by pink skin coloring and the lack of erythema.

Interventions

1. Instruct the parents to change the child's tracheostomy ties whenever they become wet and to observe the skin for rash, redness, and swelling.

2. Tell the parents to keep a shoulder roll or a rolled towel in place.

3. Have the parents clean the tracheostomy site with cotton-tipped applicators saturated in hydrogen peroxide and rinsed with saline solution or sterile water. Tell them to be especially careful to avoid getting solution into the stoma.

Rationales

1. Continuous moisture may cause skin breakdown. Redness, rash, or swelling may indicate local infection of the stoma.

2. A shoulder roll extends the neck and helps decrease the risk of skin irritation caused by the tracheostomy tube.

3. Proper cleansing rids the tracheostomy site of secretions and prevents skin irritation.

Nursing diagnosis: *Impaired gas exchange related to respiratory disorder*

GOAL: The child will maintain normal gas exchange as evidenced by a capillary refill time of 3 to 5 seconds, an oxygen saturation above 90%, and pink mucous membranes.

Interventions

1. Tell the parents to observe the child for symmetrical chest wall movement and to auscultate for bilateral breath sounds.

2. Have the parents monitor the child's heart, respiratory, and oxygen saturation rates (if the home ventilator device is capable of such monitoring). Otherwise, tell them to assess the child's skin color and capillary refill time.

3. Instruct the parents to ventilate the child manually using an Ambu bag if he has signs and symptoms of hypoxia.

Rationales

1. Symmetrical chest movements indicate that the child is receiving adequate ventilation. A decreased pitch over a lung field may indicate atelectasis.

2. Cyanosis, a decrease in oxygen saturation rate, an increase in respiratory rate, capillary refill time, and mucus production indicate early hypoxia.

3. Manual ventilation provides adequate ventilation until the unit's circuit can be checked.

Nursing diagnosis: *Potential for infection (stoma or lower respiratory tract) related to the artificial airway*

GOAL: The child will be free of infection as evidenced by the lack of foul odor and purulent drainage from the stoma and the lack of fever, coughing, and copious sputum.

Interventions

1. Instruct the parents to clean the stoma with hydrogen peroxide once or twice daily.

2. Tell the parents to suction the child using clean technique. Be sure they understand the need to avoid dropping or excessively handling the suction catheter and to keep the catheter from touching bed linens.

Rationales

1. Routine cleaning helps remove surface bacteria, thereby preventing infection.

2. Clean, rather than sterile, technique is adequate for home care because of the decreased presence of pathogens in the home setting.

Nursing diagnosis: *Altered growth and development related to the child's dependence on mechanical ventilation*

GOAL: The child will grow and develop normally as evidenced by the achievement of developmental milestones.

Interventions

1. Explain to the parents the need to provide the child with developmentally appropriate toys and activities.

2. When talking or reading to the child, have the parents maintain eye contact.

3. Help the parents to develop a communication board for the older child who cannot verbalize because of his tracheostomy or ventilator dependence.

Rationales

1. Developmentally appropriate toys and activities encourage normal growth and development without frustrating the child.

2. Language skills are enhanced by auditory stimulation and visualization of mouth movements.

3. A communication board allows the older child to express his needs and feelings, which is a normal part of developmental progression.

Nursing diagnosis: *Altered nutrition: less than body requirements related to aspiration*

GOAL: The child will maintain adequate nutritional intake as evidenced by an appropriate weight gain and lack of vomiting.

Interventions

1. When feeding the child, tell the parents to position him upright with his head flexed slightly forward.

2. Instruct the parents to add blue food coloring to foods if they suspect the child is aspirating food contents.

3. Instruct the parents to notify the doctor immediately if aspiration occurs or is suspected.

Rationales

1. This position facilitates swallowing, thereby ensuring adequate intake and decreasing the risk of aspiration.

2. This allows for easy identification of aspirated contents (blue tracheal secretions indicate aspiration).

3. The child may require nasogastric tube feedings to ensure that he receives adequate nutritional intake.

Nursing diagnosis: *Altered family processes related to the child's increased needs and the continual presence of health care personnel in the home.*

GOAL: The family will suffer minor disruptions in family processes as evidenced by the ability to carry out activities of daily living and to maintain contact with others outside the immediate family.

Interventions

1. Encourage the parents to establish house rules (such as a time schedule and smoking policy) by which all health care personnel must abide.

2. Advise the parents to establish a "family time" for family interaction and a "special time" for interaction with the child's siblings.

3. Encourage the discussion of roles and responsibilities of each caregiver (parents and other family members).

4. Encourage the training of responsible adults outside the immediate family to act as the child's caregivers.

Rationales

1. House rules help to ensure that the family maintains control of their home.

2. A regularly scheduled family time allows for the development of family unity and the reinforcement of normal family processes. A regularly scheduled special time is important because, often, the needs of siblings become lost among the demanding needs of the ventilator-dependent child, sometimes leading to emotional upsets.

3. The roles and responsibilities of each caregiver should be clearly delineated and communicated to help prevent family conflict.

4. Training others to care for the child enables the parents and other family members to be away from the child for designated periods without feeling guilty or insecure.

Documentation checklist

During the home care session, be sure to document the following:
___ the child's ongoing status
___ ventilator settings
___ signs and symptoms of infection
___ vital signs
___ respiratory status
___ parental concerns.

Peritoneal Dialysis

Introduction

In children treated for acute or chronic renal failure, acute renal disease (such as glomerulonephritis), or poisoning, home peritoneal dialysis may be necessary to remove impurities from the blood and to help maintain normal electrolyte levels.

Usually, home peritoneal dialysis involves continuous ambulatory peritoneal dialysis (CAPD) or cycled peritoneal dialysis. CAPD, which can be accomplished any time during the waking day, enables the child to remain ambulatory throughout the dialysis treatment. Cycled peritoneal dialysis, a more convenient method, relies on the use of a dialysis machine to instill and drain dialysate during the night, when the child is asleep.

Assessment

The following signs and symptoms may indicate potential complications:

Respiratory
• increased shallow respirations

Cardiovascular
• increased heart rate
• decreased blood pressure

Gastrointestinal
• abdominal distention, tightness, or pain
• anorexia
• nausea
• vomiting
• decreased bowel sounds

Genitourinary
• decreased urine output

Integumentary
• elevated temperature

Nursing diagnosis: *Knowledge deficit related to home care*

GOAL: The parents will verbalize an understanding of home care instructions.

Interventions

1. Instruct the parents on the importance of good hand-washing technique.

2. Instruct the parents on the following procedure guidelines:
• Check the dialysate solution before administration to ensure that it is the right solution and that the fluid is clear.
• Make sure that all clamps are open to the dialysis catheter and that all drainage clamps are closed.
• Begin infusing the solution (usually instilled as rapidly as the solution flows into the peritoneal cavity). If the solution is not running well, try repositioning the child.
• Monitor for signs of cramping. If cramping occurs, slow the solution rate.
• After the infusion is complete, clamp the infusion lines and allow them to remain in the peritoneal cavity (usually for 15 to 20 minutes).
• Open the drainage catheters and allow them to drain for 5 to 10 minutes.

Rationales

1. Proper hand washing is essential to decrease the risk of equipment contamination.

2. Following these guidelines helps ensure that the child receives the proper amount of dialysate solution to remove impurities from the blood.

Interventions

3. If appropriate, instruct the parents on the purpose of and procedure for CAPD. Explain that the procedure is basically the same as for regular peritoneal dialysis, except for the following:
• The procedure must be performed three or four times in a 24-hour period.
• The solution must remain in the peritoneum for several hours.
• The child will be required to wear a bag at the waist.
• The solution will be drained when the dwelling time is complete.

4. If appropriate, instruct the parents on the purpose of and procedure for cycled peritoneal dialysis. Explain that the procedure is the same as that of regular peritoneal dialysis except that the catheter is hooked to the machine as well as the drainage bag and that the machine cycles automatically during the night.

5. Instruct the parents on monitoring the child daily for signs and symptoms of peritoneal infection, including an enlarging abdomen, fever, and abdominal pain.

6. Explain the importance of using a 1:2 solution of hydrogen peroxide in water to clean any exudate from around the catheter site.

7. Teach the parents to monitor the child's daily fluid intake and output.

8. Instruct the parents on the purpose and use of all prescribed medications, including details on their administration, dosage, and potential adverse effects.

Rationales

3. Continuous ambulatory peritoneal dialysis performs the same functions as that of regular peritoneal dialysis, yet allows the child to remain ambulatory throughout the dialysis procedure.

4. This type of dialysis allows the child greater freedom and alleviates the need to periodically disconnect the catheter throughout the infiltration time.

5. Peritoneal infection may result from the introduction of bacteria into the abdominal cavity through catheterization.

6. Exudate buildup can be a source of bacterial infection and skin breakdown.

7. Such monitoring is essential to determine the amount of urine produced, as urine output is a direct indication of kidney functioning.

8. Understanding the purpose and use of all medications helps to ensure compliance with the medication regimen. Knowing the potential adverse effects should prompt parents to seek medical advice and attention, when necessary.

Nursing diagnosis: *Altered growth and development related to chronic illness*

GOAL: The child will grow and develop normally as evidenced by interacting with peers on a regular basis and developing at an age-appropriate level.

Interventions

1. Encourage the parents to allow the child's peers to visit him at home.

2. Advise the parents to encourage the child to continue with his schoolwork.

Rationales

1. Contact with peers enables the child to maintain social ties and encourages the development of age-appropriate skills.

2. Keeping up with school assignments enables the child to advance with his classmates.

Documentation checklist

During the home care session, be sure to document the following:
___ the child's ongoing status
___ abdominal girth
___ fluid intake and output
___ amount of dialysate instilled and drained
___ catheterization site
___ parental concerns.

HOME HEALTH CARE

Total Parenteral Nutrition

Introduction

Total parenteral nutrition (TPN) may be necessary for children who cannot gain or maintain optimal weight on enteral feedings alone. It involves the infusion of a solution of dextrose, proteins, electrolytes, vitamins, and trace elements in amounts that exceed the child's energy expenditure, thereby achieving anabolism. Because of the solution's concentration, TPN must be delivered into a high-flow central vein to avoid injury to the peripheral vasculature.

Assessment

The following findings are indicative of normal TPN infusion:

Gastrointestinal
• weight gain

Genitourinary
• adequate urine output

Integumentary
• good skin turgor
• insertion site that is clear, without signs of swelling or redness

---

Nursing diagnosis: *Altered nutrition: less than body requirements related to ongoing disease*

GOAL: The child will maintain adequate nutritional intake as evidenced by a stable or increased weight, good skin turgor, and a capillary refill time of 3 to 5 seconds.

Interventions

1. Instruct the parents to monitor the child's daily fluid intake (including the amount of oral and parenteral feedings) and output.

2. Instruct the parents to maintain weekly weight records

Rationales

1. Such monitoring is a direct indication of the child's fluid status and nutritional intake.

2. Weekly weight records are necessary to help determine whether the child is maintaining or gaining weight, indicating that he is receiving adequate nutrition.

Nursing diagnosis: *Potential for infection related to use of central venous catheter (CVC)*

GOAL: The child will have no signs of CVC-related sepsis as evidenced by the absence of fever and chills and by a normal white blood cell count.

Interventions

1. Instruct the parents on the use of aseptic technique when performing dressing changes and when connecting and disconnecting the CVC.

2. Instruct the parents to monitor the child's urine glucose level on a daily basis.

3. Review with the parents the signs and symptoms of infection, including redness, exudate, edema, tenderness, and elevated temperature.

Rationales

1. Aseptic technique minimizes the risk of contaminating the CVC exit site or TPN line with bacteria.

2. Glucose in the urine may indicate early systemic infection as well as intolerance to the rate of administration or concentration of the TPN solution.

3. Knowing the signs and symptoms of infection should prompt the parents to seek medical advice and attention, when necessary.

Interventions

4. Instruct the parents to cover the I.V. site with a protective covering when bathing the child.

5. Explain to the parents the importance of turning the child's head or wearing a mask when changing the child's dressing.

Rationales

4. Moisture can increase the risk of bacterial infection.

5. Taking these measures helps prevent the spread of infection through airborne contaminants.

Nursing diagnosis: *Anxiety (child and parent) related to procedure and body image changes*

GOAL: The parents and child will be less anxious as evidenced by demonstrating a degree of comfort with the TPN procedure and by verbalizing an acceptance of the child's altered body image.

Interventions

1. Develop a schedule with the home health nurse to gradually taper the number of home care visits.

2. Ensure that a primary nurse is assigned to the family to act as a liaison and a contact for questions and follow-up care.

3. Encourage the child (if appropriate) to care for his catheter and to participate in other self-care activities.

4. Encourage the family to use cycled infusion therapy (infusing TPN solutions at predesignated intervals, such as during the night when the child is asleep), when possible.

5. Introduce the parents to the parents of other children undergoing TPN therapy.

Rationales

1. Gradually tapering the number of visits (rather than abruptly stopping all visits) allows the family to begin performing the procedure on their own for a designated interval between visits, thereby increasing their confidence and lessening their anxiety about performing the procedure on their own.

2. Assigning one nurse to the family ensures that they receive consistent attention and care, which should help to ease their anxieties.

3. Performing self-care activities enables the child to develop a sense of control over his altered body image, thereby helping to decrease his anxiety.

4. Cycled therapy enables the family to maintain some semblance of a normal life-style, thereby helping to ease their anxiety.

5. Such introductions promote a sense of support and enable the parents to find ways of dealing with their altered life-style.

Nursing diagnosis: *Knowledge deficit related to home care*

GOAL: The parents will verbalize an understanding of home care instructions.

Interventions

1. Explain to the parents the purpose of all necessary equipment (including infusion pumps, I.V. pole, infusion tubing, TPN fluid, I.V. fat emulsion, and ancillary supplies), and demonstrate their use.

2. Review with the parents the proper procedures for:
• hand-washing technique
• infusing the TPN solution at the prescribed rate
• maintaining the infusion cycle time
• monitoring the infusion pump
• recording the child's intake and output
• manipulating the infusion tubing
• caring for and troubleshooting the CVC
• changing dressings.

Rationales

1. Such explanations and demonstrations enable the parents to become familiar with the function and design of all equipment so that they will know what to do when caring for the child at home.

2. Reviewing these procedures reinforces the parents' understanding of TPN and helps ensure their compliance with the treatment regimen.

Interventions

3. Instruct the parents on the following emergency procedures:
• If the catheter breaks, clamp the line.
• If air gets in the I.V. line, aspirate the air.
• If the child is bleeding from the catheter site, assess the site and place of bleeding and, if the bleeding is excessive, apply pressure to the site.

4. Explain to the parents the importance of flushing the system with saline solution if the TPN solution is not flowing through the catheter properly. Emphasize that, if the catheter is still resisting the solution, they should stop the infusion and notify the doctor.

Rationales

3. Knowing how to respond in the event of an emergency helps prevent the development of serious complications.

4. Flushing with saline solution may be necessary to clear an obstructed catheter.

Documentation checklist

During the home care session, be sure to document the following:
___ the child's ongoing status
___ catheterization site
___ vital signs
___ signs and symptoms of infection
___ parental concerns.

Tracheostomy

Introduction

Tracheostomy refers to the surgical creation of an opening into the trachea to provide a patent airway for bypassing upper airway obstruction, ensuring long-term ventilatory support, or clearing mucus secretions from the airway. Indications for tracheostomy include bronchopulmonary dysplasia, subglottic stenosis, and respiratory distress.

Assessment

The following findings indicate complications associated with a tracheostomy:

Respiratory
• crackles
• rhonchi
• respiratory distress
• stridor
• purulent mucus
• difficulty passing tracheal suctioning catheter
• cyanosis

Integumentary
• redness around the stoma
• purulent drainage
• elevated temperature

Nursing diagnosis: *Impaired skin integrity related to humidity, moisture, or mucus secretions*

GOAL: The child will have good skin integrity as evidenced by maintaining intact skin with no signs of redness, swelling, or fever and normal sputum characteristics.

Interventions

1. Instruct the parents (and child, if age-appropriate) to clean the tracheostomy site with hydrogen peroxide every 8 hours or as needed.

2. Tell the parents to keep the child's neck dry and to remove secretions, as needed.

3. Make sure the parents know to change the tracheostomy ties daily or as needed.

4. Have the parents change or clean the suction cannister, nebulizer, and other equipment every 48 hours and as needed.

5. Stress the importance of cleaning the inner cannula every 8 hours using sterile technique.

Rationales

1. Frequent cleaning decreases the irritating effects of secretions on the skin.

2. Moisture causes irritation that may lead to skin breakdown.

3. Wet ties irritate the skin and provide a warm, moist environment in which infection may develop.

4. Routine changing and cleaning decreases the risk of skin breakdown that can lead to infection.

5. Frequent cleaning using sterile technique decreases the risk of bacterial infiltration that can lead to skin breakdown and infection.

Nursing diagnosis: *Ineffective breathing patterns related to tracheal tube dislodgment or plugging*

GOAL: The child will maintain normal breathing patterns as evidenced by bilaterally equal respirations, pink and moist mucous membranes, and the absence of dyspnea, coughing, and choking.

Interventions

1. To prevent tube dislodgment, instruct the parents to keep the tracheostomy ties tied snugly in knots, not bows. Have them check the ties at least every 8 hours.

2. Explain to the parents that, when changing tracheostomy ties, they need to ensure that the new ties are in place before removing the old ties. Also explain that two people should change the ties whenever possible.

3. Emphasize the importance of keeping a spare tracheostomy tube and scissors near the child at all times.

4. Instruct the parents to change the tracheostomy tube at least monthly (weekly changes are preferable).

5. Have the parents assess the color, amount, consistency, and odor of secretions every 8 hours. Tell them to notify the doctor of any significant changes in secretions.

6. Instruct the parents to suction the child with a catheter or bulb syringe, as needed, if the child is gurgling, having difficulty breathing, or producing large amounts of secretions.

7. Have the parents instill 0.5 ml of normal saline solution directly into the tracheostomy tube to loosen thick secretions.

8. Have the parents encourage the older child to cough up secretions.

9. Explain the importance of assessing the child's breath sounds before and after suctioning.

10. Instruct the parents to provide humidified air or oxygen to the trachea, as needed.

11. Tell the parents to instill one or two drops of normal saline solution into the tracheostomy tube, as needed and when the child is away from the humidification source.

12. Tell the parents to encourage the child to drink 2 to 8 glasses (500 to 2,000 ml) of fluid (depending on the child's age) unless otherwise restricted.

Rationales

1. Bows can easily loosen or untie, increasing the risk of tube dislodgment and respiratory distress.

2. Ensuring that the new ties are in place before removing the old ties decreases the risk of accidental tube dislodgment. Having a second person assist with ties is helpful, especially if problems arise from the child's coughing or moving.

3. This allows for immediate replacement in case of plugging or accidental tube dislodgment.

4. A clean tube decreases the risk of plugging and infection.

5. Thicker, more copious secretions increase the risk of plugging and indicate the need for increased fluids or humidity (or both). A change in color or odor may indicate infection.

6. A bulb syringe helps remove secretions from the upper portion of the trachea without causing tracheal trauma. A catheter may be necessary for deep suctioning.

7. Loose, thick secretions are easier to cough up or suction out.

8. Coughing decreases the need for suctioning and the risk of tracheal trauma.

9. Such assessment is necessary to evaluate the effectiveness of suctioning in clearing secretions.

10. Humidification liquefies secretions and helps decrease respiratory distress. Most children require some humidification as long as the tracheostomy is in place; however, continuous humidification usually is not required after the first few postoperative days.

11. Normal saline solution helps to keep secretions loose and moist for easy removal, thereby decreasing the risk of respiratory distress.

12. Adequate fluids help keep secretions moist and loose for easy removal, thereby helping to decrease the risk of respiratory distress.

Nursing diagnosis: *Potential for injury (poor oxygenation) related to suctioning procedure*

GOAL: The child will remain free of injury as evidenced by maintaining good skin color and clear bilateral breath sounds (and adequate oxygen saturation, if monitored) during suctioning.

Interventions

1. Instruct the parents to ventilate the child with oxygen for 30 to 60 seconds before and after suctioning, if needed.

2. When suctioning the child, have the parents keep the catheter in place no longer than 15 seconds.

3. Tell the parents to be sure to use the correct-sized catheter when suctioning the child (usually one-half the diameter of the tracheostomy tube).

Rationales

1. Providing supplemental oxygen helps to prevent decreases in the oxygen saturation rate brought on by suctioning.

2. Keeping the catheter in place for a minimal amount of time is necessary because suctioning removes oxygen along with secretions.

3. Using too large of a catheter increases the risk of trauma to the trachea and may cause the catheter to become lodged in the tracheostomy tube.

Nursing diagnosis: *Potential for aspiration related to poor swallowing and vomiting*

GOAL: The child will not aspirate feedings as evidenced by retaining feedings without vomiting.

Interventions

1. Instruct the parents to position the child upright during each feeding.

2. Before giving the child any food or drink, have the parents suction him as needed. However, tell them to avoid suctioning the child immediately afterward.

Rationales

1. Sitting upright decreases the risk of aspiration.

2. Suctioning the child immediately after he eats or drinks may cause irritation and vomiting.

Documentation checklist

During the home care session, be sure to document the following:
___ the child's ongoing status
___ the child's vital signs
___ signs and symptoms of infection
___ equipment settings and functioning
___ parental concerns.

APPENDICES

APPENDIX A

Normal Growth and Development

Use the following chart as a general guide to some major developmental milestones. If you suspect that your patient has a developmental problem, refer him for further testing with an appropriate screening tool, such as the Denver Developmental Screening Test.

Physical development	Motor activity	Sensory ability	Social skills	Communication skills
Birth to 1 month (neonate)				
• Usually weighs between 5½ and 9½ lb (2,500 and 4,300 g) at birth, gaining about 1½ lb during first month • Usually measures 19" to 21" (48 to 53 cm) at birth, growing about 1" during the first month • Head circumference averages 12½" to 14" (32 to 36 cm) at birth • Fontanels are open; sutures may be overriding	• Can track objects and lift head for a short time • Can grasp objects placed in hands for a short time	• Becomes startled when hearing sounds • Is attentive to speech, especially mother's voice • Focuses on faces and objects when in direct line of vision	• Is completely dependent on caregivers • Establishes eye contact • Smiles briefly	• Responds to human voices • Makes small gutteral sounds • Establishes patterns of crying • Coos and expresses comfort when fed
2 to 12 months (infant)				
• Experiences rapid weight gain, especially during the first 6 months, when growth averages 1½ lb (680 g) per month; remaining 6 months, gains about ¾ lb (340 g) per month • Length increases an average of 1" (2.5 cm) per month during first 6 months, then ½" (1.3 cm) per month during remaining months • Head circumference increases about ½" (1.3 cm) per month during first 6 months, then ¼" (0.6 cm) per month during remaining months • Posterior fontanel closes completely at about 6 to 8 weeks	• Holds head erect and steady by 3 months • Sits upright by 7 months • Can maneuver from a prone to sitting position by 10 months • Can creep on hands and knees and maneuver while standing and holding onto furniture by 11 months	• Responds to hearing sounds by turning to source by 4 months; responds to hearing name by 10 months • Focuses on near objects by 5 months	• Develops sense of trust in response to having needs met • Begins developing personality • Requires continual stimulation and play • Enjoys shaking, banging, and pulling objects and demonstrating imitative behavior by 4 to 8 months • Develops stranger anxiety by 6 to 9 months	• Begins vocalizing consonants by 3 to 4 months and vowels by 4 to 6 months • Laughs aloud by 4 months • Begins mouthing words by 6 to 9 months • Associates meaning to sound, says single words, and understands the word "no" by 9 to 12 months
1 year				
• Weight since birth triples • Length since birth increases about 50% • Head and chest circumferences are equal • Can breathe through mouth when nose is occluded	• Occasionally attempts to stand alone • Walks with someone holding one hand • Uses thumb and forefinger to pick up objects; pokes at things with one finger • Sits up for prolonged time without support	• Responds to name • Localizes sounds; listens for sounds to recur • Eyes follow rapidly moving objects	• Is afraid of strange surroundings; clings to mother • Enjoys playing simple ball games • Shows emotions such as jealousy • Appears affectionate; hugs and kisses when asked to do so	• Understands simple commands such as "wave bye-bye" • Says one or two other words besides repetitive "momma" and "dadda" • Recognizes objects by names • Imitates animal sounds • Shakes head to signify no

Physical development	Motor activity	Sensory ability	Social skills	Communication skills
1 year *(continued)* • Rooting, Moro's, and tonic neck reflexes disappear • May have six to eight teeth	• Places one object after another into a container		• Plays simple interactive games such as peekaboo • Explores objects by chewing and biting on them	• Stops activity when told to do so
1 to 3 years (toddler) • Anterior fontanel is closed • Able to control anal and urinary sphincters • Height and weight increase at slower rates • Birth weight quadruples by age 30 months • Arms and legs lengthen from ossification and long-bone growth • Primary dentition complete	• Goes up and down stairs alone, by placing both feet on a step before climbing to next step • Jumps down steps without losing balance • Kicks ball forward without losing balance • Turns doorknobs • Rides tricycle • Holds crayon with fingers; copies crosses and circles	• Vision is 20/40; accommodation is complete • Hearing ability (including ability to localize sounds) fully developed	• At 15 months, feeds self with little difficulty, tolerates some separation from mother, begins imitating parents • At 24 months, feeds self well, helps undress himself, becomes possessive of toys. May achieve daytime elimination control • At 36 months, engages in parallel playing (playing in close proximity to others but without interaction), puts things away, pulls people to show them something, wants and displays increased independence from mother, begins to recognize sex differences, and knows his own sex. May achieve nighttime elimination control	• From 15 to 18 months, uses his own jargon—sounds that he understands but that aren't real words • By 24 months, uses two- to three-word phrases, and correctly pronounces vowels. Has a 270- to 300-word vocabulary • By age 3, has a 900-word vocabulary and uses 4- to 5-word sentences
4 to 5 years (preschooler) • Pulse and respiratory rates and blood pressure decrease • Height and weight gains remain constant • Height since birth doubles • First permanent teeth erupt • Right- or left-handedness established	• Walks down stairs, alternating feet • Throws and catches ball well • Ties shoelace in bow by age 5 • Hops on one foot • Uses scissors well	• Visual acuity approaches 20/20 *Note:* Amblyopia most often develops at age 4.	• At age 4, is very independent and aggressive; shows off and tattles on others. May have imaginary playmate; may live in fantasy world. • At age 5, is less rebellious, ready to accomplish tasks at hand. Cares for himself; is independent but trustworthy. Starts to understand rules and conformity; may notice prejudices; identifies with parent of same sex • Egocentric	• At age 5, can follow three commands given in a row, asks meanings of new words, has vocabulary of 2,100 words, counts and identifies coins, uses six- to eight-word sentences, describes drawings in detail
6 to 12 years (school-age child) • By age 6, height and weight gains slow; dexterity increases; child is very active • By age 7, grows at least 2″ (5.1 cm) per year; posture becomes more tense and stiff	• At age 6, is aware of using hand as a tool; draws, prints, and colors well • At age 7, repeats activities to become proficient at them; uses table knife	• Fully developed	• May become highly self-critical. Subject to depression, if unable to live up to others' expectations • Develops a strong sense of industry	• Has a 2,550- to 2,600-word vocabulary • Capable of producing all the sounds in his native language (any articulation problems present at this age need special evaluation)

(continued)

Normal Growth and Development *(continued)*

Physical development	Motor activity	Sensory ability	Social skills	Communication skills
6 to 12 years *(continued)* • By ages 10 to 12, height slows, weight gain increases; child may become obese at this age. Pubescent changes begin to appear; a girl's body lines start to become soft and rounded	• At age 8, fine motor control well developed; able to use tools such as hammers and screwdrivers		• May assume independent duties and chores • Has defined ideas and attitude toward sex • Enjoys hobbies, physical activity, and sports	• Uses complex sentence structure • Uses tone and new vocal patterns to express ideas • Uses words to express feelings, desires, and attitudes
13 to 18 years (adolescent) • Experiences significant changes in bones, muscle, and adipose tissue. Hormonal changes cause shoulder breadth, arm and leg length increases in boys; hip, pelvis, and breast development in girls. *Note:* Approximately 99% of adult height is reached by age 18	• All gross and fine motor skills are developed. Activities now serve to refine motor skills	• Fully developed	• Explores emotional needs. Frequent testing of parents' authority may cause barrier between child and parents • Explores sexuality • Feels strong need to conform with peers • May romanticize about daily life, or fantasize about death • Begins making long-range plans	• Has an adult's proficiency with language but may frequently use slang or jargon to communicate with peers

APPENDIX B

Normal Vital Sign Measurements

The following vital sign measurements are considered normal for pediatric patients.

Temperature	Heart rate	Respiratory rate	Blood pressure
Birth to 1 month 97.0° to 100.0° F. (36.1° to 37.8° C.)	70 to 180 beats/minute	30 to 80 breaths/minute	40 to 90 (systolic); 16 to 60 (diastolic)
2 months to 1 year 99.1° to 99.7° F. (37.3° to 37.6° C.)	80 to 160 beats/minute	30 to 60 breaths/minute	70 to 110 (systolic); 45 to 70 (diastolic)
2 to 5 years 98.5° to 99.1° F. (36.9° to 37.3° C.)	90 to 150 beats/minute	20 to 40 breaths/minute	75 to 115 (systolic); 45 to 80 (diastolic)
6 to 12 years 98.0° to 98.5° F. (36.7° to 36.9° C.)	60 to 110 beats/minute	15 to 30 breaths/minute	90 to 130 (systolic); 55 to 80 (diastolic)
13 to 18 years 97.6° to 97.9° F. (36.4° to 36.6° C.)	50 to 90 beats/minute	12 to 20 breaths/minute	90 to 140 (systolic); 50 to 90 (diastolic)

APPENDIX C

Physical Growth Charts

To use the growth charts* on the following pages, correlate the child's age with the appropriate growth measurement (head circumference, length/height, or weight). Consider the child's growth normal if the plotted measurement falls between the 5th and 95th percentiles; consider the child's growth abnormal if it falls below the 5th or above the 95th percentile.

Boys: birth to 36 months

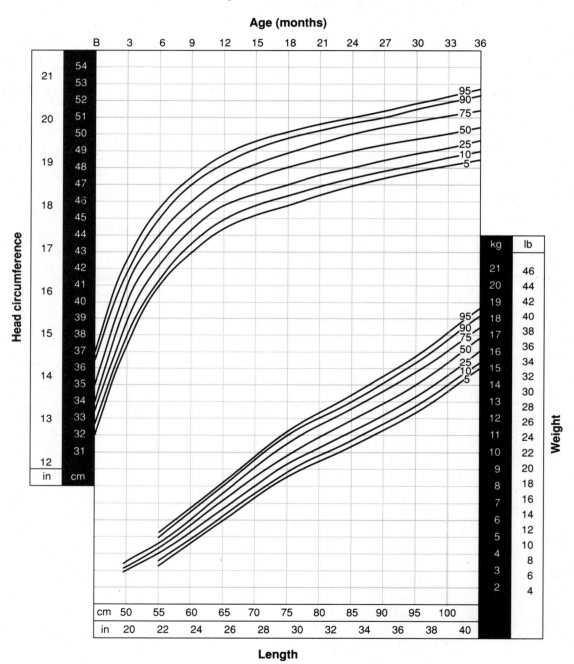

*Adapted from National Center for Health Statistics. *NCHS Growth Charts,* Rockville, Md., 1976.

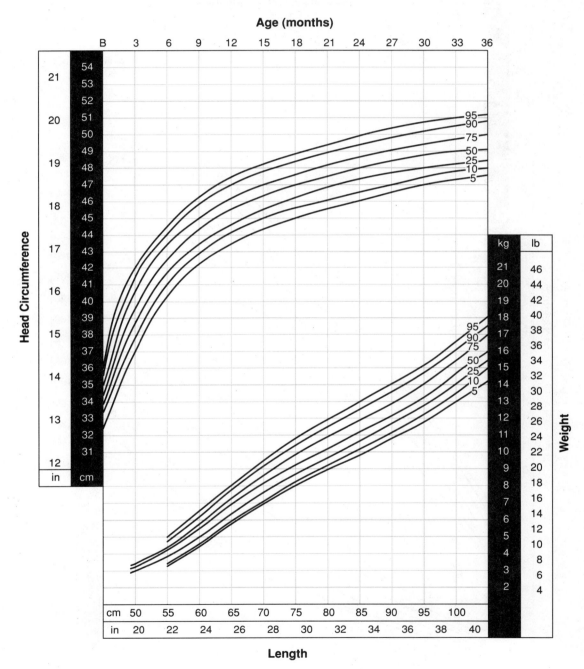

Girls: birth to 36 months

(continued)

Physical Growth Charts *(continued)*

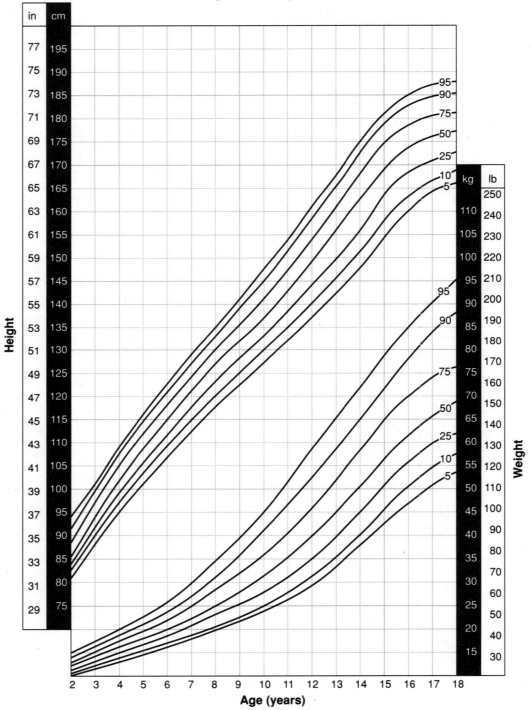

Boys: 2 to 18 years

Girls: 2 to 18 years

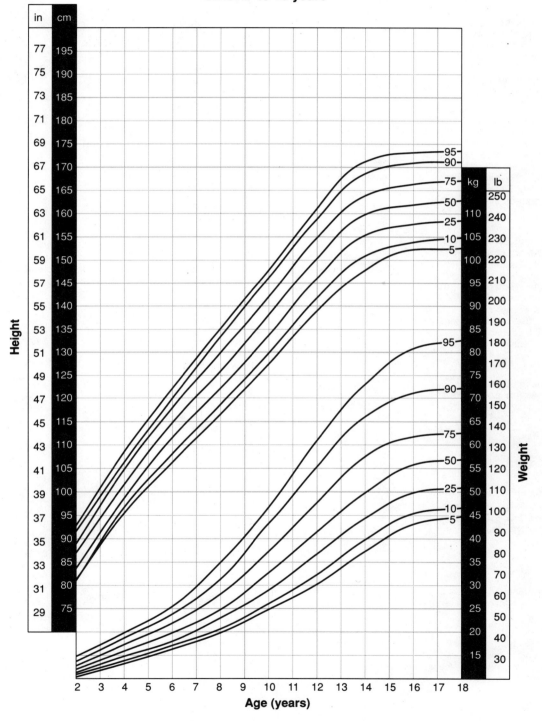

NANDA Taxonomy of Nursing Diagnoses

The North American Nursing Diagnosis Association (NANDA) has developed and adopted a taxonomy of nursing diagnoses, or diagnostic labels. The 1988 approved list appears here.

A
Activity intolerance
Activity intolerance: potential
Adjustment, impaired
Airway clearance, ineffective
Anxiety
Aspiration, potential for

B
Body temperature, altered: potential
Bowel elimination, altered: colonic constipation
Bowel elimination, altered: constipation
Bowel elimination, altered: diarrhea
Bowel elimination, altered: incontinence
Bowel elimination, altered: perceived constipation
Breast-feeding, ineffective
Breathing pattern, ineffective

C
Cardiac output, altered: decreased
Comfort, altered: chronic pain
Comfort, altered: pain
Communication, impaired: verbal
Coping, family: potential for growth
Coping, ineffective: defensive
Coping, ineffective: denial
Coping, ineffective family: compromised
Coping, ineffective family: disabled
Coping, ineffective individual

DE
Decisional conflict (specify)
Disuse syndrome, potential for
Diversional activity, deficit
Dysreflexia

F
Family processes, altered
Fatigue
Fear
Fluid volume deficit: actual (1)
Fluid volume deficit: actual (2)
Fluid volume deficit: potential
Fluid volume excess

G
Gas exchange, impaired
Grieving, anticipatory
Grieving, dysfunctional
Growth and development, altered

H
Health maintenance, altered
Health seeking behaviors (specify)
Home maintenance management, impaired
Hopelessness
Hyperthermia
Hypothermia

IJ
Incontinence, functional
Incontinence, reflex
Incontinence, stress
Incontinence, total
Incontinence, urge
Infection, potential for
Injury, potential for
Injury, potential for: poisoning
Injury, potential for: suffocating
Injury, potential for: trauma

KL
Knowledge deficit (specify)

M
Mobility, impaired physical

NO
Noncompliance (specify)
Nutrition, altered: less than body requirements
Nutrition, altered: more than body requirements
Nutrition, altered: potential for more than body requirements

PQ
Parental role, conflict
Parenting, altered: actual
Parenting, altered: potential
Post-trauma response
Powerlessness

R
Rape-trauma syndrome
Rape-trauma syndrome: compound reaction
Rape-trauma syndrome: silent reaction
Role performance, altered

S
Self-care deficit: bathing and hygiene
Self-care deficit: dressing and grooming
Self-care deficit: feeding
Self-care deficit: toileting
Self-concept, disturbance in: body image
Self-concept, disturbance in: personal identity
Self-esteem, chronic low
Self-esteem, disturbance in
Self-esteem, situational low
Sensory-perceptual alteration: visual, auditory, kinesthetic, gustatory, tactile, olfactory (specify type)
Sexual dysfunction
Sexuality, altered patterns
Skin integrity, impaired: actual
Skin integrity, impaired: potential
Sleep pattern disturbance
Social interaction, impaired
Social isolation
Spiritual distress (distress of the human spirit)
Swallowing, impaired

T
Thermoregulation, ineffective
Thought processes, altered
Tissue integrity, impaired
Tissue integrity, impaired: oral mucous membrane
Tissue perfusion, altered: renal, cerebral, cardiopulmonary,
  gastrointestinal, peripheral

U
Unilateral neglect
Urinary elimination, altered patterns
Urine retention

VWXYZ
Violence, potential for: self-directed or directed at others

APPENDIX E
Normal Laboratory Values

Below is a listing of normal laboratory values for some commonly ordered tests.

Test	Age	Normal values
Bilirubin, serum	1 to 8 days 9 days to 18 years	2 to 10 mg/dl 0.2 to 1 mg/dl
Chloride, serum	Birth to 1 month 1 month to 18 years	90 to 122 mEq/liter 98 to 130 mEq/liter
Glucose, serum	Birth to 1 month 2 months to 12 years 12 to 18 years	30 to 97 mg/dl 60 to 100 mg/dl 70 to 120 mg/dl
Hematocrit	Birth to 1 month 2 to 12 months 1 to 6 years 6 to 12 years 12 to 18 years	43% to 75% 28% to 41% 31% to 43.5% 36% to 45% Males: 37% to 54% Females: 36% to 47%
Hemoglobin	Birth to 1 month 2 to 3 months 4 to 12 months 1 to 6 years 6 to 12 years 12 to 18 years	14 to 23 g/dl 9 to 14.5 g/dl 10 to 15 g/dl 10 to 15 g/dl 11 to 15.5 g/dl Males: 13 to 18 g/dl Females: 11.5 to 16 g/dl
Platelet count	Birth to 1 month 2 months to 18 years	100,000 to 400,000/mm³ 150,000 to 400,000/mm³
Potassium, serum	Birth to 1 month 2 to 12 months 1 to 6 years 6 to 18 years	4.0 to 7.7 mEq/liter 3.4 to 5.6 mEq/liter 3.5 to 5.2 mEq/liter 3.0 to 5.2 mEq/liter
Sodium, serum	Birth to 1 month 2 to 12 months 1 to 6 years 12 to 18 years	124 to 156 mEq/liter 138 to 146 mEq/liter 138 to 180 mEq/liter 140 to 220 mEq/liter
White blood cell count	Birth to 1 month 2 to 12 months 1 to 3 years 4 to 12 years 12 to 18 years	9,000 to 30,000/mm³ 5,000 to 19,000/mm³ 6,000 to 17,000/mm³ 4,500 to 13,000/mm³ 4,500 to 11,000/mm³

APPENDIX F

Guide to Food Values

Use the information below to help meet your patient's special dietary needs.

HIGH-CALORIE FOODS

Food and amount	Calories
Apple pie (one 4″ slice)	375
Avocado (1½ cups)	245
Beef stew (1 cup)	530
Chocolate cake (one 2″ slice)	350
Chocolate pudding (1 cup)	220
Cream cheese (1 oz)	105
Custard (1 cup)	205
Eggnog (8 oz)	235
Hamburger with bun (3 oz, cooked)	330
Ice cream shake (8 oz)	420
Macaroni and cheese (1 cup)	505
Malted milk shake (8 oz)	500
Peanut butter (2 Tbsp)	95
Pumpkin pie (one 4″ slice)	330
Raisins (2 cups)	430
Shortcake with strawberries (1 cup)	400
Spaghetti (1 cup, cooked)	395
Waffle (two 4″ squares)	210

HIGH-PROTEIN FOODS

Food and amount	Protein (g)
Baked beans (1 cup)	7.5
Bean soup (½ cup)	6.0
Beef brisket (3 oz, cooked)	16.0
Beef stew (1 cup)	28.0
Chicken, fried (3½ oz)	27.0
Chicken and gravy (3 oz, cooked)	22.0
Club sandwich (3 oz)	35.5
Cottage cheese (1 cup)	22.0
Haddock, fried (3 oz)	23.5
Hamburger with bun (3 oz, cooked)	17.0
Lima beans (½ cup)	6.5
Macaroni and cheese (1 cup)	19.0
Malted milkshake (8 oz)	13.0
Oyster stew (1 cup)	15.0
Spaghetti (1 cup, cooked)	12.5
Spareribs, pork (2½ oz, cooked)	15.5
Split pea soup (½ cup)	7.0
Veal cutlet (3 oz, cooked)	24.0
Vegetable beef soup (1 cup)	6.0

LOW-FAT FOODS

Food and amount	Fat (g)
Angel food cake (one 2″ slice)	0.1
Apple cider (8 oz)	0
Apple juice (8 oz)	0
Applesauce (1 cup)	0.2
Banana (one medium)	0.2
Cantaloupe (1 cup)	0.2
Carrots (1 cup)	0.5
Cornflakes (1 oz)	0.1
Grapefruit juice (8 oz)	0.1
Grapenuts (1 oz)	0.1
Honeydew melon (1 cup)	0
Jam (1 Tbsp)	0.1
Jell-O, plain (1 cup)	0
Milk, skim (8 oz)	0.2
Orange (one medium)	0.2
Orange juice (8 oz)	0.2

(continued)

Guide to Food Values *(continued)*

LOW-FAT FOODS *(continued)*

Pancake (one 4″ cake)	1
Pears (1 cup)	0.1
Peaches, canned (1 cup)	0.1
Pineapple (1 cup)	0.1
Potatoes (1 cup)	0.1
Rye bread (1 slice)	0.3
Rye crackers (two 2″ wafers)	0.1
Sherbet (1 cup)	0
Soda, carbonated (8 oz)	0
Squash (1 cup)	0.1

HIGH-CALCIUM FOODS

Food and amount	Calcium (mg)
American cheese (1 oz)	175
Cheddar cheese (1 oz)	200
Cream-style soup (1 cup)	170
Macaroni and cheese (½ cup)	180
Milk, whole (8 oz)	290
Milk, skim (8 oz)	300
Pancakes (two 4″ cakes)	120
Pizza (2 slices)	335
Swiss cheese (1 oz)	275
Waffle (one 4″ square)	180
Yogurt, low-fat with fruit (1 cup)	345

LOW-SODIUM FOODS

Food and amount	Sodium (mg)
Apple (one medium)	1
Apple juice (8 oz)	2
Applesauce (1 cup)	5
Banana (one medium)	1
Cauliflower, cooked (1 cup)	12
Cranberry juice (8 oz)	3
Egg noodles, cooked (1 cup)	3
Flounder, baked (3½ oz)	75
Orange (one medium)	1
Popcorn, plain (1 cup)	5
Potato, boiled (1 cup)	15
Strawberries (1 cup)	1
Tuna, canned in water (3½ oz)	40

REFERENCES AND INDEX

Selected References

BOOKS

Allen, S., et al. *Home Care Instruction Manual.* Dallas: Children's Medical Center of Dallas, 1987.

Alspach, J.G., and Williams, S.M., eds. *Core Curriculum for Critical Care Nursing,* 3rd ed. Philadelphia: W.B. Saunders Co., 1985.

Bates, B. *A Guide to Physical Examination and History Taking,* 4th ed. Philadelphia: J.B. Lippincott Co., 1987.

Behrman, R.E., and Vaughan, V.C. *Nelson Textbook of Pediatrics,* 13th ed. Philadelphia: W.B. Saunders Co., 1987.

Braude, A.I., et al. *Infectious Diseases and Medical Microbiology,* 2nd ed. Philadelphia: W.B. Saunders Co., 1986.

Broadwell, D., and Jackson, B. *Principles of Ostomy Care.* St. Louis: C.V. Mosby Co., 1981.

Byrne, C.J., et al. *Laboratory Tests: Implications for Nursing Care.* Los Altos, Calif.: Addison-Wesley Publishing Co., 1981.

Diagnostic and Statistical Manual of Mental Disorders DSM-III-R, 3rd ed. Washington, D.C.: American Psychiatric Association, 1987.

Diagnostics, 2nd ed. Nurse's Reference Library. Springhouse, Pa.: Springhouse Corporation, 1986.

Diekstra, R.F., and Hawston, K., eds. *Suicide in Adolescence.* Boston: Martinus Nijhoff Publishers, 1986.

Doenges, E.M., et al. *Nursing Care Plans: Nursing Diagnosis in Planning Patient Care.* Philadelphia: F.A. Davis Co., 1984.

Garner, D.M., and Garfinkel, P.E. *Handbook of Psychotherapy for Anorexia Nervosa and Bulimia.* New York: Guilford Press, 1984.

Gordon, M. *Manual of Nursing Diagnosis: 1984-1985.* New York: McGraw-Hill Book Co., 1985.

Guide to Hospital Services. Dallas: Children's Medical Center of Dallas, 1987.

Hanak, M. *Patient and Family Education: Teaching Program for Managing Chronic Disease and Disability.* New York: Springer Publishing Co., 1986.

Hazinski, M.F. *Nursing Care of the Critically Ill Child.* St. Louis: C.V. Mosby Co., 1984.

Jarvis, L. *Community Health Nursing: Keeping the Public Healthy,* 2nd ed. Philadelphia: F.A. Davis Co., 1985.

Jeter, K. *These Special Children: The Ostomy Book for Parents of Children with Colostomies, Ileostomies, and Urostomies.* Palo Alto, Calif.: Bull Publishing Co., 1982.

Kee, J.L. *Laboratory and Diagnostic Tests with Nursing Implications,* 2nd ed. East Norwalk, Conn.: Appleton-Lange, 1986.

Levin, D.L., et al. *A Practical Guide to Pediatric Intensive Care,* 2nd ed. St. Louis: C.V. Mosby Co., 1984.

Luckmann, J., and Sorensen, K. *Medical-Surgical Nursing: A Psychophysiologic Approach,* 2nd ed. Philadelphia: W.B. Saunders Co., 1980.

Nelson, N., and Beckel, J., eds. *Nursing Care Plans for the Pediatric Patient.* St. Louis: C.V. Mosby Co., 1987.

Pallett, P.J., and O'Brien, M.T. *Textbook of Neurological Nursing.* Boston: Little, Brown & Co., 1984.

Peck, M., et al. *Youth Suicide.* New York: Springer Publishing Co., 1985.

Pediatric Laboratory Test Interpretation. Dallas: Children's Medical Center of Dallas, 1987.

Philip, A.G. *Neonatology: A Practical Guide.* Philadelphia: W.B. Saunders Co., 1987.

Pillitteri, A. *Child Health Nursing: Care of the Growing Family,* 3rd ed. Boston: Little, Brown & Co., 1987.

Redman, B. *The Process of Patient Education,* 6th ed. St. Louis: C.V. Mosby Co., 1988.

Rogers, M.C., ed. *Textbook of Pediatric Intensive Care.* Baltimore: Williams & Wilkins Publishing Co., 1987.

Roy, C. *Introduction to Nursing: An Adaptation Model,* 2nd ed. East Norwalk, Conn.: Appleton-Lange, 1984.

Schaefer, C.E., and Millman, H.L. *Therapies for Children: A Handbook of Effective Treatments for Problem Behaviors.* San Francisco: Jossey-Bass Publishing Co., 1977.

Scipien, G.M., and Barnard, M.V. *Comprehensive Pediatric Nursing,* 3rd ed. New York: McGraw-Hill Book Co., 1985.

Shoemaker, W.C., et al. *The Society of Critical Care Medicine: Textbook of Critical Care,* 2nd ed. Philadelphia: W.B. Saunders Co., 1988.

Snyder, M. *A Guide to Neurological and Neurosurgical Nursing,* 2nd ed. New York: John Wiley & Sons, 1988.

Vogt, G., et al. *Mosby's Manual of Neurological Care.* St. Louis: C.V. Mosby Co., 1984.

Whaley, L., and Wong, D. *Clinical Handbook of Pediatric Nursing,* 2nd ed. St. Louis: C.V. Mosby Co., 1986.

Whaley, L., and Wong, D. *Nursing Care of Infants and Children,* 3rd ed. St. Louis: C.V. Mosby Co., 1986.

Willet, M.J., et al. *Manual of Neonatal Intensive Care Nursing,* 2nd ed. Boston: Little, Brown & Co., 1986.

Wolman, B.B., et al., eds. *Handbook of Developmental Psychology.* Englewood Cliffs, N.J.: Prentice-Hall, 1982.

PERIODICALS

Adams, D.A., and Selekof, J.L. "Children with Ostomies: Comprehensive Care Planning," *Pediatric Nursing* 12(6):429-33, November/December 1986.

Adams, J.L., et al. "Diagnosing and Treating Otitis Media with Effusion," *American Journal of Maternal Child Nursing* 9(1):22-28, January/February 1984.

Agamalian, B. "Pediatric Cardiac Catheterization," *Journal of Pediatric Nursing* 1(2):73-79, April 1986.

Allan, D. "Management of the Head-Injured Patient," *Nursing Times* 82(25):36-39, June 18, 1986.

Bales, R. "Hypothermia: A Postop Problem That's Easy to Miss," *RN* 51(4):42-44, April 1988.

Balik, B., et al. "Diabetes and the School-Aged Child,"

American Journal of Maternal Child Nursing 11(5):324-30, September/October 1986.

Berde, C.B., et al. "Pediatric Pain Management," *Hospital Practices* 23(5):83-94, May 30, 1988.

Bergstein, J.M. "Hematuria in the Young," *Emergency Medicine* 18(17):20-34, October 15, 1986.

Birdsall, C. "How Do You Manage Peritoneal Dialysis?" *American Journal of Nursing* 86(5):592-96, May 1986.

Bowen, J. "Helping Children and Their Families Cope with Congenital Heart Disease," *Critical Care Quarterly* 8(3):65-74, December 1985.

Brucker, J.M., and Laurent, J.P. "Pediatric Craniofacial Reconstruction: An Overview of Perioperative Management," *Journal of Neuroscience Nursing* 20(3):159-68, June 1988.

Burkle, N.L. "Inadvertent Hypothermia," *Today's OR Nurse* 10(7):26-42, July 1988.

Burr, S. "Pain in Childhood," *Nursing (London)* 3(24):890-96, December 3, 1987.

Carey, B.E. "Intraventricular Hemorrhage in the Preterm Infant," *JOGN Nursing (Supplement)* 12(3):60s-68s, May/June 1983.

Cerrato, P.L. "If a Child is at Risk for Heart Disease," *RN* 51(10):93-94, October 1988.

Cotten, J.M. "A Comprehensive Nursing Approach to the Neonate with Myelomeningocele," *Neonatal Network* 2(4):7-16, February 1984.

Crawford, C., et al. "Nursing Management of the Postoperative Pediatric Patient," *Issues in Comprehensive Pediatric Nursing* 6(3):157-65, May/June 1983.

"Croup and Epiglottitis: Sudden Trouble for Young Children," *American Lung Association Bulletin* 67:9-11, March 1981.

Deegan, S. "Intermittent Catheterization for Children," *Nursing Times* 81(14):72-74, April 3, 1985.

Edwards, D. "Initial Psychosocial Impact of Insulin-Dependent Diabetes Mellitus on the Pediatric Client and Family," *Issues in Comprehensive Pediatric Nursing* 10(4):199-207, 1987.

Ellis, J.A. "Using Pain Scales to Prevent Undermedication," *American Journal of Maternal Child Nursing* 13(3):180-82, May/June 1988.

Fisk, R. "Management of the Pediatric Cardiovascular Patient after Surgery," *Critical Care Quarterly* 9(2):75-82, September 1986.

Gavin, J.R. "Diabetes and Exercise," *American Journal of Nursing* 88(2):178-80, February 1988.

Gill, B., and Page-Goertz, S. "Deep Hypothermic Arrest in Children Undergoing Heart Surgery," *Heart & Lung* 15(1):28-33, January 1986.

Gowdy, A. "Do You Know Me? The Importance of Paediatric Preoperative Visits," *NAT News: British Journal of Theatre Nursing* 25(6):19-20, June 1988.

Haire-Joshu, D., et al. "Contrasting Type I and Type II Diabetes," *American Journal of Nursing* 86(11):1240-43, November 1986.

Hausman, K.A. "Symposium on Pediatric Critical Care. Critical Care of the Child with Increased Intracranial Pressure," *Nursing Clinics of North America* 16:647-56, December 1981.

Hazinski, M. "Pediatric Home Tracheostomy Care: A Parent's Guide," *Pediatric Nursing* 12(1):41-48, 69, January/February 1986.

Heins, J.M. "Dietary Management in Diabetes Mellitus: A Goal-Setting Process," *Nursing Clinics of North America* 18(4):631-43, December 1983.

Henson, P. "Current Concepts in Renal Transplantation," *ANNA Journal* 14(6):367-68, December 1987.

Hinkle, J.L. "Treating Traumatic Coma," *American Journal of Nursing* 86(5):551-56, May 1986.

Hutchinson, A., et al. "Diabetic Control in Adolescents," *Nursing Mirror* 161(18):26-27, October 30, 1985.

Ireland, D.W. "Put Some Roar in Your Pediatric Program," *Journal of Post Anesthesia Nursing* 1(4):255-57, November 1986.

Jackson, M.M., et al. "Why Not Treat All Body Substances as Infectious?" *American Journal of Nursing* 87(9):1137-39, September 1987.

Kaktis, J.V. "An Introduction to Monitoring Intracranial Pressure in Critically Ill Children," *Critical Care Quarterly* 3:1-8, June 1980.

Kashani, I.A., and Higgins, S.S. "Counseling Strategies for Families of Children with Heart Disease," *Pediatric Nursing* 12(1):38-40, January/February 1986.

Keith, J. "Hepatic Failure: Etiologies, Manifestations, and Management," *Critical Care Nurse* 5(1):60-86, 1985.

Kershner, D.D., and Claussen, J.A. "Craniofacial Reconstruction: Perioperative Care of the Craniosynostosis Patient," *AORN Journal* 44(4):554-80, October 1986.

Lasoff, E.M., and McEttrick, M.A. "Participation Versus Diversion During Dressing Change: Can Nurses' Attitudes Change?" *Issues in Comprehensive Pediatric Nursing* 9(6):391-98, 1986.

Malinowski, P., and Yablonski, C. "Congenital Heart Disease in Infants: Nursing Assessment," *Critical Care Quarterly* 9(2):6-23, September 1986.

Manger, G., et al. "Craniofacial Surgery Nursing: An Overview," *Canadian Nurse* 83(4):18-20, 22, April 1987.

Marshall, J.G., and Ross, J.L. "Hydrocephalus: Ventriculoperitoneal Shunting in Infants and Children," *AORN Journal* 40(6):842-57, December 1984.

McFarland, K. "Pediatric Peritoneal Dialysis," *Pediatric Nursing* 14(5):426, September/October 1988.

Miller, J., and Arsenault, L. "Reye's Syndrome," *Journal of Neurosurgical Nursing* 15(3):154-64, June 1983.

Moushey, R., et al. "A Perioperative Teaching Program: A Collaborative Process for Children and Their Families," *Journal of Pediatric Nursing* 3(1):40-45, February 1988.

Nicklas, T.A., et al. "'Heart Smart' Program: A Family Intervention Program for Eating Behavior of Children at High Risk for Cardiovascular Disease," *Journal of Nutrition Education* 20(3):128-32, June 1988.

(continued)

Nugent, J. "Acute Respiratory Care of the Newborn," *JOGN Journal (Supplement)* 12(3):31s-44s, May/June 1983.

Page, G.G. "Tetralogy of Fallot," *Heart & Lung* 15(4):390-401, July 1986.

Patlak, M. "Children's All Too Common Ear Infections," *FDA Consumer* 21(10):28-31, December 1987/January 1988.

Pleasants, D. "Managing Hydrocephalus with a Ventricular Shunt," *AORN Journal* 35(5), April 1982.

Pozzi, M., and Peck, N. "An Option for the Patient with Chronic Osteomyelitis: Home Intravenous Antibiotic Therapy," *Orthopedic Nursing* 5(5):9-14, 54, September/October 1986.

Pressman, S.D. "Myelomeningocele: A Multidisciplinary Problem," *Journal of Neurosurgical Nursing* 13(6):333-36, December 1981.

Robinson, S.J. "A Nurse's Role in Preparing Children for Surgery," *AORN Journal* 30(4):619-23, October 1979.

Rosequist, C.C., and Shepp, P.H. "CE Care: The Nutrition Factor," *American Journal of Nursing* 85(1):45-47, January 1985.

Ruffle, J.M. "Induction of Anesthesia in the Pediatric Patient," *Current Reviews in Nurse Anesthetists* 9(2):11-16, 1986.

Runton, N. "Congenital Cardiac Anomalies: A Reference Guide for Nurses," *Journal of Cardiovascular Nursing* 2(3):56-70, May 1988.

Rushton, C.H. "The Surgical Neonate: Principles of Nursing Management," *Pediatric Nursing* 14(2):141-51, March/April 1988.

Sataloff, R.T., and Colton, C.M. "Otitis Media: A Common Childhood Infection," *American Journal of Nursing* 81(8):1480-83, August 1981.

Schreiner, B.J., and Travis, L.B. "When Your Child Has Diabetes: The Preteen Years," *Diabetes Forecast* 40(12):36-41, December 1987.

Schreiner, B.J., and Travis, L.B. "When Your Child Has Diabetes: The Teen Years," *Diabetes Forecast* 41(2):18-21, February 1988.

Strangio, L. "Believe It or Not: Peritoneal Dialysis Made Easy," *Nursing88* 18(1):43-46, January 1988.

Thomas, D.O. "Are You Sure It's Only Croup?" *RN* 47(12):40-43, December 1984.

Tupa, B. "Alleviating the Fears of Pediatric Patients," *Today's OR Nurse* 9(7):33-36, July 1987.

Welch, T.C. "Hypothermia: A Nursing Concern for Surgical Patients," *Today's OR Nurse* 8(4):20-22, April 1986.

Wong, D.L., and Baker, C.M. "Pain in Children: Comparison of Assessment Scales," *Pediatric Nursing* 14(1):9-17, January/February 1988.

Zeidelman, C. "Increased Intracranial Pressure in the Pediatric Patient: Nursing Assessment and Intervention," *Journal of Neurosurgical Nursing* 12(1):7-10, March 1980.

Index

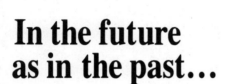

In the future as in the past...

You can rely on *Nursing* magazine to keep your skills sharp and your practice current—with award-winning nursing journalism.

Each monthly issue is packed with expert advice on the legal, ethical, and personal issues in nursing, plus up-to-the-minute...

- Drugs—warnings, new uses, and approvals
- Assessment tips
- Emergency and acute care advice
- New treatments, equipment, and disease findings
- Photostories and other skill sharpeners
- AIDS updates
- Career tracks and trends

Enter your subscription today